Moorfields
Manual of
Ophthalmology

Commissioning Editor: **Russell Gabbedy**
Development Editor: **Alex Mortimer**
Project Manager: **Rory MacDonald**
Design Manager: **Andy Chapman**
Illustration Manager: **Merlyn Harvey**
Illustrator: **Ian Ramsden**
Marketing Manager(s) (USA/UK): **Matt Latuchie/John Canelon**

Moorfields
Manual of
Ophthalmology

Timothy L. Jackson PhD, FRCOphth
Consultant Vitreoretinal Surgeon
Honorary Senior Lecturer
King's College Hospital
Denmark Hill
London

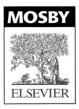

MOSBY

ELSEVIER

MOSBY
ELSEVIER

An imprint of Elsevier Limited.

First published 2008

ISBN: 9781416025726

British Library Cataloguing in Publication Data
A catalogue record for this book is available from the British Library

Library of Congress Cataloging in Publication Data
A catalog record for this book is available from the Library of Congress

Notice
Medical knowledge is constantly changing. Standard safety precautions must be followed, but as new research and clinical experience broaden our knowledge, changes in treatment and drug therapy may become necessary or appropriate. Readers are advised to check the most current product information provided by the manufacturer of each drug to be administered to verify the recommended dose, the method and duration of administration, and contraindications. It is the responsibility of the practitioner, relying on experience and knowledge of the patient, to determine dosages and the best treatment for each individual patient. Neither the Publisher nor the author assume any liability for any injury and/or damage to persons or property arising from this publication.

The Publisher

ELSEVIER your source for books,
journals and multimedia
in the health sciences
www.elsevierhealth.com

Working together to grow
libraries in developing countries
www.elsevier.com | www.bookaid.org | www.sabre.org

ELSEVIER   BOOK AID International   Sabre Foundation

The publisher's policy is to use paper manufactured from sustainable forests

Printed in China
Last digit is the print number: 9   8   7   6   5   4   3   2   1

Contents

CHAPTER 4: EXTERNAL EYE DISEASE
Guy T. Smith and John K.G. Dart

CHAPTER 5: CORNEA
Guy T. Smith and John K.G. Dart

CHAPTER 6: CATARACT SURGERY

Yashin Ramkissoon and Carol Cunningham

CHAPTER 7: GLAUCOMA

Paul J. Foster and Peng T. Khaw

CHAPTER 10: MEDICAL RETINA
Timothy L. Jackson, Catherine Egan and Alan C. Bird

CHAPTER 11: SURGICAL RETINA
Timothy L. Jackson, Lyndon Da Cruz and
Zdenek J. Gregor

CHAPTER 12: PAEDIATRICS

Adam Bates, Timothy L. Jackson and G.G.W. Adams

CHAPTER 13: STRABISMUS

Bernadette McCarry and G.G.W. Adams

CHAPTER 14: NEURO-OPHTHALMOLOGY

Ben J.L. Burton, James F. Acheson and Gordon T. Plant

APPENDICES

Bita Manzouri and Timothy L. Jackson

Contributors

James F. Acheson
14: NEURO-OPHTHALMOLOGY

G.G.W. Adams
3: ORBIT: Orbital trauma
9: OCULAR ONCOLOGY: Retinoblastoma
12: PAEDIATRICS
13: STRABISMUS

Larry Amure
OPTOMETRY AND GENERAL PRACTICE GUIDELINES

Richard Andrews
6: CATARACT SURGERY: Difficult Cases
8: UVEITIS

Keith Barton
7: GLAUCOMA: Trabeculectomy I:Surgical Technique,
Glaucoma Drainage Implants, Trans-scleral Cyclodiode Laser
Treatment

Adam Bates
9: OCULAR ONCOLOGY: Retinoblastoma
12: PAEDIATRICS

Alan C. Bird
10: MEDICAL RETINA

Jill Bloom
APPENDIX: Ophthalmic Drug Use in Pregnancy

John Brookes
7: GLAUCOMA: Congential Glaucoma

Ben J.L. Burton
8: UVEITIS: HIV
14: NEURO-OPHTHALMOLOGY

Richard O. Collin
1: OCULOPLASTICS

Helen L. Cook
10: MEDICAL RETINA: Diabetic Retinopathy

Richard H. Hart
1: OCULOPLASTICS: Congenital Eyelid Disease, Optometry and General Practice Guidelines
2: LACRIMAL: Optometry and General Practice Guidelines
3: ORBIT: Socket Disorders, Optometry and General Practice Guidelines

Hugo Henderson
1: OCULOPLASTICS: Facial Dystonias

Graham E. Holder
10: MEDICAL RETINA: Electrophysiology

John L. Hungerford
9: OCULAR ONCOLOGY

Timothy L. Jackson – Editor
10: MEDICAL RETINA
11: SURGICAL RETINA
12: PAEDIATRICS
APPENDICES
OPTOMETRY AND GENERAL PRACTICE GUIDELINES

Rajni Jain
1: OCULOPLASTICS: Congenital Eyelid Disease, Eyelid Trauma
3: ORBIT: Orbital Trauma

Peng T. Khaw
7: GLAUCOMA

Susan L. Lightman
6: CATARACT SURGERY: Difficult Cases
8: UVEITIS
10: MEDICAL RETINA: Syphilis

Natasha Lim
7: GLAUCOMA: Pharmacology of Intraocular Pressure-Lowering Drugs

Graham Macalister
OPTOMETRY AND GENERAL PRACTICE GUIDELINES

Bita Manzouri
APPENDICES

Keith Martin
7: GLAUCOMA: Steroid Pressure Response and Associated Glaucoma

Bernadette McCarry
3: ORBIT: Orbital Trauma
13: STRABISMUS

Patricia McElhatton
APPENDICES: Ophthalmic Drug Use in Pregnancy

Michael Merriman
7: GLAUCOMA: Pseudoexfoliation Syndrome, Pigment Dispersion
Syndrome, Traumatic Glaucoma

Michel Michaelides
12: PAEDIATRICS: Anterior Segment Dysgenesis, Reduced Vision
with an Otherwise Normal Examination

Moin Mohammed
10: MEDICAL RETINA: Photography

A. T. Moore
12: PAEDIATRICS: Chapter review

Prithvi Mruthyunjaya
9: OCULAR ONCOLOGY

Ian Murdoch
7: GLAUCOMA: Optometry and General Practice guidelines

Anil Nambiar
7: GLAUCOMA: Argon Laser Trabeculoplasty, Neovascular
Glaucoma, Uveitic Glaucoma

Winifred Nolan
7: GLAUCOMA: Gonioscopy

Narciss Okhravi
6: CATARACT SURGERY: Difficult Cases
8: UVEITIS: Chapter review

Carlos E. Pavesio
8: UVEITIS: Chapter review

Gordon T. Plant
14: NEURO-OPHTHALMOLOGY

Maria Papadopoulos
7: GLAUCOMA: Congenital Glaucoma, Bleb-Related Infection,
Primary Angle Closure

Poornima Rai
7: GLAUCOMA: Bleb Related Infection

Madhavan Rajan
5: CORNEA: Laser Refractive Surgery

Mahesh Ramchandani
7: GLAUCOMA: Trabeculectomy II: Post operative Care

Yashin Ramkissoon
6: CATARACT SURGERY

Marie Restori
6: CATARACT SURGERY: Biometry

Geoff Roberson
OPTOMETRY AND GENERAL PRACTICE GUIDELINES

Geoffrey E. Rose
2: LACRIMAL
3: ORBIT

Kulwant Sehmi
8: UVEITIS: Medical photography
10: MEDICAL RETINA: Medical photography

Dilani Siriwardena
7: GLAUCOMA:Optic Disc Examination, Primary Open Angle
Glaucoma, Normal Tension Glaucoma

John Sloper
12: PAEDIATRICS: Chapter review
13: STRABISMUS: Esotropia, Exotropia, Chapter review

Guy T. Smith
4: EXTERNAL EYE DISEASE
5: CORNEA
12: PAEDIATRICS: Anterior Segment Dysgenesis

Paul M. Sullivan
APPENDIX: Use of the Operating Microscope

Chris Timms
13: STRABISMUS: Chapter review

Adnan Tufail
10: MEDICAL RETINA: Age-related Macular Degeneration, Toxic Retinopathies, Retinal Laser Guidelines

Jimmy Uddin
1: OCULOPLASTICS: Chapter review

David H. Verity
1: OCULOPLASTICS

Ananth Viswanathan
7: GLAUCOMA: Interpreting Humphrey Visual Field Tests

Preface

This book was written for those who treat eye disease. It brings together the advantages of a handbook, and high quality images that are critical to a specialty that relies so heavily on pattern recognition. The chapters are organized into the main ophthalmic subspecialties. They start with any relevant background information, such as examination techniques, and go on to provide precise treatment algorithms for all the common or serious eye conditions. Key operations or procedures are given within the chapter as required. The chapters end with guidance notes for optometrists and general practitioners, to help them prioritize referrals.

Whilst maintaining this structural backbone, there is some flexibility. For example, some retinal diagnoses can be challenging and the Medical Retina chapter offers a large section dealing with the differential diagnosis of clinical signs. By contrast, the diagnosis of cataract is usually straightforward, but its removal may not be, hence an entire chapter dedicated to cataract surgery.

The main advantage of this book is that brings together a wealth of experience, with more than 60 contributors, many of whom are world-renowned experts in their field. These key authors have shown a remarkable ability to distil their knowledge into such a compact format.

It is hoped that this edition will not be the last, and I welcome any suggestions from junior or senior readers, via tim.jackson@kch.nhs.uk.

Timothy L. Jackson

'To suppose that the eye, with all its inimitable contrivances for adjusting the focus to different distances, for admitting different amounts of light, and for the correction of spherical and chromatic aberration, could have been formed by natural selection, seems, I freely confess, absurd in the highest possible degree.'

Charles Darwin

Acknowledgements

Thanks to everyone who contributed, in particular, Jill Bloom in the Medicines Information Department who checked drug dosages and usage, Patricia McElhatton at The National Teratology Information Service for reviewing the appendix on drug use in pregnancy, and David Verity and Kulwant Sehmi who both provided a large number of images from their photographic libraries. Thanks to Ian Balmer, Chief Executive, for authorising the project, and Terry Tarrant who provided the hospital with high quality retinal artwork that was used in Chapter 11. Martin Snead of Addenbrooke's Hospital reviewed the section on Hereditary Vitreoretinal Degenerations. I am grateful to all the team at Elsevier including Alex Mortimer, Andy Chapman, Merlyn Harvey, and in particular Russell Gabbedy and Rory MacDonald. Finally, special thanks to Lisa Orpwood.

To Lisa

Chapter 1
OCULOPLASTICS

Eyelid Anatomy Revision

Surface anatomy

- The upper lid margin lies 1–2 mm below the upper corneal limbus.
- The lower lid margin is at the level of the lower corneal limbus.
- The vertical palpebral fissure measures 7–12 mm.
- The upper lid peak lies just nasal to the centre of the pupil.
- The lower lid peak is just lateral to the pupil.
- The adult upper lid crease lies 7–10 mm above the lid margin on downgaze.
- The lateral angle between the two lids is about 2 mm higher than the rounded medial angle, which contains the caruncle lacrimalis, and the plica semilunaris.

Blood supply

- Dual anastomoses of the lateral and medial palpebral arteries in each lid.
- Anastomoses with the facial arterial networks.
- Posterior conjunctival artery.

Lymphatic drainage

- The lateral two-thirds of the lids drain to the superficial parotid nodes.
- The medial lids drain to the submandibular nodes.

Sensory innervation (Fig. 1.1)

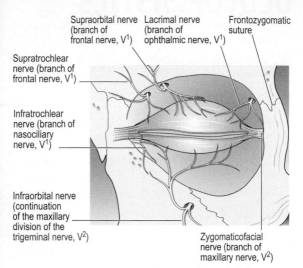

Fig. 1.1: Sensory innervation of the eyelid.

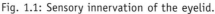

Muscle

■ The elliptical orbicularis oculi muscle consists of an orbital part which extends onto the cheek and temporal area, a palpebral part which is divided into a preseptal, pretarsal and ciliary parts, and a lacrimal part which extends into the posterior fascia of the lacrimal sac.

■ Contraction has a purse-string effect, closing the lids and drawing the muscle medially.

■ The lacrimal part dilates the lacrimal sac, contributing to the lacrimal pump mechanism.

■ Innervated by the zygomatic and temporal branches of the facial nerve.

Tarsal plates

■ Provide stability to the lids.

■ Length is 25 mm, thickness 1 mm, and maximum (central) height 10 mm (upper tarsus) and 4 mm (lower tarsus).

Canthal (palpebral) ligaments

■ Tether the tarsi to the periostium medially and laterally.

■ The medial canthal ligament has an anterior limb, which inserts anterior to the lacrimal crest, and a posterior limb, which inserts into the posterior lacrimal crest.

■ The lateral palpebral ligament attaches the lateral tarsus to Whitnall's tubercle within the orbital rim.

Orbital septum

■ Consists of planes of tough fibrous tissue which form a barrier to the spread of infection.

■ Origin: arcus marginalis at the orbital rim.

■ Insertions:

1. *Superiorly*: the levator aponeurosis;

2. *Inferiorly*: the lower lid retractors just beneath the tarsus;

3. *Medially*: the posterior lacrimal crest;

4. *Laterally*: Whitnall's tubercle.

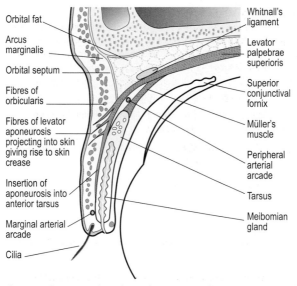

Orbital fat

Arcus marginalis

Orbital septum

Fibres of orbicularis

Fibres of levator aponeurosis projecting into skin giving rise to skin crease

Insertion of aponeurosis into anterior tarsus

Marginal arterial arcade

Cilia

Whitnall's ligament

Levator palpebrae superioris

Superior conjunctival fornix

Müller's muscle

Peripheral arterial arcade

Tarsus

Meibomian gland

Fig. 1.2: Cross-section through upper eyelid.

Upper lid retractors

◼ The striated levator palpebrae superioris (LPS) muscle is innervated by the oculomotor nerve, and has a common origin with the superior rectus muscle. Anteriorly, it becomes the levator aponeurosis as it passes anterior to Whitnall ligament, and inserts into the anterior tarsal surface. Medial and lateral extensions, or horns, insert into the periostium of Whitnall's tubercle laterally, and into the medial canthal tendon medially. A few anterior fibres pass through the orbicularis to form the skin crease. Contraction of LPS produces 12–20 mm of upper lid elevation.

◼ The sympathetically innervated Müller's muscle arises from the posterior surface of the levator muscle, and inserts into the superior border of the tarsus. Contraction elevates the lid by up to 2 mm.

Whitnall's ligament (superior transverse ligament)

◼ A fascial condensation stretching from the trochlea medially to lacrimal gland fascia laterally, 10–12 mm above the tarsus.

Lower lid retractors

◼ Arise as the capsulopalpebral head of the inferior rectus, passing forward as a fascial sheet which envelops the inferior oblique muscle and inserts into the inferior tarsus.

◼ A sympathetically innervated portion lies immediately posterior to the aponeurotic portion, arising from the fascial sheath of the inferior rectus muscle and inserting into the inferior tarsus.

◼ Contraction on down gaze results in 3–7 mm of lower lid depression.

Grey line

◼ The mucocutaneous junction situated behind the eyelashes.

◼ A grey line split opens the space between the orbicularis muscle and tarsus, dividing the eyelid into anterior and posterior lamellae.

History

Identify factors which influence disease risk, subsequent management, and prognosis. Old photographs may help determine if changes are congenital or acquired. If surgery is planned, ask about anticoagulants (NSAIDs, antiplatelet agents, warfarin) and plaster allergies. The history depends on the presenting complaint – the two commonest situations are lid lesions (Table 1.1) and lid malposition (Table 1.2).

Table 1.1: Lid lesions	
Feature	Consider
Discharge	Chalazion, abscess, mucocele, sinus disease
Pain, bleeding, change in pigmentation, sensory loss, sun exposure, previous radiotherapy	Malignancy (new or recurrent)
Rapid growth	Keratoacanthoma, infection
Slow growth	Basal cell carcinoma
Postural or diurnal variation in size	Venous anomaly
Trauma, previous surgery	Foreign body, granuloma

Table 1.2: Abnormal lid height or position	
Feature	Consider
Family history	Familial ptosis, myopathy, blepharophimosis
Eyelid movement with jaw action	Marcus Gunn jaw-wink phenomenon
Diurnal variation, diplopia, facial weakness, dysphagia, muscle weakness	Myopathy
Thyroid dysfunction (proptosis, lid retraction)	Thyroid eye disease
Red, uncomfortable eye, contact lens use, tropical medication	Ocular surface or conjunctival disease causing ptosis
Fasciculations, spasms, involuntary closure with facial movement	Blepharospasm, aberrant nerve regeneration (following facial palsy)
Neurosurgery	Facial nerve palsy (brow ptosis)
Head and neck disease, respiratory disease, thoracic surgery	Horner's syndrome
Sleep apnoea, lid eversion at night	Floppy eyelid syndrome
Lid lesion	Mechanical ptosis
Involutional facial changes	Involution ectropion and entropion

Examination

Sit directly opposite the patient. Ocular and eyelid observations must be recorded with each eye fixating in turn, or false measurement will be obtained. Note any facial asymmetry and record the following:

Best corrected visual acuity of each eye.

Margin reflex distance (MRD):

MRD 1: Upper lid margin to central corneal light reflex.

MRD 2: Lower lid margin to corneal reflex.

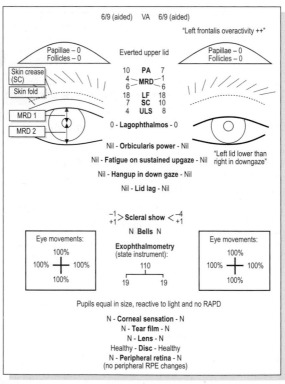

Fig. 1.3: Typical example of notes of a patient with a left aponeurosis disinsertion-type ptosis.

■ MRD gives more information than palpebral aperture (PA), the vertical distance between the upper and lower eyelid margins. For example, a patient with unilateral ectropion and ptosis may have a similar PA to the normal side.

■ In a child only PA may be measurable.

■ Where the lid contour is abnormal, record the PA at the medial and lateral limbus, and centrally.

Levator function (LF) Typically 15–20 mm in the adult.

■ Block compensatory frontalis activity when measuring LF. Hold a ruler vertically before the eye, between thumb and first finger. The second and third fingers rest firmly on the brow to overcome frontalis activity.

■ Measure the maximal vertical excursion of the upper lid, from down gaze to up gaze.

■ Note relative lid height in downgaze. In congenital levator dystrophy the lid is higher than the fellow. In acquired ptosis (aponeurotic dehiscence) the lid is lower.

Skin crease (SC) 7–8 mm in men, 9–10 mm in women.

■ Marks the fulcrum of activity of the levator palpebrae muscle on the eyelid, and is formed where levator fibres attach to the skin.

■ Measure the distance between the lid margin and skin crease(s) in down gaze.

Upper lid show (ULS) Distance between the lid margin and skin fold (not crease) in primary position. ULS asymmetry is a cause of patient dissatisfaction.

Lagophthalmos Residual interpalpebral distance with gentle closure. Ask if there is nocturnal lagophthalmos.

Scleral show (SS) Distance between the lid margin and the superior, and inferior, limbi, with each eye fixating the target in turn.

Hang up in down gaze (failure of upper lid to descend normally). May occur with levator dystrophy, previous ptosis surgery, thyroid eye disease and orbital disease.

Additional observations

■ Lid lag (phase lag on down gaze – a dynamic process).

■ Cogan's twitch (overshoot of upper lid on elevation from depression).

- Jaw movement (check for abnormal eyelid movement due to medial or lateral pterygoid synkinesis).

- Pupil reactions and size (check photopic and scotopic measurement if Horner's syndrome is suspected).

- Saccades and ductions (may be affected with myopathy or aberrant third nerve regeneration).

- Bell's phenomenon, corneal sensation (risk of corneal exposure following ptosis surgery if these are reduced).

- Take care to assess with each eye fixating in turn (e.g. apparent ptosis may be a pseudoptosis in the presence of hypotropia, or a double elevator palsy).

Record findings as shown in Figure 1.3.

Ectropion

Background Age-related ectropion is common, but exclude other causes.

Classification

- Age-related.

- Cicatricial: due to shortage of skin – may occur with ageing, trauma, previous lower lid surgery, overflow of tears/topical medication.

- Paralytic: e.g. facial nerve palsy due to any cause.

- Mechanical: from a lower lid mass such as a meibomian cyst or neoplasia.

Symptoms Epiphora, intermittent red eye, mucous discharge.

Signs Part or whole of the lower lid is everted from the globe. Other changes may be present, e.g. dermatochalasis, ptosis, punctal stenosis.

History and examination Note any previous lid surgery, trauma, and assess facial nerve power.

1. Age-related:

   - Horizontal laxity: lower lid fails to snap back when distracted from the globe.

   - Lateral and medial canthal ligament laxity: note the degree of punctal displacement with lateral traction, e.g. to the medial limbus or medial pupil.

   - Retractor laxity causing tarsal (shelf) ectropion: the tarsal conjunctiva may be inflamed/thickened from chronic exposure; punctal stenosis is commonly present.

   - Orbicularis muscle hypotony: assess for lagophthalmos, upper lid retraction, assess Bell's phenomenon, upgaze, and corneal sensation.

2. Anterior lamella cicatricial changes:

   - Ask the patient to open his/her mouth and look up. In the presence of significant cicatricial changes, the lid cannot be apposed to the globe.

   - Assess the extent of available skin in the upper lids and pre/postauricular areas as part of surgical planning.

Investigations A lower lid mass causing ectropion may require biopsy and appropriate excision.

Treatment For temporary relief place Micropore tape horizontally along the lower lid skin and then up onto the temple region to provide lift.

Surgery:

- The main principle is the correction of horizontal lid laxity, usually with a full-thickness pentagon wedge excision laterally (Box 1.1), or a lateral tarsal strip (Box 1.2).

- Medial ectropion with punctual eversion may require a medial ('diamond') tarso-conjunctivoplasty. A punctoplasty may also be indicated. The 'lazy T' procedure is a medial pentagon excision plus medial tarso-conjunctivoplasty (the posterior lamella scar forms a 'T').

- Medial ectropion due to medial canthal tendon laxity (i.e. the posterior limb) will not be addressed by repairing the anterior limb alone. Significant medial laxity may require a medial canthal fixation suture, or medial wedge excision with an anchoring suture between the medial cut end of the tarsus and the periosteum of the posterior lacrimal crest ('medial wedge'). In paralytic cases, a medial (Lee) canthoplasty helps to raise the lower lid.

Box 1.1: Pentagon wedge excision

1. Consent:

   - *Benefit*: improved lid position.

   - *Risks*: recurrence of ectropion; over- and undercorrection; scarring; inflammation; infection; suture granuloma (with nonabsorbable suture); further surgery. May produce bruising, conjunctival chemosis, and subconjunctival haemorrhage.

2. Instil topical anaesthetic into the conjuctival sac.

3. Inject 1–2 ml of 2% lidocaine with 1:200 000 epinephrine through the skin, at either end of the eyelid (27 or 28-gauge needle).

4. Use straight scissors to make a full-thickness cut through the eyelid at the junction of the lateral third and medial two-thirds of the eyelid. Overlap the cut edges to decide how much to shorten, and resect this amount, in the form of a pentagon (Fig. 1.4).

5. Haemostasis is essential before closing (Bipolar cautery).

Box 1.1: Pentagon wedge excision—cont'd

6. Pass each needle of a double 7/0 Vicryl suture through each grey line. Place the suture on traction with an artery clamp and rest this on the forehead – this aligns the tarsal edges while the tarsal sutures are placed.

7. Align the cut tarsal edges with two 6/0 Vicryl sutures. Take large bites of the tarsus; lay the knots anteriorly. Further deep sutures may be used to close the orbicularis inferior to the tarsus.

8. Now tie the 7/0 Vicryl suture through the grey line, with the knot lying within the wound. A lash line suture completes correct alignment of the lid edges. If the apposition of the lid margins is imperfect, sutures are removed and replaced.

9. Close the skin with 3–4 7/0 Vicryl sutures.

10. Apply Oc. chloramphenicol, Vaseline gauze, and eye pad for 24 hours. The absorbable skin sutures may be left in situ, although are frequently removed at first review in 10–14 days.

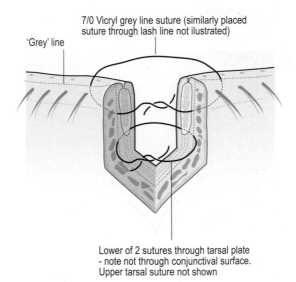

'Grey' line

7/0 Vicryl grey line suture (similarly placed suture through lash line not ilustrated)

Lower of 2 sutures through tarsal plate - note not through conjunctival surface. Upper tarsal suture not shown

Fig. 1.4: Pentagon wedge excision.

Box 1.2: Lateral tarsal strip (LTS)

1. Consent:

   - *Benefit*: improved lid position.

   - *Risks*: recurrence of ectropion; over- and undercorrection; scarring; inflammation; infection; suture granuloma (with nonabsorbable suture); further surgery. May produce bruising, conjunctival chemosis, and subconjunctival haemorrhage.

2. Inject local anaesthetic subcutaneously via a 27 or 28-gauge needle to the lateral canthal region, followed by gentle pressure.

3. Perform a lateral canthotomy by making a horizontal cut at the lateral canthus (straight scissors).

4. Ensure haemostasis

5. Grasp the lateral end of the lower lid (Adson's dissecting forceps) and perform cantholysis of the subconjunctival bandlike attachments (Fig. 1.5, arrow) between the lid and orbital rim (straight sharp scissors).

6. Dissect between orbicularis and the tarsus and divide the two by staying posterior to the grey line (straight scissors). The corresponding mucocutaneous strip of lid margin is removed.

7. Cut a tarsal strip 3–4 mm wide and ≈5 mm long, lower edge parallel to the lid margin. Pare off the conjunctiva on the strip (D15 blade).

8. Perform lateral (2 mm) upper lid grey line split to enhance subsequent vertical lift ('augmented LTS').

9. Attach the LTS to the periosteum using double-ended 5/0 undyed Vicryl. Expose the lateral orbital rim (straight or spring scissors) and spread orbicularis fibres aside (tips of the Moorfields forceps, held in the left hand, straddle the orbital rim and maintain the view of the periosteum).

10. Pass the suture ends through the inner orbital rim periosteum – 2 mm higher than the level of the medial canthus – by rolling the needle from inside the rim anteriorly.

11. Pull both ends through equally, but not completely, to leave a small loop. Place this loop over the LTS (Fig. 1.6A). Pass one needle through the end of the LTS laterally, and one medial to the loop (Fig. 1.6B). Tighten the suture to ensure a sufficiently high placement on the orbital rim and reposition if necessary.

Box 1.2: Lateral tarsal strip (LTS)—cont'd

12. Place 6/0 Vicryl grey line (buried knot) and lash line sutures (external knot) through the upper and lower lids before tying the strip suture (firm, but do not overtighten – watch the position of the lid on the globe).

13. As the LTS suture ends are pulled upwards, the noose tightens on the strip which is drawn onto the orbital rim, tucked upwards to lie within upper lid grey line split. This provides further vertical support.

14. Close orbicularis and skin with interrupted 7/0 Vicryl sutures.

15. Apply Oc. chloramphenicol, Vaseline gauze, and a firm dressing for 24 hours.

16. Review in 2 weeks for removal of skin sutures, then discharge.

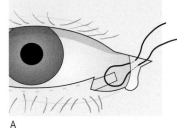

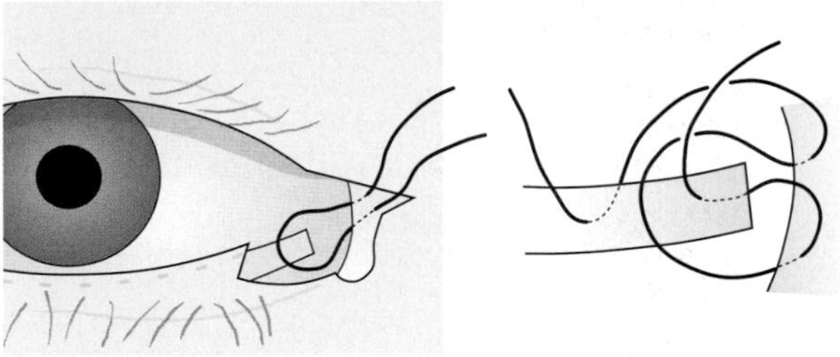

A   B

Fig. 1.5: Lateral tarsal strip.

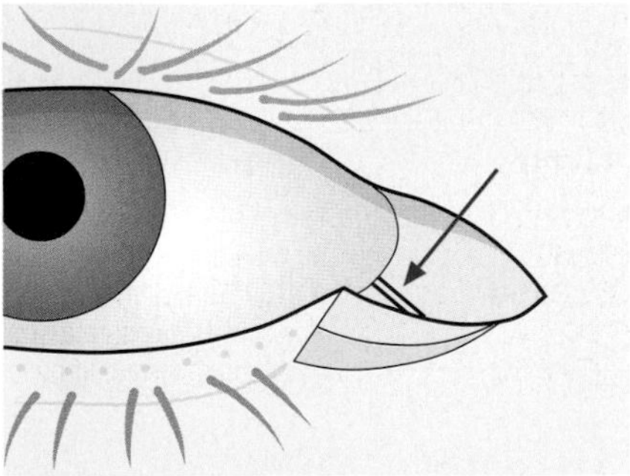

Fig. 1.6: Lateral tarsal strip.

- Tarsal, or 'shelf' ectropion requires lid shortening plus an internal retractor plication, using three 5/0 Vicryl sutures via a conjunctival approach.

- Cicatricial ectropion may respond to cessation of topical treatment, and a bland moisturising cream to the lower lid. Surgery aims to free all cicatricial bands via a wide subciliary incision, and a full-thickness skin graft, pedicle rotation, or transposition flap into the lower lid.

Floppy Eyelid Syndrome

Background Typically presents in middle-aged obese men with unilateral or bilateral chronic papillary conjunctivitis, marked upper lid tissue laxity, and spontaneous tarsal eversion at night. Frequently associated with sleep apnoea syndrome. The aetiology is unknown but histology shows decreased elastin in the tarsus.

Symptoms Irritable red eye. Upper lid eversion at night (on the sleeping side).

Signs Easily everted tarsus (Fig. 1.7) with rubbery consistency, lash ptosis, papillary conjunctivitis, and superior punctate keratitis.

History and examination The patient's partner may report heavy snoring, apnoea and lid eversion at night. Horizontal lid laxity is usually marked. Keratitis may be subtle.

Differential diagnosis Allergic conjunctivitis, chlamydial conjunctivitis, and age-related lid laxity.

Investigations Refer to a respiratory physician for sleep studies.

Treatment

- ▪ *Casualty*: Topical lubricants, mild topical steroid for keratitis.

- ▪ *Clinic*: Consider surgical options:

  1. Anterior lamellar reposition for lash ptosis.

  2. Upper lid shortening with wedge excision.

  3. Medial and lateral canthal tendon plication.

Surgical risks include inflammation, infection, scarring, and need for further lid.

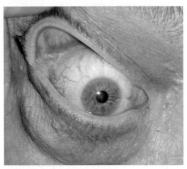

Fig. 1.7: Floppy eyelid syndrome.

Lower Lid Entropion

Background Similar aetiology to age-related ectropion (p. 9). Exclude chronic conjunctival disease and cicatrization of the posterior lamella.

Classification

- Congenital.
- Acquired: age-related, cicatricial.

Symptoms Epiphora, mucous discharge and red eye.

Signs All or part of the lower lid may be inverted. Other features include: subtarsal mucous strands, lash–cornea touch, punctate epithelial keratopathy, conjunctival cicatricial changes, punctal stenosis, skin laxity, preseptal orbicularis riding upwards ('spastic entropion').

History and examination Ask about previous lid surgery and cicatrizing disease, e.g. Steven-Johnson's syndrome, ocular mucous membrane pemphigoid (OMMP) and allergy to topical medication. Forced lid closure may elicit subtle entropion. Exclude effacement of the plica, an early sign in OMMP. Lower lid entropion may simulate distichiasis. In the former, the meibomian gland orifices are always found posterior to the lashes.

Investigations Conjunctival biopsy if OMMP suspected.

Treatment: In patients unfit for surgery, or as a temporising measure, the following may be appropriate:

- *Transverse lid sutures*: 3–4 double-ended 5/0 Vicryl sutures are passed through the lower lid just beneath the tarsus, brought out through the skin, and tied to create a slight ectropion. Sutures may be left to absorb.
- *Everting sutures*: Pass 3 double-ended 5/0 Vicryl sutures through the lower fornix and out through the skin. Shorter-acting than transverse lid sutures (Fig. 1.8).
- *Botulinum toxin A*: Inject into the preseptal orbicularis (3 injections of Dysport 20 units, 1 cm from the lower lid margin). May need to be repeated.

Surgery:

- Horizontal lid laxity must be addressed (lateral tarsal strip or pentagon wedge excision, p. 10–13) to reduce the risk of recurrence. Everting sutures, or, in more severe cases, plicating sutures to the lower lid retractors (Jones procedure), are placed at the same time. The Weiss procedure involves a full-thickness horizontal lower lid incision and does not address horizontal laxity.

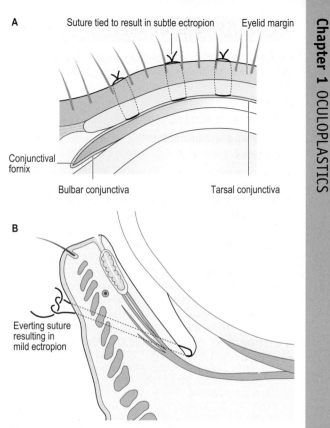

A Suture tied to result in subtle ectropion   Eyelid margin

Conjunctival fornix

Bulbar conjunctiva   Tarsal conjunctiva

B

Everting suture resulting in mild ectropion

Fig. 1.8: Everting sutures **(A and B)**.

- The Quickert operation is effectively a Weiss procedure with horizontal lid shortening.

- The Jones procedure directly plicates the lower lid retractors to the tarsus and anterior lamella via an incision level with the lower border of the tarsus. Avoid lower lid retraction from overtightening. Use adjustable sutures if surgery is under general anaesthesia.

- Posterior lamella graft (e.g. buccal mucosa) is indicated in cicatricial cases. Aggressive control of conjunctival inflammation should precede surgery in cases of OMMP. Quiescent OMMP cases should also receive peroperative oral and topical steroids.

Upper Lid Entropion

Background Upper lid entropion is frequently due to a posterior lamella cicatricial process, e.g. chronic conjunctivitis, trachoma, ocular mucous membrane pemphigoid (OMMP). In sockets, it is usually due to a shortage of lining.

Symptoms Ocular irritation, epiphora.

History and examination Ask about trauma, and chronic ocular surface inflammation (e.g. OMMP). Exclude blepharospasm, posterior lamella cicatricial changes, and corneal pannus or epithelial changes.

Differential diagnosis Lash ptosis without lid entropion, e.g. floppy eyelid syndrome.

Management For mild cases, an anterior lamella reposition may suffice. A skin crease incision is made down to the tarsus, and three double-armed 5/0 Vicryl sutures are placed through the upper tarsus, brought out through the skin above the lashes and tied. With all procedures, recession of the retractors off the anterior tarsal plate, with or without division of the lateral horn, may also be required. Greater eversion is achieved with a grey line split, and, if required, a horizontal wedge excision of the anterior tarsus. More severe cases may require a lamella division, i.e. splitting the anterior and posterior lamellae via the grey line as far as the superior fornix and recessing the retractors. Where there is keratin on the posterior aspect of the tarsus, a terminal tarsal rotation may be required.

Trichiasis

Eyelash follicles are in a normal position (unlike distichiasis) but directed towards the globe (Fig. 1.9). Causes include chronic lid margin disease and conjunctival cicatricial diseases, e.g. Stevens-Johnson syndrome and ocular mucous membrane pemphigoid. Treat small numbers of lashes with electrolysis (Box 1.3), but up to half may re-grow, and treatment may cause tarsal scarring and further trichiasis. Full-thickness lid excision with repair of the defect is a more permanent treatment for localized trichiasis. Manage more extensive areas with cryotherapy (Box 1.4), but be aware that this may cause localized skin depigmentation in dark-skinned patients; electrolysis and correction of any lid margin malposition may be preferable in such patients.

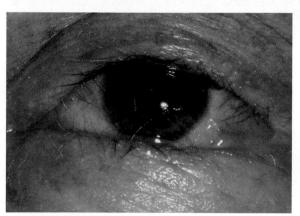

Fig. 1.9: Trichiasis.

Box 1.3: Electrolysis

1. Inject local anaesthesia and use a microscope.

2. Grasp the lid margin with large toothed forceps (e.g. Adson's forceps) and direct the fine electrolysis needle alongside the hair shaft down to the lash follicle.

3. Deliver the current until gentle blanching occurs. Power and time settings differ from one unit to another, e.g. the Ellman Surgitron radiofrequency device uses 'cut/coagulation' setting with power <1 unit.

4. Adequately treated lashes are then easily epilated and the hair bulb visualized.

Box 1.4: Cryotherapy

1. Some units have a thermocouple needle that is inserted into the tissue to check temperature, but this is not essential, if the average time it takes to reach −20°C has been assessed on a previous series of patients using the same cryo probe.

2. Inject local anaesthesia and protect the eye with a plastic lid guard.

3. Use the lid cryoprobe to apply a double freeze–thaw cycle (to −20°C) with spontaneous thawing between treatments.

4. Prescribe topical antibiotic ointment for 5–7 days.

Distichiasis

Clinical features

In contrast to trichiasis, distichiasis is a congenital disorder in which a separate and more posterior row of metaplastic lashes exists (often growing out of the meibomian gland orifices). The lid margin is in a normal position (Fig. 1.10).

Management

▨ If only a few lashes are affected, evert the eyelid with a meibomian clamp, use a microscope and incise the shaft of the eyelash through the partial thickness of the tarsus to the hair bulb. Electrolyse it under direct vision.

▨ More extensive areas can be treated by splitting the lid at the grey line, freezing the posterior lamella, and suturing the lamella back together. The posterior lamella must be advanced to compensate for the shrinkage after cryotherapy, which could lead to subsequent entropion formation.

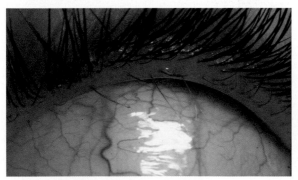

Fig. 1.10: Distichiasis.

Facial Nerve Palsy

Background Bell's palsy accounts for 75% of cases but is a diagnosis of exclusion.

Aetiology

- Idiopathic facial nerve palsy (IFNP, Bell's palsy):

    1. Commoner in the elderly (>70 years).

    2. Spontaneous recovery occurs in 75% of cases.

    3. Exposure keratopathy is unusual.

- Central or peripheral nervous system lesions.

- Trauma, including iatrogenic causes such as surgery for acoustic neuroma, and facial or parotid surgery.

- Systemic infections and inflammations.

- Herpes zoster oticus (Ramsay Hunt syndrome).

- Middle ear disease.

- Mastoiditis.

- Parotid tumours.

Symptoms Related to corneal exposure, failure of the lacrimal pump mechanism, and facial asymmetry.

Signs Include facial weakness (including brow ptosis and droop of the angle of the mouth), upper lid retraction, and lower lid atony (Fig. 1.11).

History Ask about prodromal viral illness, earache, previous facial palsy, trauma, middle ear disease, headache, and dysphonia.

Examination Examine for underlying causes (see Aetiology above). Regeneration syndromes may be missed. Differentiate between lower and upper motor neurone (central) lesions. Central lesions spare the frontalis action due to bilateral innervation. Actively exclude vesicles in the external auditory canal (Ramsay Hunt syndrome) because of the risk of CNS complications with immunosuppression. Test corneal sensation and check Bell's phenomenon and upgaze (the corneal prognosis is guarded if any are abnormal). Examine cranial nerves.

Investigations Consider neuroimaging for patients with:

- Concomitant focal neurology.

- Nonresolving facial nerve paresis after 3 months.

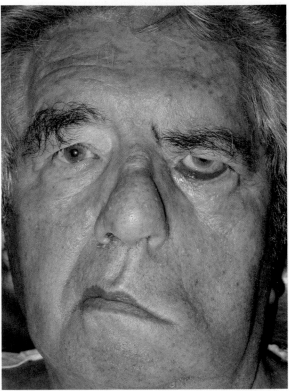

Fig. 1.11: Left facial nerve palsy.

Complications

- Exposure keratopathy and corneal perforation. Contributing factors include upper lid retraction due to unopposed levator activity, lower lid ectropion, lagophthalmos, and failure of tear drainage.

- Lower lid atony leading to horizontal laxity and ectropion.

- Aberrant nerve regeneration syndromes including gustatory epiphora, and facial synkineses, e.g. narrowing of the palpebral aperture with lower facial movement.

Treatment

■ Systemic

1. Medical management of IFNP is controversial. Cochrane Database reviews indicate no significant benefit from either systemic steroids (2002) or aciclovir (2001).

■ Ocular

1. Corneal protection

   a. Topical lubricants, e.g. G. Viscotears hourly and Oc. Lacrilube nocte.

   b. Botulinum toxin to the upper lid to induce temporary ptosis (5 iu Botox with a short, 27-gauge needle either transconjunctivally at the upper border of the tarsus, or transcutaneously through the skin crease).

   c. Temporary tarsorrhaphy with sutures, cyanoacrylate glue, or surgery. A medial (pillar) surgical tarsorrhaphy is preferable to a lateral tarsorrhaphy, because the peripheral visual field is maintained.

   d. Lower lid tightening (lateral tarsal strip, which may be 'augmented', i.e. placed higher on the orbital rim to aid tear drainage).

   e. Lower lid elevation with autogenous fascia lata passed through the length of the lid and sutured medially to the medial canthal tendon, and laterally to the orbital rim periosteum.

   f. Medial (Lee) canthoplasty, medial canthal fixation suture, or medial wedge resection (placing anchoring suture to the periosteum of the posterior lacrimal crest).

   g. Upper lid loading with a gold weight (typically for nocturnal lagophthalmos).

   h. Upper lid lowering (Müller's muscle excision for 1–3 mm retraction, or posterior or anterior approach levator recession for larger degrees of retraction).

   i. Sural nerve grafting to improve facial tone.

2. Epiphora

   a. Residual epiphora is managed once ectropion or lid laxity has been addressed.

   b. Gustatory epiphora: botulinum toxin to the lacrimal gland (Dysport 20 units transcutaneously, in three divided doses in one clinic visit), or direct surgical denervation of the orbital lobe of the lacrimal gland.

  c. Dacryocystorhinostomy (DCR) to reduce lacrimal outflow resistance.

  d. Lester Jones tube if the patient remains symptomatic at least 9 months following DCR.

3. Aberrant regeneration syndromes

  a. These often respond to low-dose botulinum toxin injections.

4. Cosmesis

  a. External direct brow pexy (skin and muscle excision with anchoring suture to the periosteum) or endoscopic brow lift (incision above the hair line).

  b. Lower lid blepharoplasty if there is tissue laxity and oedema.

  c. Angular sling to raise the mouth.

  d. Temporalis muscle transfer to create an encircling sling of fascia, passing laterally to medially in both lids.

  e. Facial reanimation may be achieved by cross nerve anastomosis.

Follow-up If there is no recovery of Bell's palsy within 6 weeks reconsider the diagnosis: 10% of patients with acute facial nerve palsy have a treatable lesion.

Discharge only when all factors contributing to corneal exposure have been addressed and the patient is stable on topical lubricants. This may take months to decades.

Ptosis

Background Ptosis describes a low position of the upper lid on the globe. It is not a diagnosis. *Children with ptosis are at risk of amblyopia if the eyelid covers any part of the pupil, and may require urgent brow suspension.*

Aetiology

- *Congenital*: Congenital levator dystrophy, congenital Horner's syndrome.

- *Hereditary*: Myopathic (myaesthenia gravis, ocular myopathy, systemic myopathy).

- *Acquired*: Trauma, involutional (aponeurosis dehiscence), oculomotor nerve disease, ocular surface disease or orbital inflammation (e.g. chronic contact lens wear, dacryoadenitis), iatrogenic (lid/orbital surgery), mechanical (upper lid mass), and as part of the postenucleation socket syndrome.

- *Pseudoptosis*: Aberrant facial nerve regeneration, blepharospasm, habit spasm, enophthalmos, hyperglobus, contralateral upper lid retraction or proptosis.

Symptoms Heavy lid, restricted visual field and brow ache (frontalis overaction).

Signs These include excess frontalis contraction, raised skin crease, deep upper sulcus, other involutional changes (e.g. dermatochalasis, lower lid ectropion), and abnormal head position. Lid height on downgaze relative to the healthy fellow lid is low in aponeurosis dehiscence and high in congenital (myogenic) ptosis. There is a high prevalence of strabismus and refractive errors in congenital cases.

History Ask about: duration; jaw wink; variability; fatigue; diplopia; previous lid surgery; trauma; facial palsy; family history.

Examination In addition to a full lid examination (p. 6) check the following: corneal sensation; Bell's phenomenon; orbicularis power; frontalis action; eye movements (risk of postoperative corneal exposure); pupil size/responses; exophthalmometry; peripheral fundal examination.

Investigation Arrange sympathetic chain imaging in Horner's syndrome (head, neck and upper thorax). Check antiacetylcholine receptor antibody screen and electromyographic studies in suspected myopathy. In ocular myasthesia gravis, antibodies may be absent in 40% of patients.

Management Children at risk of amblyopia require a frontalis sling procedure within 2–4 weeks. If the upper lid obscures *any* part of the upper visual field, then consider early intervention, because a full visual field is required for normal visual development. Where there is a mild to moderate ptosis without risk of amblyopia, correction may be delayed until the age of awareness (4–5 years). Otherwise, surgery may reasonably be delayed until early adult years. In adults, bilateral ptosis may cause functional blindness, and warrants early intervention. Surgical techniques depend on the cause:

- *Congenital ptosis with levator function (LF) ≥5 mm:* levator muscle advancement on the tarsus (anterior or posterior approach).

- *Congenital levator dystrophy with poor LF (<5 mm):* brow suspension with autogenous tissue in children >4 years of age (e.g. autogenous fascia lata). For the younger patient, use synthetic material, e.g. Nylon (Supramid) in children of a few months old, mersilene mesh in children up to 4 years old.

- *Congenital levator dystrophy associated with jaw wink:* bilateral levator disinsertion and autogenous fascia lata brow suspension. Informed discussion with the parents/carers is essential. Unilateral surgery may cause asymmetry.

- *Involutional ptosis:* repair/advancement of the levator aponeurosis onto the tarsus.

- *Myopathy including chronic progressive external ophthalmoplegia and myaesthenia gravis*: brow suspension if LF < 8 mm (<5 mm in children) because of the risk of corneal exposure with an aponeurosis advancement (due to orbicularis weakness, reduced Bell's phenomenon, and reduced upgaze). Use local anaesthesia ± sedation, with nonautogenous material, due to the risk of cardiac conduction defects with general anaesthesia. If the patient has reasonable frontalis effort, brow suspension with mersilene mesh may be performed. Aim to leave the lid height similar to the preoperative level, allowing for frontalis lift to raise the lids above the visual axis. In the patient with a third nerve palsy, or any situation where there is a risk of diplopia in lifting the lid, silicone may be used because of its ease of removal.

Consent Risk of over- or undercorrection, corneal exposure, lid oedema, infection, and asymmetrical skin creases.

Postoperative care G chloramphenicol q.d.s.; Oc. chloramphenicol nocte; p.r.n. topical lubricant.

Follow-up One week for removal of sutures, then 3 months. Consider early revision if overcorrected. Manage mild overcorrection with gentle lash traction twice daily.

Chalazion

Chalazion

Background Lipogranulomatous inflammatory lid reaction to retained sebaceous secretions (meibomian glands or glands of Zeiss). Histology shows focal or diffuse involvement which may involve the whole lid. May become secondarily infected leading to abscess formation. Associated with lid margin disease (blepharitis), acne rosacea, and seborrhoeic dermatitis.

Differential diagnosis *Sebaceous gland carcinoma is notorious in masquerading as recurrent chalazion or unilateral blepharoconjunctivitis.* Also consider Merkel cell tumour (rare). Other infective lesions around the eyelids include acute staphylococcal infection of the meibomian gland, and infections of a lash follicle and associated gland of Zeiss or Moll. These present as tender swellings which may resolve spontaneously or discharge. Any swelling in the region above the medial canthal ligament suggests neoplasia of the lacrimal sac and requires urgent investigation (CT and biopsy).

History Lump in one or both eyelids. May resolve spontaneously or become intermittently inflamed.

Examination Focal or diffuse lesion(s) within the lid (Fig. 1.12), often with lid margin and tear film changes. Lid eversion may reveal an exophytic inflamed conjunctival granuloma.

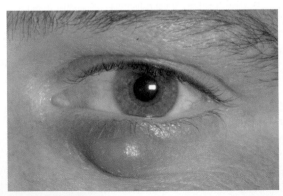

Fig. 1.12: Chalazion.

Medical management

Options include:

- Twice daily warm compresses to the lids, and lid margin hygiene to improve the flow of meibomian gland secretions.

- Topical antibiotic ointment (Oc. chloramphenicol or Oc. fucithalmic b.d.).

- Oral doxycycline if rosacea is present (50 mg o.d. for 3 months).

- Intralesional steroid injection (0.1 mL triamcinolone with a 30-gauge needle).

Surgical management (incision and curettage)

1. Mark the skin over the lesion with a surgical pen to aid localization.

2. Apply topical conjunctival anaesthesia then inject local anaesthetic into the lid (1 mL of lidocaine 2% with 1 : 200 000 epinephrine). Injecting slowly reduces patient discomfort.

3. Position a cyst clamp over the lid and tighten firmly before everting the lid.

4. Make a vertical incision (E11 blade) into the tarsus, no closer than 2 mm to the lid margin.

5. Curette out the granuloma, which may be firm. Larger lesions may require a cruciate incision with excision of tarsus.

6. Send material to histopathology in recurrent or atypical cases.

7. Instil Oc. chloramphenicol and cover the eye with a Vaseline gauze and an eye pad for 4–6 hours. Prescribe Oc. chloramphenicol q.d.s. 1 week.

Follow-up Not required for routine cases

Necrotizing Fasciitis

Background A group A streptococcus infection of the subdermal tissue planes with necrosis of the overlying skin. Complications include septicaemia, systemic organ failure, and death. Early recognition and prompt intervention are critical.

History Determine the risk factors. These include old age, trauma, and immunosuppression, including diabetes.

Examination Look for skin discoloration, or frank necrosis with sloughing tissue (Fig. 1.13). Check vital signs.

Differential diagnosis Preseptal cellulitis (without progression to orbital cellulitis or necrotizing fasciitis), chronic dacroadenitis (oedema limited to the periorbital region, tenderness in superotemporal quadrant, no skin necrosis).

Investigations FBC, acute-phase inflammatory markers, renal and hepatic profiles.

Management Start high-dose intravenous penicillin and ciprofloxacin, and debride necrotic tissue down to healthy (bleeding) tissue. Repeat surgical debridement if required. Send tissue for culture and sensitivity. Co-manage patients with a physician in the presence of systemic signs.

Subsequent reconstructive approaches include laissez faire (granulation), local myocutaneous flaps, and full-thickness skin grafting.

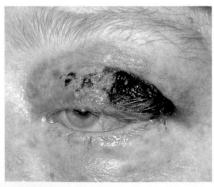

Fig. 1.13: Necrotizing fasciitis.

Benign Lid Lesions

Epithelial lesions

- *Squamous papilloma*: a sessile or pedunculated lesion of viral origin (Fig. 1.14). Manage by shave excision biopsy.

- *Seborrhoeic keratosis* (senile verucca): single or multiple plaques or pedunculated lesions occurring in middle-aged to older adults (Fig. 1.15). Perform excision biopsy.

- *Keratoacanthoma*: solitary, subacute nodule of possible viral origin characterized by a keratin-filled crater, or horn (Fig. 1.16). The differential diagnosis includes squamous cell carcinoma, basal cell carcinoma and seborrhoeic keratosis. Where there is no indication of spontaneous resolution, perform an excision biopsy which must include deep tissue.

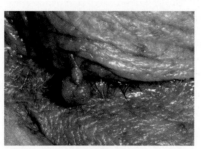

Fig. 1.14: Squamous papilloma.

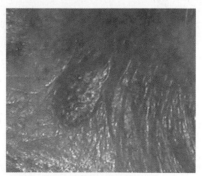

Fig. 1.15: Seborrhoeic keratosis of the lower eyelid.

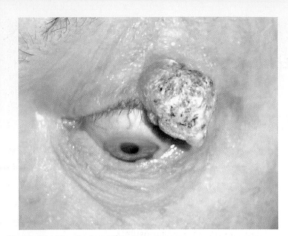

Fig. 1.16: Keratoacanthoma.

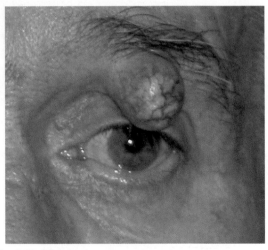

Fig. 1.17: Pilar cyst.

■ *Pilar cyst*: also called sebaceous or epidermoid cyst. Presents as a mobile subcutaneous or dermal mass containing desquamated cells and keratin (Fig. 1.17). Manage with complete excision with preservation of overlying skin.

■ *Molluscum contagiosum*: single or multiple periocular lesions which shed poxvirus particles and may present as a chronic follicular conjunctivitis (Fig. 1.18). Manage by direct excision.

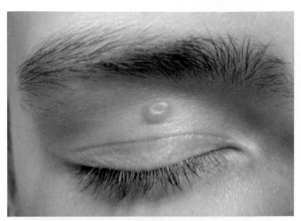

Fig. 1.18: Molluscum contagiosum.

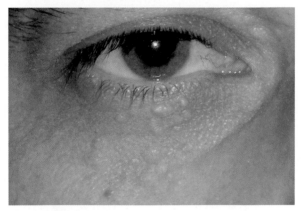

Fig. 1.19: Syringomata.

Adnexal lesions

▨ Lesions originating from eccrine sweat glands include sudiferous cysts, which may occur as solitary or multiple lesions on the eyelids, and syringomata (Fig. 1.19) which present as multiple small pale papules on the lower lids. Manage by surgical excision or carbon dioxide laser.

▨ Lesions of the apocrine glands of Moll include apocrine hidrocystoma which presents as a small fluid-filled cyst on the eyelid margin (Fig. 1.20), and cylindroma, a dome-shaped

33

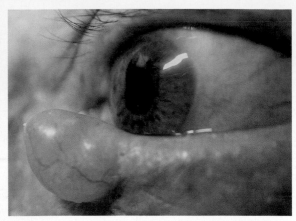

Fig. 1.20: Large cyst of Moll (apocrine hidrocystoma).

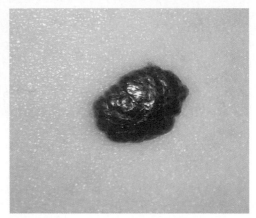

Fig. 1.21: Capillary haemangioma (strawberry naevus).

pink nodule. Extensive involvement of the scalp is described as a turban tumour. Excise intact if troublesome.

■ Lesions of hair follicles include trichoepithelioma, trichofolliculoma, trichilemmoma and pilomatrixoma. All require excision biopsy.

Vascular lesions

■ *Capillary haemangioma*: superficial 'strawberry naevi' (Fig. 1.21) are the most common, but deeper, orbital lesions can occur (p. 92). An oscillatory decay pattern precedes complete involution within the first decade. Larger lesions may cause astigmatism and mechanical ptosis. Where there is a risk of amblyopia, treatment (p. 92) may be required.

▪ *Naevus flammeus* ('port wine stain'): this flat red-purple vascular lesion is formed of dilated capillaries, is usually unilateral in distribution, and does not blanch with pressure (unlike a capillary naevus). In addition, it does not involute spontaneously, and is associated with other ocular and leptomeningeal vascular lesions in the Sturge-Weber syndrome (Fig. 1.22).

▪ *Pyogenic granuloma*: occurs after trauma (Fig. 1.23). Histology shows nongranulomatous inflammatory cells, fibroblasts and blood vessels. Treatment is surgical excision.

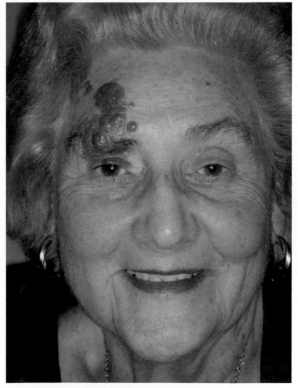

Fig. 1.22: Naevus flammeus associated with Sturge-Weber syndrome.

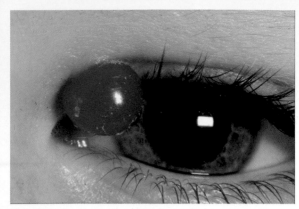

Fig. 1.23: Pyogenic granuloma.

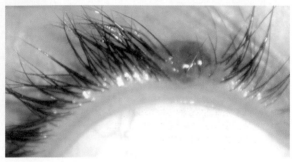

Fig. 1.24: Intradermal naevus with localized lash loss (excision biopsy required).

Pigmented lesions

▧ *Pigmented naevi*: common lesions that do not require excision in the absence of atypical features such as growth, change in pigmentation, or lash loss (Fig. 1.24). Note that basal cell carcinomas may be pigmented, and melanomata may lack pigmentation.

▧ *Naevus of Ota* (oculodermal melanocytosis): see page 392.

Xanthomatous lesions

▧ *Xanthelasma*: presents in the medial upper and lower lids in middle-aged adults (Fig. 1.25), and is associated with hyperlipidaemia in ≈50% of cases. Treatment options include surgical excision, carbon dioxide laser, and topical trichloroacetic acid.

■ *Juvenile xanthogranuloma*: presents within the first 2 years of life with raised nodules, typically in the head and neck region, which regress spontaneously within a few years. Associated iris involvement may cause glaucoma, uveitis and spontaneous hyphaema.

Neural lesions

■ *Eyelid neurofibroma*: may be isolated or associated with neurofibromatosis type I. Lesions may occur as a solitary fleshy mass or diffuse lid infiltration with mechanical ptosis (plexiform neuroma) (Fig. 1.26). Complete excision is difficult to achieve and recurrence is common.

Miscellaneous

■ *Exophytic conjunctival granuloma*: a posterior lid lesion associated with chalazia or previous posterior lid surgery (Fig. 1.27). Treat with shave excision biopsy.

■ *Cutaneous sarcoid granuloma*: May require repeated intralesional long- plus short-acting steroid injection (intralesional depomedrome 40 mg/mL, and perilesional dexamethasone 5 mg/mL).

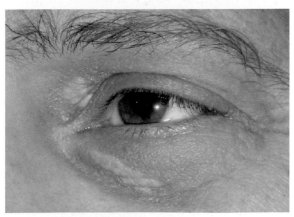

Fig. 1.25: Xanthelasmata.

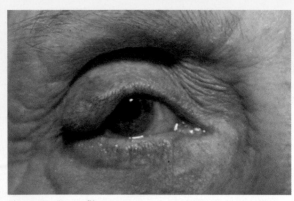

Fig. 1.26: Neurofibroma.

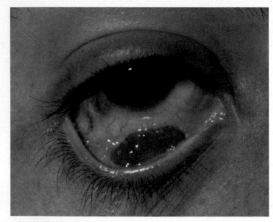

Fig. 1.27: Conjunctival granuloma.

Neoplastic Lid Lesions

Background There are no pathognomonic features of neoplasia, but a careful history may identify a gradually enlarging lid lesion, crusting, bleeding, irritation, red eye, and epiphora due to mechanical ectropion, corneal irritation, or involvement of the lacrimal drainage system. A biopsy is indicated to exclude malignancy.

Premalignant disease

- *Actinic keratosis*: 20% of cases may progress to squamous cell carcinoma. Lesions may be widespread and a dermatology opinion may be required. Treat by excision or cryotherapy (Fig. 1.28).

- *Bowen's disease* (intraepithelial neoplasia): cellular atypia is present at the level of the basement membrane, but no deeper. Progresses to squamous cell carcinoma in 2–3% of cases; most advocate complete excision unless there is limited tissue, such as around the canaliculi (Fig. 1.29). Such cases are managed by debulking and cryotherapy, with full excision in cases of malignant transformation.

- *Lentigo maligna*: slowly spreading macular lesion, with irregular border. Become infiltrative in 33% of cases. Complete excision is preferable, but where this is impractical, the area needs to be monitored closely, with excisional biopsy, performed on any enlarging or suspicious areas (Fig. 1.30).

Primary eyelid malignant disease

- *Basal cell carcinoma* BCC accounts for >90% of all neoplastic eyelid lesions, being most prevalent in fair-skinned individuals.

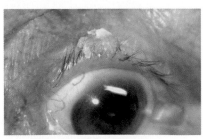

Fig. 1.28: Actinic keratosis.

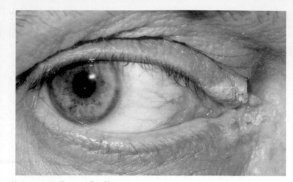

Fig. 1.29: Bowen's disease.

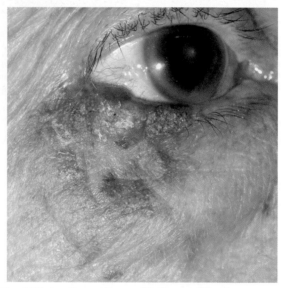

Fig. 1.30: Lentigo maligna with focal infiltrative changes.

Subtypes are described as nodular, ulcerative, cystic, sclerosing, pigmented or morphoeiform, the latter being the most difficult to manage. Lesions occur most commonly on the lower lid and medial canthus (Fig. 1.31), and may be raised (e.g. nodular) or flat (e.g. morphoeiform). Other features include destruction of the lash follicles, a raised pearly edge

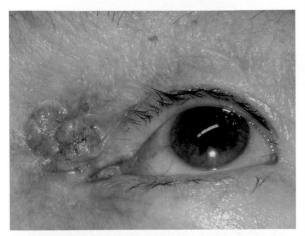

Fig. 1.31: Basal cell carcinoma.

with telangiectatic vessels, ulcerated centre, cyst formation, and pigmentation.

Complete excision with minimal sacrifice of healthy tissue is achieved by Mohs' micrographic surgery, where available. Margin control may also be achieved with frozen section or fast paraffin. Close communication with the histologist is essential. Reconstruction may entail direct closure for small margin tumours, local sliding myocutaneous flaps, and/or full-thickness skin grafting for anterior lamella defects. Posterior lamella defects may be reconstructed with local conjunctival advancement, free tarsoconjunctival graft from the upper lid, hard palate graft, and nasal mucosal or labial mucosal grafts. Very small eyelid lesions, and those in elderly, frail patients, may be managed with cryotherapy. Local radiotherapy is not useful; subsequent lesion recurrence may be as high as 20% and may be difficult to control. Chemotherapy plays no role. Distant metastases are exceptionally rare.

■ *Squamous cell carcinoma* SCC represent ≈5 % of all eyelid malignancies. Lesions occasionally develop from preexisting areas of actinic keratosis or Bowen's disease. Typically present as a thickened, erythematous scaly lesion (Fig. 1.32), but may also resemble BCC. Surface keratinization may be marked. SCC is more aggressive than BCC, with ≈5% of patients developing local periocular recurrence despite histologically complete excision.

Excision and reconstruction principles are similar to BCC. SCC has a metastatic potential; mortality is due to local

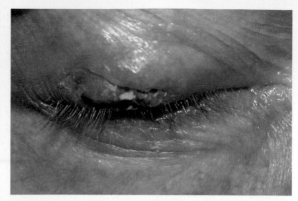

Fig. 1.32: Squamous cell carcinoma.

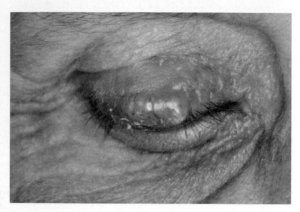

Fig. 1.33: Sebaceous gland carcinoma.

perineural spread to the CNS (≈2 %). The alternative to surgical excision includes cryotherapy which is good for small lesions, particularly those close to the lacrimal drainage apparatus. Radiotherapy is effective but is preferably avoided on the upper lid, because of the risk of inducing an irritable eye from keratin production on the tarsal conjunctiva, and for lesions at the medial canthus, which may extend deeply.

■ *Sebaceous gland carcinoma:* A rare, aggressive tumour which commonly arises from the meibomian glands (Fig. 1.33). It carries a high morbidity due to local, haematogenous, and lymphatic spread. A history of presumed recurrent chalazion or a chronic unilateral blepharoconjunctivitis should raise suspicion.

Early diagnosis and complete excision is essential. Mapping biopsies of the superior and inferior tarsal and bulbar conjunctiva are performed to exclude multicentric origin and pagetoid spread. The histologist should be alerted to use the appropriate lipid stains. Orbital exenteration is indicated in patients with diffuse involvement of the lid or conjunctiva. Radiation therapy plays a palliative role.

- *Melanoma:* represents <1 % of eyelid neoplasms. Lesions are irregularly pigmented (Fig. 1.34), but a large minority may lack pigmentation. Other features include inflammation and bleeding. Clinical forms include lentigo maligna, superficial spreading, and nodular melanoma. Metastases are common in the latter two forms. The Breslow thickness predicts the average time to metastasis. The cure rate for lesions <0.75 mm thick approaches 100%.

  Excise lesions <1.5 mm thick with wide margins and reconstruct. Lesions >1.5 mm require additional neck lymph node scintigraphy and biopsy. Involve nuclear medicine, and

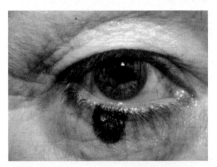

Fig. 1.34: Melanoma.

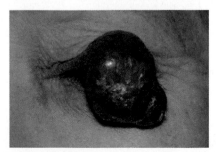

Fig. 1.35: Large Merkel cell tumour.

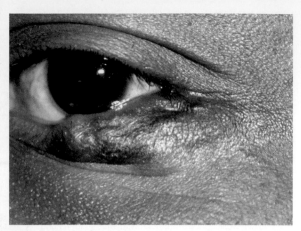

Fig. 1.36: Kaposi's sarcoma.

head and neck or plastic surgery colleagues. Distant metastasis may occur even with clear histological margins.

■ *Merkel cell tumour:* a small-cell undifferentiated/ neuroendocrine carcinoma which characteristically presents as a firm, painless nodule with overlying violet skin changes (Fig. 1.35). Growth is rapid, metastases common, and the prognosis poor. Early diagnosis and aggressive, histologically guided surgical excision are important.

Secondary malignant disease

■ *Metastatic disease*: eyelid involvement is rare. Primary sites include breast and bronchus. Involve physicians.

■ *Lymphomatous deposits*: refer to oncology for systemic investigation and management.

■ *Kaposi's sarcoma* (Fig. 1.36): presents as a purplish or red/ brown non pruritic nodule or macule which commonly affects the face, in particular the tip of the nose, eyelids and conjunctiva. It develops in the presence of Kaposi's sarcoma-associated herpes virus (HHV-8), which is associated with HIV infection and other lymphotrophic disorders. Local control may be achieved with radiation. Management is of the underlying immune deficiency.

Facial Dystonias

Clinical features The facial dystonias include benign essential blepharospasm and hemifacial spasm. Increasingly frequent blinking and periocular spasms may lead to social embarrassment, anxiety, depression, and, ultimately, functional blindness.

Examination Record the position and degree of spasm or fasciculation diagrammatically. Perform a full ocular and cranial nerve examination (including corneal sensation). Note any lid margin disease or tear film abnormalities.

Investigations Refer patients with hemifacial spasm, recent or rapid onset blepharospasm, or blepharospasm with other neurological features (e.g. reduced corneal sensation) to a neurologist for assessment and neuroimaging. Those with longstanding, stable symptoms and without other neurological signs do not require investigation.

Management overview Botulinum toxin injections improves symptoms in >90% of patients. An empirical approach is required to identify the optimum dose: more than one set of injections may be required for adequate control of spasms. Where toxin injections do not control symptoms without causing side effects, a protractor myectomy is effective, although toxin injection may continue to be required. A frontalis sling may be helpful in patients with pretarsal apraxia (that is, inability to open the eyelids due to spasms of the pretarsal orbicularis), once the spasm has been controlled by toxin injections. Surgery (protractor myectomy or brow suspension) is indicated in about 10% and 4%, respectively. Protractor myectomy will relieve symptoms in about two-thirds of patients, and brow suspension in >90%.

Botulinum toxin injections All volumes and dosages given below are for Dysport and are not applicable to other preparations of toxin. Reconstitute one vial of Dysport with 2.5 mL 0.9% sodium chloride BP for injection, yielding a solution of 20 units per μL (according to the manufacturer's instructions).

Complications Ptosis, diplopia, entropion, ectropion, exposure keratitis, and allergy.

Contraindications Known hypersensitivity, history of myopathy, bleeding disorders, pregnancy/lactation.

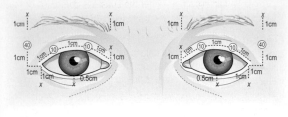

x = 20 units dysport
⑩ = 10 units dysport
㊵ = 40 units dysport

Fig. 1.37: Botulinum toxin injections for blepharospasm and hemifacial spasm.

Week 1 (first clinic visit):

1. Blepharospasm and hemifacial spasm:

    Dysport is given in six locations around the eye, all locations receiving 20 units (Fig. 1.37) with the exception of the lateral upper lid, where 40 units is given.

    For patients with evidence of pretarsal spasm 10 units of Dysport is given in two locations on the upper lid (topical anaesthetic cream may be required).

2. Aberrant facial nerve regeneration and myokymia: lower initial doses.

3. Treat dry eye or blepharitis.

4. Inform patients about support groups, e.g. The Dystonia Society, and provide information leaflet if available.

Week 2:

1. Spasm controlled: continue the same regimen every 3–4 months as required.

2. Spasm not controlled: further injection(s) to muscles that remain in spasm. Reviewed 1 week later (Week 3).

Week 3:

1. Spasm controlled: review in 3 months. If further botulinum toxin is indicated, the dose given is the sum of the previous two injections.

2. Spasm not controlled: further injection(s) to muscles that remain in spasm. Review 1 week later (Week 4).

Continue this cycle until either the spasm is controlled or the side effects of treatment become intolerable.

Surgery

- Offer protractor myectomy (extended blepharoplasty via a cosmetic blepharoplasty incision) to patients in whom toxin injections are ineffective and/or induce intolerable side effects (ptosis, facial droop, rectus muscle paralysis, or allergic response).

- Facial nerve avulsion is a shorter operation with lower perioperative morbidity, and is reserved for the elderly and infirm. The duration of effect is shorter and the procedure carries more complications than protractor myectomy.

Further management

- Induced ptosis as side effect of controlling pretarsal spasm: trial of ptosis props.

- Ptosis props not tolerated due to dry eyes or a spastic Bell's phenomenon: avoid brow suspension.

- Ptosis props tolerated: offer brow suspension. Use supramid prolene suture or silicone rod, which can easily be reversed if surgery is not tolerated.

- Spastic Bell's phenomenon (eyeball rolls under upper eyelid despite adequate control of spasm): offer systemic centrally acting medication e.g. clonazepam.

Congenital Eyelid Disease

Blepharophimosis-ptosis-epicanthus inversus syndrome

Clinical features An autosomal dominant disorder (gene defect on chromosome 3), characterized by a variable degree of ptosis with poor levator function, epicanthus inversus, blepharophimosis (narrowing of the horizontal palpebral aperture), telecanthus (canthal displacement due to soft tissue anomaly), hypertelorism (canthal displacement due to a wide nasal bridge), and lower lid ectropion. Other associated features include hypoplasia of the tarsal plate, prominent vertical brow hair, a flat brow, and female infertility.

Management Urgently prevent amblyopia (p. 26); otherwise elective surgery may be deferred until age 3–4, when nasal bridge growth begins, the tissues are larger, and the epicanthic folds reduce in size. A mild epicanthic fold is corrected with a Y–V plasty over the medial canthal tendon (MCT). A Z-plasty alone over the epicanthic fold(s) is indicated where there is no telecanthus. Telecanthus is corrected by resecting the middle portion of the MCT and suturing the ends together. A transnasal wire, which draws the MCTs toward the midline, may be indicated in hypetelorism, and in severe cases of telecanthus, where medial canthal bone requires removal in addition to medial canthal soft tissue. Ptosis surgery is carried out after the medial canthoplasty, and usually requires brow suspension with autogenous fascia lata. A full-thickness skin graft to the upper and lower lids may also be required.

Eyelid coloboma

Clinical features Eyelid colobomas may be idiopathic, or associated with developmental 1st arch or clefting syndromes. Upper lid colobomas are more common, representing a spectrum from a small localized absence of the tarsus and associated lashes, to complete absence of the upper lid with corneal exposure. Ocular and systemic associations include forniceal conjunctival bands and foreshortening, anophthalmos, cryptophthalmos, limbal dermoids, and Goldenhar's syndrome. Lower lid colobomata may be associated with lower facial clefting syndromes.

Management Complete ocular, orthoptic, and systemic evaluation are required. Corneal exposure is treated aggressively, and is an indication for urgent upper lid surgery. Small to medium-size defects (<50% of lid width) may be repaired by pentagon wedge excision of the anomalous tissue with direct closure, with or without lateral cantholysis. Larger defects require staged surgery with a lower to upper lid switch flap and subsequent division of the flap. A forced duction test is performed, conjunctival traction bands are excised, and forniceal foreshortening is managed with buccal mucous membrane graft(s). Monitor for amblyopia.

Distichiasis

See page 21.

Epiblepharon

Clinical features An excess fold of skin and muscle in the lower lid. In severe cases, lash–globe contact may occur.

Management The majority of cases resolve spontaneously. Where there is no entropion, everting sutures are indicated. Where the lower lid is turned in, excision of a strip of skin and muscle is performed.

Eyelid Trauma

Background Broad groups of eyelid injury are recognized, but any combination may occur:

■ Lacerating trauma.

Uncomplicated:

± lid margin laceration.

Complicated by injury to: levator complex, lacrimal apparatus, globe, orbit, sinuses, cranium.

± retained lid or orbital foreign body (FB).

■ Blunt trauma (contusion, avulsion of lid).

■ Chemical injury.

History A carefully documented history is often medicolegally important. Note the following:

■ The time and nature of an alleged assault or FB, as well as the distance and trajectory.

■ Whether parts or all of the FB have been recovered.

■ Other ocular symptoms.

■ ENT symptoms including epistaxis and CSF rhinorrhoea.

Examination

■ Record VA.

■ Accurately document or preferably photograph the extent of any wound, noting if it is partial or full thickness. Note any involvement of the lid margin(s), lacrimal drainage apparatus, or posterior lamella.

■ Exclude anterior segment, (p. 205), posterior segment (p. 551), and orbital injury (p. 101).

Investigations Imaging is chiefly to exclude bony injury, retained FB, gas, and pus. A plain skull X-ray is quick and readily available but ultrasound and CT may be appropriate. Avoid MRI if metal FBs are suspected.

General principles of repair

■ Most systemic and ocular injuries take priority over eyelid repair.

- Extensive lid, globe, orbital, and even intracranial injury may occur through a small eyelid laceration.

- Primary canalicular repair is easier within 24 hours of injury, but other lid injuries may wait 48 hours. Provide antibiotic cover if repair is delayed.

- Involve paediatricians if children are injured. Nonaccidental injury, though uncommon, should be considered. Children with traumatic ptosis are at risk of amblyopia and may require urgent brow suspension.

- Provide tetanus toxoid cover.

- Animal bites may be closed primarily but cover with a suitable oral antibiotic, e.g. co-amoxiclav 375 mg t.d.s. p.o..

- Corneal protection is a key objective in any repair.

- Repair under general anaesthesia unless there is limited injury to the lid alone.

- Thoroughly clean all dirty wounds.

- *Do not discard tissue unless necrotic or infected.*

- Primary repair aims to approximate tissue planes – posterior lamella, tarsus and skin. Complex procedures (e.g. skin grafting) are undertaken secondarily.

- Avoid vertical shortening as tissue contracture leads to ectropion.

- In most situations use a standard 2-1-1 knot: draw the suture in opposite directions with each throw and tie knots anteriorly to avoid corneal abrasion.

- Use deep 5/0 absorbable sutures to draw planes together and anchor tissues. Skin sutures should not bear tension.

- *Skin*: Use 7/0 Vicryl continous, or 6/0 Vicryl interrupted ± 6/0 Nylon continuous. Use a rapidly absorbing suture in children (e.g. Vicryl rapide).

- *Tarsus*: Use 5/0 Vicryl × 2–3.

- *Grey line and lash line*: Use buried 7/0 Vicryl.

- Remove skin sutures at 1 week.

- Avoid silk sutures.

Specific injuries

■ *Lid margin*: Repair using the same principles as a pentagon wedge excision (see page 10).

■ *Levator palpebrae complex*: thoroughly clean the wound and approximate corresponding tissue as accurately as possible. Do not extend the wound to identify further structures because spontaneous resolution of the ptosis may occur, up to 6 months post-injury and the ptosis may in part be due to a neuropraxia.

■ *Medial canthal tendon*: even in cases of avulsion, a residual stump of deep tissue may often be grasped with toothed forceps, and approximated to the medial cut end of the tarsus using a 5/0 suture (absorbable or nonabsorbable) on a fish-hook or half-circle needle.

■ *Canaliculus*: controversy exists regarding the repair of injury to a single canaliculus, as adequate tear drainage may occur via the healthy fellow canaliculus, and the failure rate is high due to ring contracture. However, if repair is undertaken, a monocanalicular self-retaining silicone stent may be placed (shorten the stent before insertion). Identification of the cut proximal end of the canaliculus within the wound is aided by application of 10% epinephrine on a cotton bud (the transected end appears as a pale ring), or by syringing through the fellow canaliculus with fluorescein or air. The bell-shaped end of the stent fits in the punctal ampulla flush with the punctum. The stent does not require suturing and may easily be removed at 2–3 weeks as epithelialization occurs within a few days. The presence of a stent will not prevent tissue contracture, which occurs over many months. This technique avoids the use of the pigtail probe, which, depending on the design of the probe and the experience of the surgeon, may lead to injury of the healthy canaliculus. Alternatively, if sufficient distal canaliculus is present, this can be opened along its posterior surface by a few millimetres, and marsupialized into the conjunctival sac with an 8/0 absorbable suture. Where both canaliculi are injured, repair by an experienced surgeon is indicated. A silicone rod may be used and tied in the nose. The risk of failure is high. If subsequent dacryocystorhinostomy with retrotubes fails, a Lester Jones tube may be indicated.

Optometry and General Practice Guidelines

Children with any eyelid abnormality should be referred early to detect and manage amblyopia. Adult eyelid malpositions (entropion/ectropion) may be managed routinely unless there is ocular surface irritation either from a stagnant tear film or aberrant lashes. Half-inch micropore tape applied along the lower lid and brought up onto the temple will tighten the lid and provide a temporary correction of lid laxity.

The majority of cases of facial palsy are idiopathic (Bell's palsy) and will not require tarsorrhaphy, but should be referred urgently to determine other risk factors for corneal exposure (e.g. reduced corneal sensation or Bell's phenomenon). Similarly, corneal exposure from any cause of lid malposition (e.g. entropion) should be dealt with urgently. Look for staining with 2% fluorescein dye in the exposed corneal areas. Refer suspected tumours urgently.

Any patient with presumed eyelid infection with breakdown or frank necrosis of the overlying skin should be given intravenous antibiotic (e.g. penicillin V or co-amoxyclav) and referred immediately. Necrotizing fasciitis is rare but has a high mortality.

Injuries to the eyelids require urgent attention, in particular upper eyelid trauma where there may be a risk of corneal exposure, and a risk of undetected globe, orbital, or even intracranial injury. The risk of corneal exposure is higher where there is eyelid margin injury. Patients with canalicular trauma should also be referred urgently, because a successful anatomical union becomes more difficult after 24–36 hours.

The following guidelines for hospital referral urgency are not prescriptive, as clinical situations vary.

Immediate

Same day

Urgent (within 2 weeks)

Soon (within 1 month)

Routine

Chapter 2
LACRIMAL

The Watery Eye

Anatomy and Physiology The tear film provides corneal lubrication, nourishment and protection, has anti-infective properties, aids removal of bacteria, cells, and debris, and optimizes the optical interface between air and cornea. It is triphasic, comprising a *mucoid layer* (from goblet cells), *aqueous layer* (primarily lacrimal glands but also accessory glands of Krause and Wolfring), and *lipid layer* (meibomian glands).

Symptomatic watering results from reduced tear removal (by evaporation and drainage) and/or overproduction. Obstructive epiphora refers to reduced tear drainage. Tear distribution is also important, as is eyelid movement ('lacrimal pump') and position. Patient tolerance of watering varies widely.

Consider the lacrimal drainage system as three compartments:

1. Tear lake.

2. Lacrimal sac.

3. Nasal cavity.

Relatively high-resistance conduits connect these compartments; the canaliculi (connecting compartments 1 and 2), and nasolacrimal duct (2 and 3) (Fig. 2.1):

■ *Canalicular obstruction* produces 'flow' symptoms: 'Eyes well up with water', blur on downgaze, e.g. reading. 'Volume' symptoms are minimal or absent.

■ *Nasolacrimal duct obstrucition* (NLDO) produces 'volume' symptoms due to backwash from the lacrimal sac. These include: recurrent conjunctivitis; morning stickiness; mucus debris in the tear film; dacryocystitis; lacrimal sac mucocele or abscess.

History Assess severity – symptoms indoors are more significant than those outdoors in cold, windy weather. Ask about onset, time relationships, duration, and site of tear spillover. Medial spillage suggests impaired drainage; lateral spillage may relate to lower lid laxity, or upper lid dermatochalasis contacting the tear film with chronic skin wetting by capillary action. Reflex

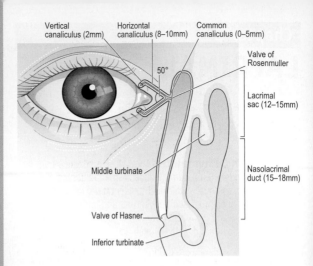

Fig. 2.1: Lacrimal drainage anatomy. The angle between the horizontal and common canaliculi in the axial plane is approx. 135 degrees. Therefore, one must pull the lid laterally when probing the common canaliculus (during intubation, e.g. at DCR) to straighten out this angle to 180 degrees, thus preventing a 'false passage' and canalicular perforation.

NB: When performing *diagnostic outpatient syringing*, advance the cannula not more than 5–6 mm into the horizontal canaliculus to avoid common canalicular injury.

watering from tear-film deficiency is often worse in dry, warm conditions, bright light, or when blinking is reduced, e.g. concentrating on reading, computer use, and Parkinson's disease. Simultaneous runny nose suggests overproduction. Bloody tears suggests a sac tumour (rare), canaliculitis, or trauma to the canaliculi/sac (including iatrogenic injury). Ask about surface irritation or itch (atopy), a history of facial/nasal trauma, and previous nasal or lacrimal surgery. 'Crocodile tears' are associated with facial palsy and involve neurogenic reflex watering, often sudden, from the thought of food, eating, or chewing. Lacrimal sac swelling may be secondary to a dacryocele (a congenital cyst), mucocele (see below), pyocele, dacryocystitis (painful), tumour (usually painless ± bloody tears), or occasionally air (± pain).

Examination Examine for causes of overproduction or impaired drainage.

■ *Overproduction*: Look for:

1. Lid or lash malposition – trichiasis, distichiasis, entropion.

2. Lid margin disease (p. 113).

3. Tear film deficiency – perform Schirmer's test (p. 147) and tear film break-up time (p. 157).

4. Corneal or subtarsal foreign body.

5. Conjunctivitis – look for allergic papillae, follicles.

6. Corneal disease, especially superficial punctate keratopathy from tear film anomalies or exposure keratopathy, and early dendritic keratitis.

7. Uveitis, scleritis.

■ *Impaired drainage*: Look for:

1. Eyelid laxity or malposition of the lower lid or punctum particularly ectropion.

2. Punctal or canalicular stenosis-cicatrizing conjunctivopathy, systemic chemotherapy, especially 5 FU and trauma (including iatrogenic).

3. Canaliculitis (see p. 67).

4. Fistula – congenital, or acquired (following dacryocystitis).

5. Lacrimal pump failure – especially facial palsy.

6. Lacrimal sac mucocele – this is a chronic collection of mucopurulent material due to low grade colonization/ infection of stagnant tears. Pressing on the sac produces mucus or pus reflux (Fig. 2.2). A dacryocystorhinostomy (DCR) is often required for associated epiphora.

7. Lacrimal sac mass – consider tumour or tense mucocoele. In general, a mass below medial canthal tendon (MCT) originates from the sac; lesions above the MCT indicate non-sac origin.

8. Dacryocystitis – active or resolved (p. 68).

9. Nasal obstruction, e.g. mass, inflammation, scarring. If it is possible to gently pass a cotton bud alongside the lateral wall of the nose, this suggests a reasonable nasal airway is present; if not, consider endoscopy.

10. Altered facial/lid relationship – this may include prominent eyes, lower lid sag and hypoplastic midface.

11. Prior surgery or trauma – look for scars.

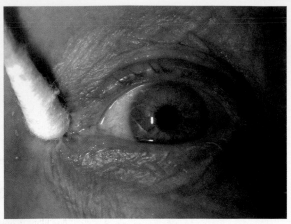

Fig. 2.2: Mucocele with mucous reflux.

Clinical tests

- *Fluorescein disappearance test (FDT)*: Instil a tiny drop of fluorescein 2% in both eyes at the start of history taking. After approximately 5 minutes, look for asymmetry in the tear film height.

  High + diluted = overproduction.

  High + undiluted = impaired drainage.

- *Syringing*: Perform a diagnostic lacrimal syringing in *all* patients with epiphora, except those with acute dacryocystitis in whom the procedure is usually painful. Consider patient comfort and use a reclining chair with head support. Be very gentle to avoid canalicular trauma. In experienced hands the procedure is painless, even without topical anaesthesia. If necessary, dilate the punctum (after topical anaesthetic), but avoid tearing the fibrous annulus and avoid sharp dilators. Keep the lower lid under firm lateral tension to eliminate the angle between the horizontal and common canaliculus and hence prevent canalicular perforation ('false passage'). Gently inject saline using a 2.5 mL syringe with a lacrimal cannula, inserted no more than 5 mm into the horizontal canaliculus. It is seldom necessary to check for 'hard' or 'soft stops' by pushing the cannula up against the nasal bones. Lower canalicular reflux suggests obstruction proximal to common canaliculus. Upper canalicular reflux with fluorescein or mucus reflux which suggests a mucocele nasolacrimal duct obstruction (NLDO). Early reflux via the upper canaliculus without fluorescein suggests common canalicular obstruction.

- *Jones I dye test*: Assesses physiological drainage. Instil fluorescein 2%, then insert a cotton bud under the inferior turbinate – if there is dye on the cotton bud, the test is positive. Nasal endoscopic visualization is more accurate. A negative result indicates nonpatency, partial patency, or functional NLDO. The test is most useful following DCR; otherwise, it is less reliable.

- *Jones II dye test* (nonphysiological): As per Jones I but after syringing. Jones II dye test is not needed if Jones I is positive.

Investigations

- *Dacryocystogram* (DCG): Indications include a failed DCR or trauma without mucocele (surgery for post-traumatic or recurrent mucocele is relatively straightforward in experienced hands so DCG is not needed), suspected functional NLDO (shows delayed clearance from sac on late erect films), bloody epiphora, and unusual craniofacial syndromes.

- *CT*: Perform if suspected sinonasal disease, lacrimal tumours, and in some cases following trauma, especially if metallic implants are suspected.

- *Scintigraphy*: Can distinguish between delayed drainage between compartments 1 and 2 (impaired 'pick up' of tears), and 2 and 3 (anatomic/functional obstruction).

- *Nasoendoscopy*: Occasionally required.

Management

- *Overproduction*: Treat the underlying cause, e.g. lid hygiene, lash removal, topical lubricant, steroid, or antibiotic.

- *Impaired drainage*:

  Lid malposition – surgical correction.

  Punctal stenosis – punctoplasty (Box 2.1).

- *Canalicular stenosis*:

  Proximal: DCR + retrograde canaliculostomy (canaliculi are intubated from within the opened lacrimal sac and a 'cut-down' performed distal to the site of obstruction).

  Distal: canalicular-DCR (C-DCR; canaliculi are anastomozed to sac flaps after excision of intervening scar tissue, *or* scar is excised from within the sac until the probes are seen – stents passed directly into the sac) ± lacrimal canalicular bypass, e.g. Lester Jones tube (LJT).

- *Canaliculitis*: See page 67.

Box 2.1: Punctoplasty ('3-snip' or posterior ampullectomy)

1. Dilate lower punctum with a punctum dilator, e.g. Nettleship.

2. Make two parallel cuts (medial and lateral) in the posterior wall of the vertical canaliculus (ampulla) and join at the bottom with fine, straight scissors (e.g. Vannas).

3. Incise 2–3 mm along horizontal canaliculus from the conjunctival surface.

4. Excise 'triangle' of ampulla and conjunctiva between these two incisions.

5. Gently cauterize conjunctiva at wound edges.

6. Prescribe G. chloramphenicol q.d.s. and mild topical steroid q.d.s. for 2 weeks.

7. Review in 2–3 weeks.

■ *Acute dacryocystitis* (lacrimal sac abscess): See page 68.

■ *Mucocele or functional NLDO*: DCR (see below).

■ *Lacrimal sac tumour*: Biopsy sac; if discovered intraoperatively, abandon DCR and excise the sac.

■ *Lacrimal pump failure* ('atonic canaliculi'): Difficult to treat. Tighten/shorten lid ± punctoplasty ± DCR ± lacrimal bypass (e.g. LJT).

■ *Nasal congestion*: Prescribe a nasal decongestant, e.g. xylometazoline hydrochloride nasal spray 0.1%, 1 spray per nostril, 2–3 times daily for 2–4 weeks. Beware interactions with monoamine oxidase inhibitors, etc., and avoid use over 5–7 consecutive days to avoid rebound rhinorrhoea. Also prescribe steroid, e.g. beclamethasone dipropionate/Beconase nasal spray 50 mcg/metered spray, 2 sprays per nostril b.d. for 2–3 weeks. Consider an ENT opinion.

■ *Congenital NLDO* see page 65.

Dacryocystorhinostomy

Background Aims to create a mucosal-lined anastomosis between the sac and nose using an external (open) or endoscopic approach. External DCR remains the 'gold standard' with larger rhinostomy, and first-intention flap healing. An external approach is absolutely indicated if sac tumour is suspected (if confirmed, biopsy the sac but do not complete DCR), and for canalicular disease. For technique see Box 2.2.

Consent

■ *Benefit*: External DCR success rate is 90–95%; endoscopic surgical, 80%; endoscopic laser, 70–80%. Success varies

---

Box 2.2: Dacryocystorhinostomy (DCR)

1. Select general anaesthetic (GA) or local anaesthetic (LA) with sedation (lignocaine 2% and bupivicaine 0.5% with 1:200 000 epinephrine in side of nose, medial peribulbar, infraorbital nerve block, plus cocaine 10% intranasally).

2. Haemostasis is assisted by head-up position, BP control, intranasal 0.1% epinephrine moistened cotton buds or cocaine 10% nasal pack.

3. Stat cefuroxime 750 mg i.v. reduces the postoperative infection rate.

4. Make a straight incision 1 cm anterior to the medial canthus, approx. 1.5 cm long, raise skin flap and expose MCT using blunt dissection (Rollet's rougine).

5. Dissect MCT and periosteum from anterior lacrimal crest, release sac, especially superiorly, and mobilize laterally.

6. Start rhinostomy by opening suture between nasal and lacrimal bones with Traquair periosteal elevator. Use bone punch, e.g. Kerrison's rongeurs, to extend as far superiorly and anteriorly as possible, inferiorly (level with inferior orbital rim) and posteriorly (to the posterior lacrimal crest). Rhinostomy should measure about 2–3 cm in diameter (Fig. 2.3). Protect nasal mucosa from inadvertent perforation.

7. Perform anterior ethmoidectomy with curved haemostat or bone nibbler.

8. Fully open sac from fundus to duct and fashion sac and nasal mucosal flaps, using all available rhinostomy space. Incise nasal mucosa >3 mm anterior to root of middle turbinate – anterior nasal mucosal flap should be larger than posterior (Fig. 2.4). Suture flaps with 6/0 Vicryl. 'Suspend' anterior flaps to overlying orbicularis.

9. Insert O'Donoghue tubing or similar stent. Tie tubing in the nose and place a marker stitch, e.g. 5/0 silk to aid later stent removal.

10. Carefully close skin with 6/0 nonabsorbable suture. Keep closure flat and avoid 'bow-stringing'.

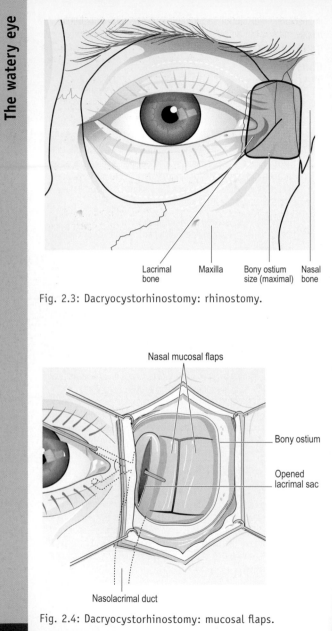

Fig. 2.3: Dacryocystorhinostomy: rhinostomy.

Fig. 2.4: Dacryocystorhinostomy: mucosal flaps.

with definition (anatomic versus symptomatic), symptoms (≈100% cure from mucocele stickiness with correctly performed external DCR), and underlying disease (mucocele > functional NLDO ≈ 70–80% > canalicular block ≈ 60–80%).

■ *Risk*: With a correctly placed external DCR incision, 2–3% have a visible scar at 1 year; 1–2% have significant postoperative epistaxis that might require nasal packing, admission, and monitoring for hypovolaemia.

Postoperative care No hot drinks for 12 hours; no nose blowing for 1 week. Prescribe chloramphenicol 0.5% and prednisolone 0.3% drops, both q.d.s. 2 weeks, then b.d. 2 weeks. If bilateral surgery or major infection, add cephalexin 250 mg q.d.s. p.o. 1 week.

Follow-up Remove sutures at 7–10 days and stent at 4–6 weeks, unless C-DCR (2–3 months) or retrograde canaliculostomy (2–3 weeks).

Lester Jones Tube

Provides a permanent fistula connecting the conjunctival sac to nose. Requires prior DCR and carunculectomy. Use a 'bull-horn' dilator followed by passage of the LJT down the dilated tract; place the LJT just behind the medial canthus, angled slightly inferiorly (Fig. 2.5). Avoid abutting the nasal septum. Avoid nose blowing for 1 week postoperative because of the risk of the tube coming out, and review at 6 weeks. Advise the patient to place finger over the tube if sneezing or blowing nose, and perform daily 'sniff' test to confirm patency (inhale through nose with ipsilateral nostril blocked; sniffing water into nose may aid cleaning by 'rinsing' effect). Attend within 1–2 days if tube dislodges when replacement without GA is sometimes successful. Review annually for internal cleaning and saline irrigation.

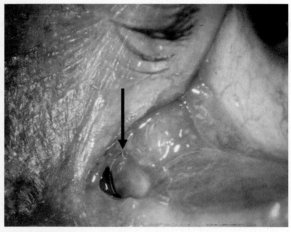

Fig. 2.5: Lester Jones tube (arrow).

Congenital Nasolacrimal Duct Obstruction

Background The lacrimal system usually canalizes at 8 months of fetal life. In the first year postpartum, 96% of cases of nasolacrimal duct obstruction resolve; a further 60% resolve in the second year with some slow resolution thereafter.

Examination Perform the fluorescein disappearance test (p. 58). Check for an expressible mucocele and dacryocele (a tense, bluish sac swelling usually in the first month of life). Look for fistulae, typically in the medial lower lid; these may drain fluorescein (Fig. 2.6).

Differential diagnosis

- Watery eye: atopy, punctal atresia (rare), conjunctivitis.
- Lacrimal sac mass: dermoid; haemangioma; meningoencephalocele; rhabdomyosarcoma (all very rare).

Management Explain the natural history. Massage the sac six times daily by firm pressure on medial upper lid, behind anterior lacrimal crest; demonstrate to parents. Use topical antibiotics for episodes of conjunctivitis. Defer probing until 12 months, unless acute/recurrent dacryocystitis, but only probe when the acute episode has resolved (Box 2.3).

Follow-up Review as required if first probing, 6–8 weeks if redo. Consider intubation if multiple endoscopically monitored probings fail.

Box 2.3: Syringe and probe (probing) procedure

1. Explain the procedure:
   - *Benefit:* Complete symptom resolution: >90% if done age 1 year, 90% at 2 years, 80% at 3 years, 70% at 4 years, 40% at 5 years.
   - *Risk:* False passage, bleeding, failure, bronchospasm.
2. Examine (under GA) lids, conjunctiva, puncta, look for fistulae, and expressible mucocele.
3. Perform dacryocystogram if redo to clarify anatomy.
4. Inject saline and fluorescein mixture using a lacrimal cannula. Feel for resistance. If not able to easily introduce cannula, dilate puncta gently. Place a fine suction catheter up nose to look for fluorescein.

Box 2.3: Syringe and probe (probing) procedure—cont'd

5. Consider probing even if patent to syringing, e.g. if significant symptoms or prior failed probing. Try to start with a '0' Bowman for lower punctum, '00' for upper. Try to avoid smaller probes or sizes larger than '1'.

6. Insert probe vertically (2 mm) then horizontally with lid on lateral traction. Feel for 'hard stop' as probe contacts medial sac wall against nasal bones. Otherwise, compressed tissue results in a 'soft stop'.

7. Direct probe vertically down into the nasolacrimal duct (NLD), angled slightly posteriorly and medially. Feel for a 'pop' as the probe perforates the membrane of a nonpatent NLD.

8. Check probe is below inferior turbinate – feel using large probe along floor of nose or look with an endoscope.

9. Repeat syringing. This also assists sac washout.

10. Prescribe prednisolone 0.1% and chloramphenicol drops, both q.d.s. 2–3 weeks.

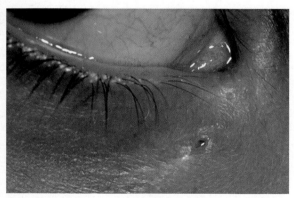

Fig. 2.6: Accessory lacrimal opening (Courtesy D. Verity).

Canaliculitis

Background Canaliculi become grossly dilated with intraluminal deposits caused by low-grade infection, classically *Actinomyces*, but also fungi.

Symptoms Chronic discharge. Epiphora is often mild but worse in mornings.

Signs Swollen inflamed lid medial to prominent 'pouting' punctum. Features may be subtle (Fig. 2.7).

Management Canaliculotomy: dilate and open 5 mm of horizontal canaliculus. Use a fine chalazion curette to remove deposits. Send for microbiology. Prescribe G. chloramphenicol q.d.s. 1–2 weeks ± penicillin 250 mg p.o. q.d.s. for 1–2 weeks if severe. Penicillin G drops (100 000 U/mL) may be used if there is a poor response to surgery, but canalicutomy is all that is required for most patients.

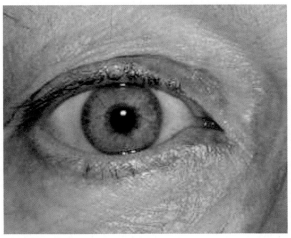

Fig. 2.7: Canaliculitis (*Actinomyces*).

Acute Dacryocystitis/ Lacrimal Sac Abscess

Background A purulent lacrimal sac infection/abscess with surrounding cellulitis, often associated with nasolacrimal duct obstruction. Caused by superinfection of a mucocele. May fistulize to skin.

Clinical features Tense, painful erythematous swelling below the medial canthal tendon, often with a history of stickiness and epiphora (Fig. 2.8).

Management Hot compresses 4–6 times daily, G. chloramphenicol q.d.s. until resolved, and cephalexin 250– 500 mg p.o. q.d.s. 1–2 weeks or until cellulitis resolve. If febrile or acutely unwell treat as preseptal cellulitis (p. 85). Incise and drain if fails to respond to above measures after 5–7 days, or if worsens. Apply topical skin anaesthetic (e.g. EMLA) for 30 minutes, then inject LA slowly around the abscess. This is often very painful, so consider GA. Incise with a blade, drain, send pus to microbiology and pack with ribbon gauze if large abscess. Arrange definitive treatment with dacryocystorhinostomy when cellulitis resolves.

Children with nonresolving acute dacryocystitis or infected dacryocele require systemic antibiotics, examination under anaesthesia, and drainage via nasal cavity.

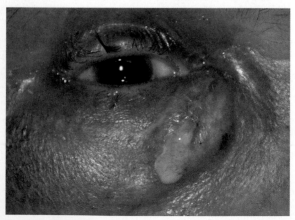

Fig. 2.8: Acute dacryocystitis.

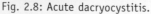

Optometry and General Practice Guidelines

Most lacrimal problems are nonurgent. Reassure patients who have very mild watering, e.g. only outdoors in cold, windy weather. In those with troublesome epiphora, treat or refer any sinonasal disease (e.g. rhinitis, polyps, mass) before referral to an ophthalmologist, preferably one experienced in lacrimal disorders. Also consider epiphora secondary to eye disease and ask if the eye becomes red and painful or if vision is blurred. Treat or refer any readily identifiable ocular surface problem (e.g. tear film deficiency, blepharitis, allergic conjunctivitis, trichiasis). Look specifically for eyelid/lash malpositions, e.g. lower lid ectropion/entropion.

A firm, nonreducible mass below the medial canthal tendon (for anatomy see p. 1) or blood-stained tears suggest lacrimal sac neoplasm, so refer urgently. Any swelling presenting in the region above the medial canthal tendon is neoplasia until proven otherwise.

Instruct parents of children with congenital nasolacrimal duct obstruction to massage firmly over the nasolacrimal sac (not the side of the nose) six times daily. Refer if symptoms fail to resolve after a year, or sooner if episodic conjunctivitis is present.

The following guide to referral urgency is not prescriptive, as clinical situations vary.

Same day

- Canalicular injuries p. 50
- Acute dacryocystitis/lacrimal sac abscess (commence G. chloramphenicol q.d.s. and systemic antibiotics, e.g. cephalexin 250–500 mg p.o. q.d.s.) p. 68

Urgent (within 1 week)

- Epiphora with blood stained tears p. 55
- Noncompressible lacrimal sac mass (mucoceles are compressible) p. 57

Routine

- Isolated epiphora p. 55
- Epiphora with recurrent conjunctivitis (treat episodes with G. chloramphenicol q.d.s. 1 week) p. 55
- A child with epiphora since birth warrants routine referral unless suspected dacryocele, recurrent problematic conjunctivitis, or any dacryocystitis p. 65
- Suspected canaliculitis (prescribe G. chloramphenicol q.d.s. 2 weeks) p. 67
- Lacrimal sac mucocele p. 57

Chapter 3

ORBIT

Anatomy

Bones of the orbit

■ Frontal, zygoma, maxilla (thin), sphenoid (greater and lesser wings), ethmoid (thin), lacrimal (thin), palatine.

Anatomic relations of the bony orbit

■ Roof: Anterior cranial fossa, frontal sinus.

■ Medial: Ethmoid air cells, sphenoid sinus.

■ Floor: Maxillary antrum.

■ Lateral: Temporalis fossa, middle cranial fossa.

Orbital septum

■ Separates the lids from the orbit and acts as barrier to the spread of infection; encloses the lacrimal sac which straddles the pre- and postseptal spaces.

Surgical spaces

■ Subperiosteal (potential space), extraconal, intraconal, and sub-Tenon's (Fig. 3.1).

Lacrimal gland

■ The larger orbital lobe is separated from the palpebral lobe by the lateral horn of the levator aponeurosis; ductules pass through the palpebral lobe to the fornix.

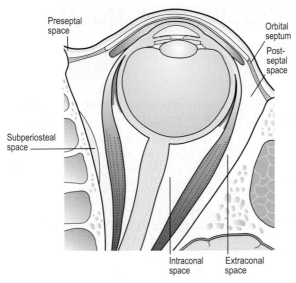

Preseptal space

Orbital septum

Post-septal space

Subperiosteal space

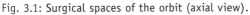

Intraconal space

Extraconal space

Fig. 3.1: Surgical spaces of the orbit (axial view).

History and Examination

History

Ask about the following:

1. **P**roptosis.

2. **P**ain: causes include inflammation, infection, acute pressure changes (e.g. haemorrhage), and bony / neural invasion.

3. **P**rogression: symptoms may occur over minutes (e.g. haemorrhage); hours–days (e.g. inflammation); weeks–months (e.g. malignancy); months–years (e.g. benign tumour).

4. **P**ast medical history: in particular thyroid disease, malignancy, and sinusitis.

5. (**P**erceptual) visual problems: diplopia, blurring, altered colour perception and refractive change.

6. **P**alpable or visible mass.

7. **P**eriorbital abnormalities: including sensory change (paraesthesiae, numbness), redness, tenderness, watering, and lid anomalies.

Examination

Note the following:

1. General inspection ('**P**anoramic'): note facial scars, asymmetry, swellings/masses, and goitre or thyroidectomy scar. Old photos (e.g. driver's licence) may clarify disease onset.

2. Visual function ('**P**erception'): VA, colour vision (Ishihara), red desaturation, reduced brightness perception and confrontation testing/formal perimetry if relevant.

3. **P**upils: Test for RAPD.

4. Exophthalmometry (**P**roptosis?): For a rough estimate look from above and behind the patient, but perform exophthalmometry as follows if proptosis or enophthalmos is suspected:

   ■ Check the location and symmetry of the lateral orbital rims (often recessed following orbitofacial fracture).

   ■ Rest an exophthalmometer gently against each lateral orbital rim and note the distance between the calipers (base distance) from the rule.

- Ensure the eye being tested is fixating on the examiner's eye and record the anterior corneal position, avoiding parallax error.

- Record the instrument make and base distance for subsequent readings.

  Average upper limit of normal:

  a. Caucasian: 20 mm (equator just in front of the lateral orbital rim, e.g. on CT scan);

  b. African-Caribbean: 22 mm.

  Asymmetry ≥2 mm is abnormal. Beware pseudoproptosis from high myopia/contralateral microphthalmos, or gross facial asymmetry. Axial proptosis suggests thyroid eye disease or an intraconal mass. Enophthalmos suggests an expanded orbital volume (e.g. blowout fracture) or contracted orbital contents (e.g. scirrhous metastatic breast carcinoma). A change with Valsalva or head-down posture suggests a low-flow vascular malformation. The differential diagnosis of nonaxial proptosis is given below.

5. Nonaxial globe displacement: using a horizontal clear plastic ruler, measure from the midline to the corneal reflex of the fixating eye on both sides to look for a difference. Compare the vertical positions of each *fixating* eye against a horizontal axial plane. Distinguish the following:

   - Telecanthus: increased distance from the midline to the medial canthus (normal is 15–17 mm).

   - Hypertelorbitism (hypertelorism): increased separation of otherwise normally sized orbits.

   - Pseudohypertelorbitism: lateral displacement of the medial walls with normally located lateral walls (narrow orbits).

   Causes of nonaxial displacement include:

   - Inferior displacement: lacrimal gland mass, frontal sinus mucocele, encephalocele, sphenoid wing meningioma, orbital roof fracture, nerve sheath tumour.

   - Superior: maxillary sinus tumour and lymphoproliferative disorders.

   - Lateral: ethmoid sinus mucocele/tumour and subperiosteal collection.

   - Medial: lacrimal gland enlargement.

6. **P**alpation: examine orbital rim, soft tissues, and feel for masses (note location, shape, size). Gently palpate all quadrants using little finger.

7. **P**ulsation: check for globe pulsation, thrill, or bruit using the bell of the stethoscope over a closed eye.

8. Full ocular examination: check conjunctival fornices. Note choroidal folds from retrobulbar mass or disc collaterals, e.g. optic nerve sheath meningioma.

9. Ocular motility: distinguish neuropathic, myopathic, and mechanical dysmotility. Consider formal documentation (e.g. Hess chart), especially in thyroid eye disease and orbital fracture.

10. **P**eriorbital examination: skin; lids position (retraction and/or lateral eyelid flare in thyroid eye disease); regional lymph nodes; and cranial nerves V and VII. Note fullness of the periorbital regions, nose, abnormalities, or facial asymmetry.

Imaging

Patients with proptosis require imaging, with a few exceptions such as mild thyroid eye disease. When viewing an orbital mass consider the following:

1. Physical characteristics: size, shape (round suggests benign), and internal structure (e.g. fluid level).

2. Location: tissue of origin and surgical space.

3. Biologic behaviour: longstanding benign masses may induce bone remodelling or 'scalloping', whereas malignant lesions often destroy tissue, producing irregular bony erosion.

Plain X-ray Redundant when CT is available. Blowout fracture is a clinical diagnosis and easily missed on plain X-ray.

Computed tomography (CT) First-line imaging modality for orbital disease. Indications include proptosis, orbital masses, bony lesions, trauma and hyperacute haemorrhage. CT is relatively cheap, readily available, and good for showing bone and metal foreign bodies. Main disadvantages are radiation exposure and contrast reactions. Contrast is often helpful, especially with tumours, but is contraindicated in patients with iodine allergy, dehydration, cardiac failure, hyperthyroidism, or renal impairment. Diabetics have a ≈9% risk of contrast-induced renal failure. Request fine axial cuts (2 mm for orbit, 1 mm for optic canal) and direct or reformatted coronal sections ± reformatted sagittal sections. View bone using bone 'windows', looking for hyper- and hypo-ostotic lesions, bony erosion, or fractures. Use soft tissue 'windows' to systematically examine extraocular muscles, optic nerve, lacrimal gland, fat, vessels, extraorbital structures (brain, sinuses, nose), any mass lesions, or vascular changes. 3D reconstructions are useful in trauma cases. CT angiography is mainly useful for neuro-ophthalmic problems.

Magnetic resonance imaging (MRI) Mainly indicated for disease at the orbitocranial junction, e.g. optic sheath tumours. Orbital MRI requires fat-suppression to allow delineation of soft tissue structures. Cortical bone has a very low signal intensity and appears black. Cancellous bone has a moderate signal intensity. MRI is contraindicated if metal foreign bodies are suspected (See also p. 629)

Ultrasound Internal tumour reflectivity may aid diagnosis. Doppler flow studies may help diagnose and monitor vascular lesions such as haemangiomas.

Other tests

Blood tests As appropriate, e.g. thyroid function tests.

Perimetry Useful for assessing optic nerve function and temporal change.

Biopsy In general, it is preferable to obtain tissue by open biopsy (incisional or excisional), rather than CT or ultrasound-guided fine-needle aspiration cytology, as histology gives better structural representation than cytology, and multiple stains are available.

Congenital Disorders

Dermoid and epidermoid cysts

Background A choristoma (normal tissue in abnormal location) arising from surface ectoderm trapped at sites of embryologic folding. Cysts are classified by their contents and lining:

■ Epidermoid: squamous epithelial lining only with associated keratin.

■ Dermoid: lined by squamous epithelium and dermis. Hairs, sebaceous glands/oil, and keratin may be present.

■ Conjunctival: conjunctival lining with mucus contents.

Epidermoid and dermoid cysts may have intra- and extraorbital components (temporalis fossa, CNS, nose) with an interconnecting 'stalk' traversing bone, a so-called 'dumb-bell' configuration.

Clinical features Typically, a firm, mobile, nontender lump is noted soon after birth in the superotemporal quadrant (STQ) (Fig. 3.2) or less commonly, superonasal quadrant (SNQ), sometimes attaching to the zygomaticofrontal or frontonasal suture. Patients may have episodes of inflammation following trauma, or skin discharge with very superficial, ruptured or incompletely excised lesions. Deep orbital lesions can present in adulthood with proptosis and recurrent orbital inflammation.

Investigations CT is not required unless it is not possible to palpate behind the equator of the cyst.

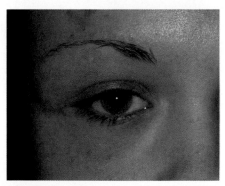

Fig. 3.2: Superotemporal quadrant dermoid with temporal fossa extension.

Management Arrange nonurgent intact excision before school age, when the risk of trauma increases. Removal may require periosteal dissection ± bone removal (e.g. 'dumb-bell' cyst). The preferred approach for STQ/SNQ lesions is via the upper lid skin crease. If deep extension is found unexpectedly and the surgeon is not familiar with removal of complex lesions, leave the cyst intact, close the wound, and refer to an experienced orbital surgeon: *do not remove lesions incompletely*. If accidental rupture occurs, perform a thorough washout of the surgical field to remove proinflammatory cyst contents.

Dermolipoma

Background A choristoma of dermal elements (ectopic skin) occurring on the ocular surface, typically the STQ.

Clinical features Discharge and irritation from abnormal conjunctival wetting and surface hairs, and poor cosmesis. Look for a STQ firm, immobile, pale-yellowish mass closely applied to the globe (Fig. 3.3).

Differential diagnosis Orbital fat prolapse, lacrimal gland prolapse, and subconjunctival lipoma (all mobile under the conjunctiva).

Management Conservative microsurgical excision by an experienced surgeon, avoiding damage to the lacrimal gland

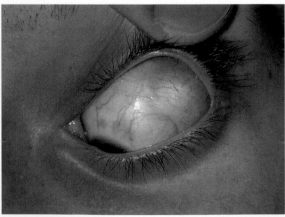

Fig. 3.3: Dermolipoma.

ductules and lateral rectus. Careful conjunctival closure without tension helps prevent ocular motility restriction.

Corneolimbal (epibulbar) dermoid

A choristoma of conjunctival origin, often protruding over the cornea (Fig. 3.4). May produce discomfort, exposure, or astigmatism. May be associated with Goldenhar's syndrome that may also feature eyelid colobomas, accessary auricular appendages, poor hearing, hemifacial microsomia, and vertebral abnormalities. Manage symptomatic dermoid lesions with topical lubricants/steroids or excision (superficial sclerokeratectomy/ lamellar keratoplasty). Asymptomatic conjunctival lesions tend to be stable and excision is rarely required.

Microphthalmos and anophthalmos

Background Rare, often sporadic, idiopathic disorder of multifactorial aetiology. May be associated with: hemifacial microsomia (e.g. Goldenhar's syndrome); renal, cardiac, and cerebral abnormalities; CHARGE and other rare congenital syndromes; cleft palate; and polydactyly.

Clinical features An absent or small eye is noted soon after birth. Microphthalmos may be associated with a variably sized cyst arising from the eye or its vestigial remnant; reduced lid and orbit

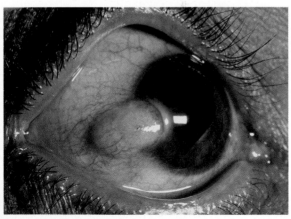

Fig. 3.4: Limbal dermoid.

growth; microcornea; colobomata; cataract; glaucoma and aniridia.

Management Leave cysts intact to stimulate orbital and lid growth, unless excessively large. In the absence of a cyst, insert progressive orbital and socket expanders, either as serial solid shapes or expanding implants. Once final orbital and lid growth is achieved, further expansion of the orbit (orbital implants, bony grafts), fornices (mucous membrane grafts), and lids is often required.

Thyroid Eye Disease

Background An idiopathic autoimmune disorder resulting in an active orbital inflammatory phase (months–years) and subsequent 'inactive' fibrotic phase, largely involving extraocular muscles and connective tissues. There is a female preponderance with peak incidence at age 30–50 years. Severe cases are more common in older patients, males, and smokers. Usually associated with hyperthyroidism, but patients may be hypo- or euthyroid. A minority of cases develop sight-threatening optic neuropathy or exposure keratopathy.

Classification

The 'Clinical Activity Score'[1] measures *activity* and scores 1 for each of 10 features:

- Pain: (i) retrobulbar, (ii) on eye movement.

- Redness: (iii) lid, (iv) conjunctiva.

- Swelling: (v) lids, (vi) conjunctiva, (vii) caruncle, (viii) ≥2 mm increase in proptosis over 1–3 months.

- Loss of function: (ix) ±5° decrease in eye movement over 1–3 months, (x) loss of ≥1 Snellen line over 1–3 months

'NOSPECS'[2] classifies *severity* as:

- **N**o symptoms or signs.

- **O**nly lid retraction ± lid lag.

- **S**oft tissue involvement (lid, conjunctival inflammation).

- **P**roptosis.

- **E**xtraocular muscle involvement ± diplopia.

- **C**orneal disease.

- **S**ight-threatening optic neuropathy.

Symptoms include injection, redness dryness/watering, photophobia, ache, visual loss (colour, VA, fields), and diplopia. Ask about smoking, family history of thyroid eye disese (TED) or other autoimmune disorder and past thyroid problems.

Signs Look for proptosis (usually axial); optic neuropathy (reduced VA; colour vision; RAPD; field loss); exposure keratopathy; upper lid retraction (Fig. 3.5); lid 'lag' on downgaze (descent of upper lid slower than that of the globe); lagophthalmos; increased IOP on (typically) upgaze, but also

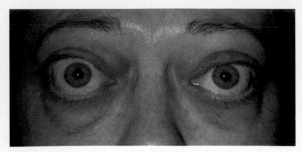

Fig. 3.5: Moderately severe, inactive, thyroid eye disease.

primary position; conjunctival inflammation and chemosis; caruncle oedema; superior limbic keratoconjunctivitis; lid inflammation; orbital fat prolapse; ocular dysmotility. The most commonly affected muscle is the inferior rectus, followed by medial, superior, then lateral rectus. Elderly patients may present with relatively inactive orbitopathy and progressive, typically vertical, strabismus.

Differential diagnoses Consider idiopathic orbital inflammatory disease and other orbital inflammatory disorders; lymphoproliferative disorders, especially reactive lymphoid hyperplasia; and caroticocavernous fistula (enlarged superior ophthalmic vein on imaging). Consider myasthenia gravis in elderly males with inactive TED.

Investigations Request thyroid function tests. CT (Fig. 3.6) is indicated if orbital decompression is planned, for uncertain an diagnosis, or asymmetry >2 mm on exophthalmometry. Consider thyroid autoantibodies (antithyroid peroxidase, antithyroglobulin, thyroid microsomal antibodies, thyroid stimulating antibodies) although these have poor sensitivity and specificity.

Management

■ *Casualty*: Refer as follows.

Sight-threatened: same-day orbital opinion.

Active: orbital clinic in 2–4 weeks.

Inactive: routine referral (preferably to a specialist orbital clinic).

■ *Clinic*: Urge smokers to stop. Achieve and maintain euthyroidism and avoid sudden fluctuations in thyroid hormone levels. Consider endocrinology referral.

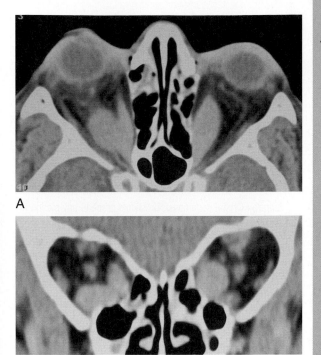

A

B

Fig. 3.6: Thyroid eye disease: axial **(A)** and coronal **(B)** CT scans showing marked right inferior rectus and left medial rectus enlargement.

Conservative: ocular lubricants, elevation of head at night, and sunglasses.

Immunosuppression: Consider steroids if active inflammation coexists with: optic neuropathy; sight-threatening exposure keratopathy; significant soft tissue signs; or ocular dysmotility. Start with enteric-coated prednisolone 1 mg/kg/day but reduce dose if less severe. Consider ranitidine 150 mg b.d. p.o. For optic neuropathy review at 1 week and if responding reduce to 20 mg/day over 2–3 weeks and refer for urgent orbital radiotherapy; if not responding, arrange urgent surgical decompression. For marked soft tissue disease or diplopia, reduce from 1 mg/kg/day to 20 mg/day over 2 weeks and review; if responding, refer for nonurgent radiotherapy; if not, consider decompression. Gradually reduce steroids over 1–3 months depending on presentation and response. Note baseline tests, side effects, and monitoring required for patients on oral steroids (p. 343). Consider steroid-sparing agents (e.g. azathioprine, ciclosporin) if steroid intolerant or contraindications, and co-manage with physicians. Consider admission and methylprednisolone i.v. for severe sight-threatening disease not responding to oral steroids.

Radiotherapy (XRT): The evidence base is uncertain, but consider low dose (20–24 Gy) lens-sparing orbital irradiation in cases of sight-threatening disease or significant soft tissue inflammation, including ocular dysmotility. For adjunctive use with immunosuppression, maintain prednisolone at approximately 20 mg/day.

Surgery: Orbital decompression should precede any planned strabismus surgery, which should precede lid surgery.

Orbital decompression should be considered when TED is inactive and stable, unless the sight is threatened. The main indication is facially disfiguring, non-sight-threatening proptosis. Bony decompression for >24 mm proptosis involves three walls (medial and lateral walls, floor) or two and a half walls (only medial half of floor) if <24 mm. *Benefit*: mean 7–8 mm of globe retroplacement. *Risks*: visual loss (<1 : 1000), new diplopia (≈15%), other risks are low (permanent infraorbital nerve numbness, haemorrhage, infection, late overcorrection or 'imploding antrum syndrome', troublesome scar, redo surgery). Fat decompression may be considered, but is less effective and probably associated with an increased risk of restrictive motility disorder.

Strabismus surgery generally involves recessions, once orthoptically stable for ≥ 6 months.

Lid surgery:

Upper lid retraction: retractor recessions are often required and may use a spacer (e.g. auricular cartilage, hard palate mucosa, Alloderm). Consider tarsorrhaphy if this fails.

True lower lid retraction (as opposed to displacement from proptosis): retractor release with spacer.

Cellulitis

Background Preseptal and orbital cellulitis constitute a medical emergency, requiring immediate administration of high-dose, broad-spectrum systemic antibiotics before imaging or referral to an orbital specialist. Orbital cellulitis may be life-threatening if it spreads to the intracranial space. Possible sources of infection include paranasal sinuses, oropharynx, skin, foreign bodies, trauma (including iatrogenic), and haematogenous spread. Bacteria are the commonest cause, especially, streptococci, staphylococci and *Haemophilus influenzae*. Anaerobes and other Gram-negative organisms are less common. Consider rare causes in immunocompromised patients, especially mucormycosis, aspergillosis, tuberculosis, and viruses, e.g. herpes zoster.

Clinical features Preseptal cellulitis produces fever, pain, swelling, ptosis, tenderness and redness (Fig. 3.7). Orbital cellulitis is similar but with chemosis, reduced eye movements ± diplopia, vision loss, RAPD, and proptosis.

History and examination Ask about sinus disease, trauma, surgery, skin infection, immunocompromise, and diabetes. Perform exophthalmometry, and check temperature, general status (hydration, etc.), eye movements, colour vision, confrontation fields, RAPD, and full ocular examination noting optic disc appearance. Mark the extent of skin inflammation to determine if it is subsequently improving or worsening.

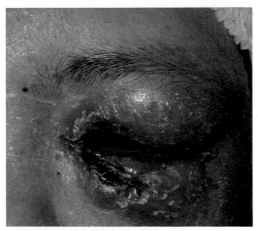

Fig. 3.7: Preseptal cellulitis.

Investigations Investigate all cases except mild preseptal cellulitis responding to treatment. Request CT (sinus disease, orbital or intracranial abscess), MRI if suspected organic foreign body, FBC (neutrophilia), blood culture if systemically septic, and blood glucose. Swab any sources of pus for microbiology.

Management Start treatment immediately. Doses given are for adults.

■ Preseptal cellulitis

Mild: Co-amoxiclav 500/125 mg p.o. t.d.s. or flucloxacillin 500 mg p.o. q.d.s., both for 10 days. Review daily until there is a definite improvement, then every 2–7 days until complete resolution. Treat as severe (see below) if the patient fails to respond, or is ≤5 years old, septic, or potentially noncompliant.

Severe: Admit for ceftriaxone 1–2 g i.v. daily in divided doses until responding (1–2 days), then treat as for mild.

■ Orbital cellulitis

Admit: Monitor orbital and visual functions 2–3 times daily. Give ceftriaxone 1–4 g i.v. daily plus flucloxacillin 1–2 g i.v. q.d.s. (beware cholestatic jaundice). In adults (>10 years old) with chronic sinonasal disease add metronidazole 500 mg i.v. t.d.s. Continue i.v. treatment for 3–5 days, provided condition improves. Request CT, blood glucose, FBC, ± blood culture (if septic). Refer to ENT if sinus disease is detected. Repeat CT to exclude abscess if any deterioration occurs. Arrange urgent neurosurgical referral if there is neurologic deterioration or intracranial abscess. Change to oral antibiotic (see Preseptal cellulitis above) when there is definite improvement. Review every 2–5 days after discharge until complete resolution.

■ Orbital abscess

Drain if patient >10 years old *or* clinical/visual deterioration *or* failed medical therapy. Consider surgical decompression if the orbit is very tense or not responding to antibiotics. Consider systemic steroids if visual loss occurs despite the above measures.

Idiopathic Orbital Inflammatory Disease

Background Inflammation is not a diagnosis, but a tissue response to trauma, infection, tumour necrosis, ischaemia, toxins, allergy, etc. Idiopathic orbital inflammatory disease (IOID) is, by definition, a diagnosis of exclusion and in most cases a biopsy is required. Avoid the term 'pseudotumour' which implies a diagnosis. Any orbital tissue can be involved and presentation varies from acute to chronic.

Corticosteroids alter both the clinical course and histopathologic findings in a number of inflammatory processes, including IOID, lymphoma, and metastatic carcinoma. Use steroids only after a tissue diagnosis is established, with the following exceptions:

- Superior orbital fissure (Tolosa-Hunt) syndrome,
- Classic orbital myositis,
- Classic thyroid eye disease, or
- Sight-threatening orbital inflammatory disease awaiting urgent biopsy.

Clinical features Inflammation produces:

- Rubor: redness of lids, conjunctiva, and extraocular muscle insertions.
- Dolor: pain on eye movement ± tenderness.
- Calor: warmth.
- Tumor: lid swelling, mass or enlarged lacrimal gland.
- Loss of function: ptosis, diplopia and restricted eye movement, visual loss, sensory loss.

Take a careful general medical history for underlying systemic diseases and arrange full medical examination as required.

Differential diagnoses includes infective cellulitis; haematologic or lymphoproliferative disorders (leukaemia, lymphoma); sinus disease; autoimmune disease, including thyroid eye disease, sarcoidosis and Wegener's granulomatosis; caroticocavernous fistula; primary or secondary orbital malignancy.

Investigations Arrange orbital CT (or MRI). Consider the following tests: FBC; ESR; CRP; U&E; autoantibodies; sACE; Ca^{2+}; CXR; CT chest.

Management Attempt to determine the underlying aetiology. See the following pages for management of specific inflammatory conditions (dacryoadenitis, p. 89, orbital myositis, p. 90, superior orbital fissure syndrome, p. 91). Consider referral to a physician or oncologist. In the absence of a classic presentation of orbital myositis or superior orbital fissure syndrome, consider NSAIDs, e.g. flurbiprofen 100 mg p.o. t.d.s. for 2 weeks, then 50 mg t.d.s. for 1–2 months; warn of side effects including GI upset and bleeding, and consider prophylaxis with omeprazole 20 mg p.o. daily, or ranitidine 150 mg p.o. b.d. If no response to NSAIDs, arrange orbitotomy ('opening of the septum') and biopsy for histopathology ± microbiology. Systemic steroids (typically prednisolone up to 1 mg/kg/day) may be commenced after biopsy. Taper over 1–3 months, monitoring for response. Be aware of steroid side effects and required monitoring (page 343). If inflammation recurs, repeat the biopsy before increasing prednisolone. Low-dose, lens-sparing orbital radiotherapy (20 Gy per orbit) may be considered in refractory cases after a negative biopsy.

Dacryoadenitis

Background Lacrimal gland inflammation is most commonly idiopathic, but may be associated with infection (mostly viral, e.g. mumps, Epstein Barr virus, cytomegalovirus, varicella-zoster), sarcoidosis, Sjögren's syndrome, and lymphoproliferation. Persistent lacrimal gland inflammation should raise the suspicion of carcinoma.

Clinical features Typically, pain, erythema, swelling ± ptosis of lateral upper lid, and disturbed tear production (Fig. 3.8). Sensory loss or paraesthesiae are rare and if present suspect carcinoma.

Differential diagnosis Consider lacrimal gland carcinoma (p. 98). Consider sarcoidosis if: bilateral; respiratory disturbance; rash; hilar lymphadenopathy on CXR; raised serum Ca^{2+} and ACE.

Investigations CT for symptoms >2–3 weeks. Biopsy is indicated if there is a poor response after several weeks treatment, >3–4 weeks of pain, or a persistent lacrimal fossa mass at 4 months.

Management Treat as idiopathic orbital inflammatory disease (p. 87)

Follow-up for 6 months then discharge if there is complete resolution and no suspicious features (persistent pain or mass; sensory disturbance).

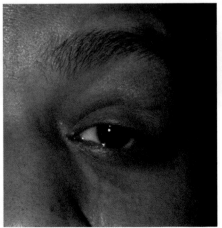

Fig. 3.8: Dacryoadenitis.

Orbital Myositis

Background Idiopathic inflammation of the extraocular muscles.

Clinical features Prodrome of periorbital ache exacerbated by eye movement, followed 2–3 days later by diplopia. Symptoms are worst looking away from the field of action of the affected extraocular muscle (EOM). Patients may have proptosis, redness over EOM insertions, upper or lower lid retraction, or ptosis. Repeated attacks may cause fibrosis and a permanent squint.

Investigations CT shows EOM enlargement, classically (but not reliably) involving the insertion (thyroid eye disease classically spares the EOM insertion) (Fig. 3.9).

Differential diagnosis Includes metastasis, vascular malformation, and lymphoproliferative disease. Typically only one EOM is affected; if >2 consider thyroid eye disease (p. 81), which may overlap, as may idiopathic orbital inflammatory disease (p. 87).

Management For *classic* presentation, prednisolone up to 1 mg/kg/day usually produces a response within 24 hours. Gradually taper over 2–4 weeks. Biopsy if there is a poor response to treatment or recurrence. Radiotherapy is helpful if cases are recurrent, chronic, or for failed medical treatment with 'negative' (i.e. inflammatory change only) biopsy.

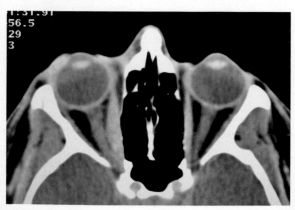

Fig. 3.9: CT of right medial rectus myositis.

Superior Orbital Fissure Syndrome (Tolosa-Hunt Syndrome)

Background Idiopathic inflammation involving the superior orbital fissures (SOF) region. May also involve the cavernous sinus.

Clinical features May include retrobulbar ache, ophthalmoplegia, periorbital sensory loss/disturbance (V_1 & V_2), and visual loss.

Investigations CT shows an infiltrative mass at the orbital apex and loss of the normal fat pad at the SOF (applies to any infiltration at the SOF).

Differential diagnosis Exclude intracranial spread and lymphoma. Trauma may produce similar signs (see page 103), as may tumours and granulomus at the orbital apex.

Management Treat with high-dose prednisolone 1 mg/kg/day if tolerated, tapering according to response. Expect a rapid and good response. Biopsy in recurrent or suspicious cases carries high risk of visual loss, permanent ophthalmoplegia, or sensory loss. Radiotherapy may be appropriate.

Orbital Vascular Lesions

Classification

■ *Proliferations* are usually absent at birth, and result from endothelial proliferation followed sometimes by involution. They are well circumscribed, may cause mass effect, and connect to otherwise normal vascular channels.

■ *Malformations* are present at birth but may be subclinical. They are classified further by their haemodynamics: high flow (arterial/arteriovenous), low flow (venous, a.k.a. 'varices') and 'no flow' (lymphatic a.k.a. 'lymphangioma'). These lesions grow commensurately with the patient.

■ *Shunts* are abnormal communications between arterial and venous circulations. They may be congenital (including malformations) or acquired (e.g. traumatic).

Proliferations

Hamartomatous (haemangioma) (Fig. 3.10) Presents in early months of life with rapid growth over weeks to months, and gradual involution, typically resolving before age 10 years. Superficial, dermal, 'strawberry naevi' account for 90% (p. 34); 10% are deeper. Mass effects include ptosis, astigmatism, globe displacement, and ocular dysmotility. Hematomas may be associated with haemangiomata elsewhere; extensive lesions may cause red blood cell or platelet sequestration and circulatory stress. Lesions may pulsate (unusual), or enlarge with Valsalva manouvre (e.g. crying). CT may be required to determine the depth and usually shows well-defined, enhancing lesions. Arrange serial Doppler ultrasound scans (USS) to monitor size and internal flow rates. Careful visual monitoring for amblyopia is essential for periocular lesions. Treat amblyopia as necessary, and monitor and reassure about the natural history. Larger lesions or failure of amblyopia therapy may necessitate treatment with intralesional corticosteroids, e.g. dexamethasone 4 mg in 1 mL to periphery of lesion + Depomedrone 40 mg in 1 mL to centre of the lesion. Review in 4–6 weeks and consider a further 1–2 injections. Explain the small risk of blindness and scalp ischaemia from vaso-oclusion. Systemic steroids are sometimes required: if so refer to a paediatrician. Excision can be considered but risks haemorrhage.

Neoplastic lesions include haemangiopericytoma, angiosarcoma, and Kaposi's sarcoma (see p. 394).

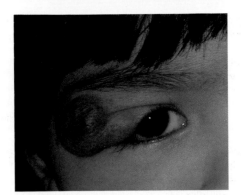

Fig. 3.10: Haemangioma.

Malformations

High-flow or arteriovenous malformations

(AVMs) Comprises arterial feeding vessels, an arterialized vascular network, and venous drainage. May produce pulsatile proptosis, bruit, conjunctival arterialization, chemosis, lid swelling, pain from thrombosis or haemorrhage, impaired vision, and dysmotility. CT or MRI show irregular, rapidly enhancing mass, flow voids (MRI), with high flow on Doppler USS. Angiography provides precise anatomic delineation. Treated by interventional radiology (e.g. intravascular coils, glue) followed by excision where possible.

Low-flow vascular malformations

■ *Arteriovenous (a.k.a. 'cavernous haemangioma')* Formed by small arterial feeders with thin-walled vessels and venous drainage, commonest in middle-aged females. May present as an incidental finding on imaging, or with slowly progressive axial proptosis ± globe indentation, producing hypermetropia and choroidal folds. Apical lesions may cause retrobulbar ache, visual loss (including gaze-evoked amaurosis), and ocular dysmotility. Imaging shows a well-defined, round, irregularly enhancing mass. May be soft and compressible on USS. Traditionally, nonapical lesions not affecting vision are observed; however, excision of small lesions has low morbidity and confirms the diagnosis.

■ *Venous (a.k.a. 'varices')* These irregular venous dilatations enlarge with dependent posture or Valsalva manoeuvre.

Lesions may ache, and cause pain and proptosis if they bleed. Superficial lesions have visibly dilated veins (Fig. 3.11). Repeated haemorrhages and scarring may cause enophthalmos due to fat atrophy. There may be involvement of contiguous structures (CNS, face, sinuses, temporalis fossa). Static CT or MRI shows multiple irregular masses, often along the course of a vein ± signs of prior bleeding. There may be a thin hyperdense rim on CT. Angiography is rarely required. Dynamic CT, MRI, or USS may show filling with Valsalva. USS shows cystic spaces. Management may involve amblyopia therapy or surgical excision for unremitting pain, severe cosmetic disfigurement, or massive expansion. Surgical risks include haemorrhage and recurrence. Drainage of acute haemorrhage ('chocolate cysts') is possible. Interventional radiologic techniques and injection of a sclerosants such as glue may reduce lesion size.

No-flow malformations (a.k.a. 'lymphangiomas')

Superficial lesions (Fig. 3.12) produce intermittent swelling, ecchymoses, and disfigurement of the lids and conjunctiva; deeper lesions produce intermittent haemorrhage or thrombosis, with episodic swelling, visual disturbance, or dysmotility. May be extraorbital, especially involving the face and oropharynx. Imaging and treatment are similar to low-flow malformations, but lesions are nondistensible and more infiltrative.

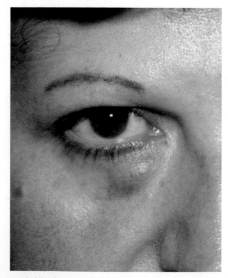

Fig. 3.11: Orbital varix.

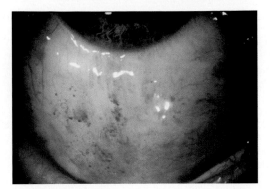

Fig. 3.12: Lymphangioma.

Arteriovenous shunts (carotid cavernous fistula)

See page 675.

Other vascular lesions

Aneurysm; orbital venous thrombosis (postinflammatory, idiopathic); spontaneous orbital haemorrhage (elderly, haemorrhagic diathesis, anticoagulants).

Orbital Lymphoproliferative Disorders

Background Orbital lymphoproliferations are divided into reactive lymphoid hyperplasia, intermediate lymphoproliferation (atypical lymphoid hyperplasia), and lymphoma. Orbital T-cell lymphoma is extremely rare. B-cell lymphoma is histologically divided into low and high grade, the former being much more common. The most common B-cell lymphoma is marginal zone type. The orbit may be involved secondarily from adjacent or distant B-cell lymphoma. Conversely, orbital lymphoma may spread to extraorbital sites, e.g. CNS.

Clinical features The typical presentation is a gradual onset of a painless infiltrative mass in the sixth and seventh decades, often with nonaxial proptosis. Disturbed ocular motility may occur, but neurovascular or visual compromise is uncommon (Fig. 3.13). Conjunctival involvement (≈20%) is classically 'salmon patch' in colour and texture. Lacrimal gland involvement is common. High-grade tumours produce a more rapid, infiltrative course.

Investigation Distinguish from non-neoplastic or idiopathic inflammatory disorders (p. 87). CT typically shows a well-defined, enhancing, 'moulding', extraconal, homogeneous, soft-tissue mass. Calcification is uncommon. Biopsy, sometimes repeated, is mandatory, and immunohistochemistry ± gene rearrangement studies (Ig heavy chain PCR) are usually required. A fresh specimen may be required for flow cytometry.

Management

- *Reactive lymphoid hyperplasia*: Extraorbital, especially lymph node, involvement is not uncommon. Progression to lymphoma

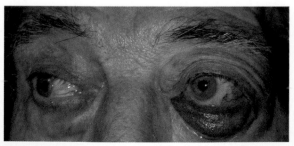

Fig. 3.13: Orbital lymphoma with restricted adduction of the left eye.

occurs in ≈10% of cases. The response to prednisolone is generally excellent; low-dose radiotherapy (XRT) may be required for functional disturbance; debulking or decompressive surgery may be required for gross mass effect or proptosis.

■ *Intermediate lymphoproliferaton*: Behaves similar to low-grade B-cell lymphoma. A systemic immunoregulatory disorder may coexist. The response to prednisolone may be poor, requiring immunosuppression or XRT.

■ *B-cell lymphoma*: Refer all patients to a haematologist/ oncologist for systemic investigation. The risk of systemic disease varies with site (eyelid > orbit > conjunctiva) and is higher with bilateral disease. About 25% have prior or concurrent systemic disease, and 50% subsequently. Low-grade lymphoma is treated with XRT (≈24 Gy), or systemic disease with chemotherapy (e.g. chlorambucil) often with good response. Higher-grade, systemic disease generally requires chemotherapy and or XRT (30–35 Gy). Alternatives exist, e.g. monoclonal antibodies and allogeneic transplants. As the prognosis is generally good, consider the risk versus benefit of treatment.

Lacrimal Gland Tumours

Pleomorphic adenoma

Background The commonest benign lacrimal gland tumour. May involve the orbital (majority) or palpebral lobe of the lacrimal gland.

Clinical features Classically presents in the second to fifth decades as very slowly progressive proptosis, inferomedial globe displacement, and superotemporal quadrant lid swelling. Ocular indentation may cause blurred vision, choroidal folds, and a hypermetropic shift. Ocular dysmotility may occur. Pain, sensory disturbance, and inflammation are uncommon and suggest malignancy.

Investigations CT typically reveals a round or bosselated, well-circumscribed, enhancing mass indenting the globe and lacrimal fossa. Calcification occurs in 3%.

Differential diagnosis (of superotemporal quadrant masses) Other benign lacrimal gland tumours (rare), malignant lacrimal gland tumours, lymphoproliferation, neural tumours (e.g. neurofibroma), idiopathic orbital inflammatory disease, Sjögren's syndrome, sarcoidosis, Wegener's granulomatosis, dermoid or lacrimal cysts, extrinsic tumours.

Management Refer routinely to an experienced orbital surgeon. Clinicoradiologic features should suggest the diagnosis. Incisional biopsy is contraindicated as it increases the risk of recurrence and malignant transformation. Complete excision with an intact pseudocapsule is required, often via a lateral orbitotomy. Keratoconjunctivitis sicca may occur postoperatively, even with preservation of the palpebral lobe.

Follow-up: 5–10 years to exclude malignant transformation that may occur despite histological clearance. If histological foci of malignant change are found, extend follow-up and consider radiotherapy as for lacrimal gland carcinoma.

Lacrimal gland carcinoma

Background Primary lacrimal gland malignancies have a high mortality. The commonest is adenoid cystic carcinoma; *de novo* adenocarcinoma, squamous and mucoepidermoid carcinomas occur less frequently. Carcinoma may arise from a pleomorphic adenoma, so-called 'malignant mixed tumour'.

Differential diagnosis Similar to pleomorphic adenoma (see previous section), which must itself be excluded clinicoradiologically. Consider carcinoma in cases of nonresolving dacryoadenitis.

Clinical features Typically, a brief (<1 year) history of a superotemporal quadrant mass with pain, sensory loss, and paraesthesiae. Inflammation may occur.

Investigations CT classically shows an infiltrative tumour moulding to the globe with finely irregular bony erosion, and calcification in 33%.

Management Refer to an experienced orbital surgeon for urgent incisional biopsy to confirm the diagnosis. Treatment of most well-defined tumours then involves complete local excision, occasionally exenteration or radical craniofacial resection, followed by radiotherapy.

Follow-up Review lifelong to treat the inevitable dry eye, radiation-induced cataract, and monitor for local or systemic recurrence, particularly pulmonary.

Rhabdomyosarcoma

Background The commonest primary malignant mesenchymal tumour of childhood. May be spontaneous (majority) or familial.

Clinical features Orbital involvement typically presents in the first decade with rapid proptosis (weeks), superotemporal swelling with globe displacement, lid swelling, erythema, and ptosis. Pain, visual loss, and watering are uncommon. A small number arise from extraorbital sites with secondary orbital spread. May rarely present in the elderly.

Differential diagnosis Consider inflammatory disorders (e.g. orbital cellulitis), haemangioma, lymphangioma, aggressive neurofibroma, and poorly differentiated tumours (e.g. neuroblastoma, Ewing's and other sarcomas).

Investigations CT usually shows a homogeneous, well-defined, enhancing, soft tissue mass without bony destruction – typically not including the muscles. Biopsy (incisional or excisional) is required for histologic typing.

Management Treat with excisional biopsy. Refer to a paediatric oncologist for staging and multiagent chemotherapy, which generally results in a good prognosis. Radiotherapy may be required.

Fibrous Histiocytoma

The commonest adult mesenchymal orbital tumour. Usually presents in middle age with a slow-growing, firm, superonasal mass, proptosis, and visual loss. Dysmotility, pain, lid swelling, and ptosis are less common. Infiltration and local recurrence are typical but metastases rare. Treatment involves complete local resection, and occasionally radical excision or exenteration to prevent local recurrence. Radiotherapy is unhelpful and the role of chemotherapy unclear.

Orbital Trauma

Background The commonest orbital injury is a 'blowout' fracture, typically involving the floor and/or medial wall. If the injury results from an alleged assault or workplace injury, make detailed notes documenting timing and circumstances of the injury: measure or preferably photograph all injuries. For traumatic optic neuropathy see page 661.

History Ask about the nature of the injury, any visual symptoms including diplopia, blurred vision or field loss, periorbital sensory loss, dental malocclusion, and trismus (inability to open the mouth).

Examination Check VA, RAPD, colour vision, infraorbital sensation, ocular motility, exophthalmometry (note any nonaxial globe dystopia), and bony orbital rims. Perform a careful head, ocular, and general assessment to exclude other injuries.

Mangement Consider the following diagnoses:

■ *Orbital floor fracture* Features include: periorbital ecchymoses; subconjunctival haemorrhage (SCH); enophthalmos; limited eye movement, especially upgaze (from inferior rectus entrapment, bruising, oedema or neurapraxia); infraorbital nerve hypoaesthesia/numbness/pain; subcutaneous emphysema. Children may have a 'greenstick' fracture with significant muscle entrapment but minimal bruising ('white eye blowout') and nausea and vomiting, especially on upgaze.

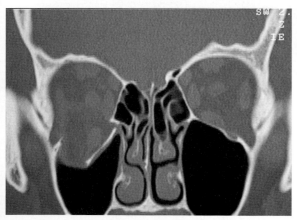

Fig. 3.14: CT of a right orbital blowout fracture.

Request CT (same or next day) (Fig. 3.14) with fine cuts of orbits and face (axial, coronal ± sagittal). Consider plain X-rays if CT is unavailable, and skull and cervical X-rays as indicated. Ban nose-blowing for 10 days.

Surgery is required in the following situations:

■ Child: a white-eye blowout requires surgery within 48–72 hours.

■ Enophthalmos >2 mm and symptomatic: this may become apparent weeks after injury.

■ Greater than 50% of the floor area involved, as there is a high risk of late enophthalmos.

■ Diplopia that fails to resolve after 2–3 weeks.

Monitor diplopia carefully with serial Hess charts. Some diplopia on extreme up- or downgaze may persist, but if restriction affects the primary position or the field of binocular vision at 2–3 weeks then consider orbital exploration, and fracture repair. Persistent diplopia may require inferior rectus recessions, and/or Faden procedures of the superior rectus and inferior rectus of the unaffected eye. Ipsilateral inverse Knapp procedure can be helpful after about 6 months if improvement has stopped. In general, results are often disappointing. Consider decompressing the infraorbital canal if there is significant pain in the inferior orbital nerve territory. Options for repair include alloplastic material (e.g. porous polyethylene) or autogenous material (e.g. cranial bone).

■ *Medial orbital wall fracture* Often has subcutaneous emphysema, variable ecchymoses, medial rectus (MR) dysfunction, enophthalmos, or proptosis. Repair if there is significant MR entrapment causing pain, diplopia, or if enophthalmos >2 mm. Otherwise observe. Ban nose blowing for 10 days.

■ *Lateral orbital wall and roof fracture* Isolated lateral wall fractures are rare and are usually associated with zygomatico-orbitomaxillary complex fractures. Small, undisplaced roof fractures may be monitored for neurologic and ophthalmic complications with broad-spectrum antibiotic cover (e.g. Co-amoxiclav).

■ *Orbital haematoma* May occur in blunt trauma, bleeding diatheses, or vascular anomalies. Features include: severe orbital or ocular pain; proptosis; ptosis; restricted eye movements, periorbital oedema; progressive visual loss and optic neuropathy; marked subconjunctival haemorrhage;

elevated IOP. Most cases are mild and are observed. If there is moderate to severe visual loss and or optic neuropathy, admit and consider urgent lateral cantholysis, orbitotomy, and evacuation of the haematoma. Formal bony orbital decompression may rarely be required. Consider the following, after consultation with an orbital surgeon, if there is no response to surgical decompression: mannitol (0.5–2 g/kg i.v. over 30–60 minutes), acetazolamide (500 mg i.v.), high-dose corticosteroids (e.g. methylprednisolone i.v. 0.5–2 g b.d.). Consider prophylactic antibiotics in cases associated with sinus fracture. Monitor visual and orbital function regularly (up to 2–3 times a day), depending on the response to treatment.

- *Superior orbital fissure syndrome* Severe impact to the lateral wall may produce oedema, haemorrhage, or bony compression of adjacent soft tissues with subsequent ophthalmoplegia (cranial nerves III, IV, VI), ptosis (III), mydriasis, efferent pupillary defect (III), loss of accommodation (III), and V_1 sensory loss (including cornea). Management includes high-dose corticosteroids, e.g. i.v. methylprednisolone for 48 hours (up to 8 g/day in 1–2 divided doses or infusion), then prednisolone 1 mg/kg/day rapidly reducing (beware steroid side effects and contraindications, p. 343). Reduction of significantly displaced fractures may be considered. Superior orbital fissure syndrome may also occur with orbital apex tumours, granulomas, and idiopathic orbital inflammation (p. 91).

- *Orbital apex syndrome* This consists of superior orbital fissure syndrome with optic neuropathy. Management includes high-dose steroids (as above) and bony decompression.

- *Orbital foreign bodies* These occur in up to 3% of orbital trauma. A clear history of penetrating trauma may not be forthcoming, especially in children. Look for small entry wounds. Request CT, or MRI if organic matter is suspected. Avoid MRI if metallic objects are suspected. Beware intracranial and intraocular penetration. Removal is indicated if organic (e.g. wood), copper containing, infective (e.g. associated with an abscess, discharging sinus), or for a functional deficit (e.g. optic neuropathy, ocular motility disturbance).

Eye Socket Disorders

Post-enucleation socket syndrome (PESS) Caused by an absent or small implant following enucleation or evisceration; attempted correction with a large, heavy prosthesis may result in poor prosthetic retention, rotation, and instability. Clinical features form the mnemonic, PESS: *P*tosis, *E*nophthalmos, deep upper lid *S*ulcus, lower lid *S*ag (Fig. 3.15). Patients may also develop upper lid entropion with lagophthalmos.

Consider a larger artificial eye, but this may worsen lower lid sag, retention, and stability problems. If no implant is palpable, augment volume with a secondary ball implant. If an implant is present, exchange for larger ball implant, add orbital floor implant (e.g. silicone, Medpor, cranial bone graft), or autogenous material to the socket and/or postseptal upper lid sulcus (e.g. dermis-fat, micro-fat graft).

Discharge is a common and often minor problem, relating mainly to the presence of the prosthesis. Regular prosthetic care, including polishing, helps reduce proteinaceous surface biofilm. Evert the lid to exclude giant papillary conjunctivitis, and if present treat with topical steroids, e.g. G. Maxitrol q.d.s. for 1 month. Exclude exposed sutures or implants – these generally require removal of exposed material (± later reinsertion of implant or graft). True socket infection is rare and relates to bacterial contamination at the time of implant insertion, implant exposure, and host factors e.g. prior radiotherapy, diabetes or immunosuppression.

Implant exposure generally relates to inadequate surgical implantation. Failure to widely open the posterior orbital space and dragging of anterior tissues leads to insufficiently posterior placement. Restitution of dragged tissues further shallows the

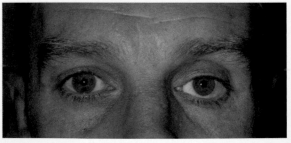

Fig. 3.15: Left postenucleation socket syndrome.

implant. Other factors include poor host conditions (e.g. prior radiotherapy), insufficient socket lining (limiting closure over implant), disproportionately small, bony socket (e.g. prior radiotherapy, microphthalmos/anophthalmos), and possibly use of nonabsorbable sutures.

Poor prosthetic motility is common after eye removal ± orbital implantation, especially in horizontal gaze (shorter fornices). It is less common after evisceration than enucleation. Distinguish motility of the socket (often poor after trauma, multiple surgeries) from that of the prosthesis. Optimize prosthetic fitting and volume augmentation. The use of pegged implants may improve motility but has a high complication rate (≈50%), e.g. granuloma, exposure, infection, peg extrusion, 'clicking' noise, poor prosthesis retention.

Procedures

Box 3.1: Enucleation

1. Obtain fully informed consent and agreement from two consultant ophthalmologists. Mark the side.

2. Avoid if there is endophthalmitis, as infection may spread to the orbit and brain.

3. Surgery is usually performed under GA, but retrobulbar LA with sedation is possible.

4. *Confirm the side* by examining the eyes, notes, and consent form.

5. Perform 360° peritomy using spring scissors and blunt dissect Tenon's capsule from the globe.

6. Preplace 5/0 Vicryl in the recti near their insertion, then disinsert. Disinsert obliques (may reattach the inferior oblique)

7. Divide the optic nerve using enucleation scissors or snare. Gently handle the eyes with ocular tumours to minimize the risk of seeding. Send the eye for histopathology.

8. Obtain central retinal artery haemostasis using bipolar cautery and pressure.

9. Select an implant, typically 22 mm size. Acrylic is much cheaper than other choices. For implants other than porous polyethylene (Medpor), a wrap (e.g. Vicryl mesh) is required for muscle attachment. Donor sclera is generally avoided because of the risk of prion transmission.

10. Insert the implant behind posterior Tenon's capsule using a 'no-touch' technique, e.g. insert into a surgical glove finger and glide into place through a hole cut in the end of the finger.

11. Suture the recti to the implant/wrap using the preplaced sutures.

12. Close Tenon's capsule (interrupted 5/0 Vicryl) and conjunctiva (continuous 7/0 Vicryl).

13. Insert the largest possible conformer into the fornices, leaving 2–3 mm lagophthalmos. Apply antibiotic ointment.

Box 3.1: Enucleation—cont'd

14. Apply a pressure dressing for 5–7 days and prescribe broad-spectrum antibiotics, e.g. cephalexin 250 mg p.o. q.d.s. 7 days.

15. Review in 5–7 days. Early complications include orbital haemorrhage, oedema, and infection. Late complications include postenucleation socket syndrome, implant extrusion, exposure or malposition, and lining deficiency (p. 104).

16. Refer for an ocular prosthesis in 3–4 weeks.

Box 3.2: Evisceration

1. Consent, precautions, anaesthesia and peritomy are similar to enucleation (Steps 1–5 above).

2. Perform a 360° limbal keratectomy (blade then spring scissors).

3. Remove the intraocular contents using a metal scoop.

4. Carefully debride all uveal tissue with a cotton bud. Avoid alcohol as this may cause scleral necrosis. Cauterize the vortex veins and any bleeding vessels.

5. Split sclera diagonally across the macula into two halves (each with two recti attached).

6. 'Islandize' the optic nerve with a small scleral rim. This prevents neuroma.

7. Insert an unwrapped implant into the posterior orbit via a 'glide'. As per enucleation, avoid the implant contacting the surgeon or lids. Unlike enucleation, an implant wrap is not required.

8. Close the sclera (5/0 Vicryl) with a 4–5 mm overlap, avoiding closure under tension over the implant.

9. See 'Enucleation', points 12–16.

Optometry and General Practice Guidelines

Infection of the skin and the eye is not uncommon, but it is important to distinguish minor soft tissue infection from preseptal cellulitis, and especially orbital cellulitis (infection behind the orbital septum). Reduced visual acuity, eye movements, diplopia, and proptosis suggest orbital cellulitis.

Orbital cellulitis requires immediate referral to a specialist to exclude life- or vision-threatening complications. Commence broad-spectrum intravenous antibiotic therapy (cefuroxime, and in patients over 10 years old, metronidazole) *immediately*, before investigation or referral. This measure may be sight and life saving.

Orbital trauma also requires urgent assessment; small penetrating entry points may be hard to detect or absent. Exclude and stabilize other injuries to head, neck, and spine before arranging ophthalmic review.

The following guide to referral urgency is not prescriptive, as clinical situations vary.

Immediate

■ Pre- or postseptal orbital cellulitis   p. 85

■ Necrotizing fasciitis suggested by violaceous
   skin discoloration or frank necrosis   p. 30

■ Trauma   p. 101

Urgent (within 1 week)

■ Proptosis with visual dysfunction   p. 73

■ Proptosis with corneal exposure keratopathy
   (commence G. hypromellose 0.3% 2 hourly)   p. 73

■ Orbital inflammation (exclude cellulitis)   p. 87

■ Structural and congenital lesions where there
   is suspicion of globe displacement, reduced
   vision, or incipient amblyopia, e.g. paediatric
   orbital capillary haemangioma   p. 77–80, 92

Routine

■ Chronic proptosis (months to years) without
   visual dysfunction   p. 73

■ Structural and congenital lesions with
   documented normal acuity   p. 77–80, 92

References

1. Mourits MP, et al. Clinical activity scores as a guide in the management of patients with Graves' ophthalmopathy. Clin Endocrinol (Oxf) 1997; 47(1):9–14.
2. Werner SC. Modification of the classification of the eye changes of Graves' disease: recommendations of the Ad Hoc Committee of the American Thyroid Association. J Clin Endocrinol Metab 1977; 44(1):203–204

Chapter 4

EXTERNAL EYE DISEASE

Conjunctival Anatomy

- The conjunctival epithelium includes goblet cells that produce the mucous layer of the tear film.

- The conjunctival stroma comprises a superficial adenoid layer and a deep fibrous layer. The former contains lymphoid tissue that results in follicle formation with appropriate stimuli (it is undeveloped in infants who cannot develop a follicular response). The tarsal conjunctiva is firmly anchored to the tarsus, resulting in papillae when there is conjunctival infiltration, whereas the bulbar conjunctiva is only loosely attached to the globe and papillae are not seen except at the limbus.

- Lymphatics drain to the submandibular and preauricular lymph nodes.

- The accessory lacrimal glands of Wolfring and Krause are located in the conjunctival stroma at the superior margin of the upper tarsus and the superior fornix, respectively.

- The meibomian glands open posterior to the grey line.

- The conjunctiva has comparatively few pain fibres from the trigeminal nerve (ophthalmic division), so pain is poorly localized.

History and Examination

History Key symptoms include redness, surface irritation, itch, discharge, watering, conjunctival swelling, and mildly blurred vision if the tear film is disturbed. More severe visual loss may indicate corneal or other disease.

Examination Systematically examine the lid margin and position, lashes, meibomian gland orifices, punctae, fornices, tarsal plates, tear film, limbus, cornea, and conjunctiva. Note and ideally draw the following:

- Conjunctival injection (hyperaemia): may be diffuse or localized.

- Subconjunctival haemorrhage: may be fine punctate haemorrhages, larger blotches, or a solid sheet.

- Discharge: note if serous or watery (viral, toxic aetiology), mucopurulent (bacterial conjunctivitis), or stringy (allergic).

- Chemosis: oedematous conjunctiva appears milky and may swell beyond the lid margins.

- Follicles: focal lymphoid hyperplasia over the tarsus produces rounded, avascular, whitish-grey centres with small vessels encircling the base (Fig. 4.1). Differentiate from papillae.

- Papillae: inflammatory exudates accumulate in the fibrous layer, heaping the conjunctiva into mounds. There is a central tuft of vessels (Fig. 4.2). When small, papillae produce a

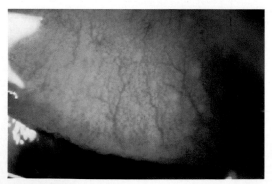

Fig. 4.1: Follicles.

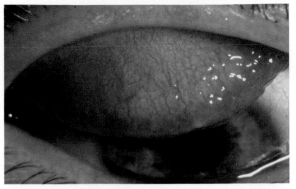

Fig. 4.2: Papillae (Courtesy of DH Verity).

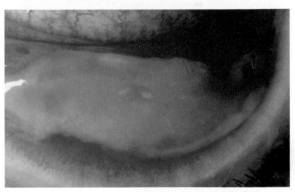

Fig. 4.3: Pseudomembrane (Courtesy of DH Verity).

smooth velvety appearance. 'Giant papillae' have a cobblestone appearance. At the limbus, giant papillae appear as gelatinous mounds, usually in the palpebral aperture.

- Pigment: assess the extent and whether this is associated with increased conjunctival thickness.

- Pseudomembrane: coagulated exudate that adheres to the tarsal or forniceal conjunctiva. It is easily peeled off and the bed underneath does not bleed, unlike a true membrane. In practice, these may be indistinguishable (Fig. 4.3).

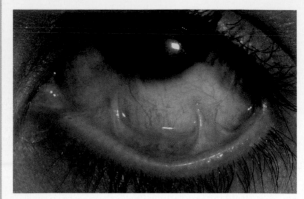

Fig. 4.4: Symblephara (Courtesy of DH Verity).

- Symblepharon: identify the position (medial, lateral, or superior fornices) and extent (Fig. 4.4).

- Punctal orifice: note as normal, occluded, absent, stenosed, or if there is a plug in situ.

Anterior Blepharitis

Background Includes two main types that may coexist: seborrhoeic and staphylococcal. Commonly complicated by meibomian gland dysfunction. See also posterior blepharitis (p. 114) and ocular rosacea (p. 116).

History Ask about ocular irritation, burning sensation, and lid margin erythema.

Examination

- Staphylococcal: dry, scaly lash debris, lid margin erythema, and pinpoint lid margin ulceration.
- Seborrhoeic: greasy lash debris (Fig. 4.5) and seborrhoea of the scalp, brows, and ears.

Treatment Advise *lid hygiene*: clean away the lash debris once or twice daily with a cotton-tipped bud dipped in boiled or sterile water (e.g. contact lens solution) or use proprietary lid cleaning pads made for the purpose. For staphylococcal disease prescribe Oc. chloramphenicol or Oc. fucithalmic b.d. to the lid margins for 3 weeks.

Follow-up One month if there is corneal involvement; otherwise, not routinely required.

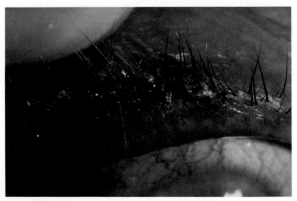

Fig. 4.5: Anterior blepharitis.

Posterior Blepharitis

Background A spectrum of disease from meibomian seborrhoea, through meibomianitis and meibomian conjunctivitis, to meibomian keratoconjunctivitis (ocular rosacea; next section). Bacterial enzymes (*S. epidermidis*, *S. aureus*, *Propionibacterium acnes*) produce excessive free fatty acids and abnormal tear lipids that cause inflammation and irritation. Altered meibomian gland secretions contribute to meibomianitis. See also anterior blepharitis (p. 113) and ocular rosacea (p. 116).

History Chronic, non-specific symptoms include crusting of lashes (80%), ocular redness (80%), foreign body sensation (65%), chalazia (60%), blurred vision (45%), tearing (40%), and burning sensation (40%). The symptoms of meibomian seborrhoea are worse than the signs.

Examination

- Lids: meibomian seborrhoea has excessive meibomian secretions with little inflammation. With meibomianitis there are dilated, prominent meibomian gland orifices (100%), meibomian gland plugs (100%) and pouting meibomian gland orifices (35%) (Fig. 4.6). With time, partial lash loss (60%), lid notching (45%), and telangiectasia develop.

- Conjunctiva: diffuse injection (100%), papillary hypertrophy (100%), rose bengal uptake (100%), tear film debris (55%), reduced tear break up time (100%), and foamy tear film (60%).

- Cornea: in meibomian keratoconjunctivitis there is superficial punctate keratopathy (SPK) of the lower cornea (100%).

- Skin: look for seborrhoeic dermatitis, acne rosacea, or seborrhoeic sicca.

Treatment Emphasize that this is a chronic condition with no known cure and that indefinite treatment is often required. Advise lid hygiene:

1. Fill a wash basin with hot water. Soak a facecloth until comfortably hot, make into a ball and press firmly over the closed eye. Re-warm the face cloth as it cools. Continue for 5 minutes. Then;

2. Express stagnant meibomian gland secretions by massaging from top to bottom along the length of the upper lid (massage up in the lower eyelid). Then;

3. Clean debris out of lashes. See anterior blepharitis (p. 113).

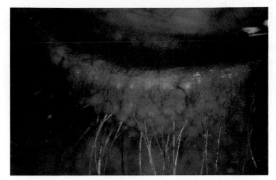

Fig. 4.6: Posterior blepharitis.

A course of antibiotic ointment (e.g. chloramphenicol or fucithalmic b.d. to the lid margins for 3 weeks) may help. For corneal involvement prescribe doxycycline 100 mg o.d. p.o. for 8 weeks to thin meibomian gland secretions and reduce excessive free fatty acids (contraindications include age <8 years and pregnancy). Alternatively, use erythromycin 250 mg q.d.s. p.o. for 8 weeks. Warn about the risk of sunburn when on tetracyclines. Consider short-term topical corticosteroids, e.g. prednisolone 0.5% b.d. 2 weeks in severe cases. Treat any dry eye and skin disease.

Follow-up For moderate to severe disease review routinely in clinic. Expect improvement in 2–3 months, then reduce lid hygiene to the minimum required to prevent symptoms.

Ocular Rosacea

Background A form of severe blepharo-keratoconjunctivitis more commonly seen in light-skinned people. See also anterior and posterior blepharitis (pp. 113 and 114).

History Similar to posterior blepharitis. May have facial flushing with alcohol or spicy food.

Examination The skin shows erythema, telangiectasia and pustules over the cheeks, nose, and forehead with thickening of the skin over the nose (rhinophyma) in the later stages (Fig. 4.7). The eye is involved in 60% of cases:

- Lids: posterior blepharitis, chalazia.

- Conjunctiva: variable diffuse injection ± small grey nodules on the bulbar conjunctiva near the limbus. These may ulcerate.

- Cornea: involved in 5% with superficial punctate keratitis and peripheral ulceration that may progress to perforation, ± superficial and deep neovascularization, ± lipid keratopathy.

Treatment Eliminate spicy food and alcohol that exacerbate acne rosacea. Treat as for severe meibomian keratoconjunctivitis (p. 114).

Follow-up Depends upon the severity and response to treatment. Review corneal vascularization fortnightly until quiescent.

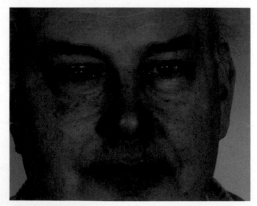

Fig. 4.7: Rosacea.

Bacterial Conjunctivitis

Background Bacterial conjunctivitis is most commonly caused by Staphylococcal and Streptococcccal spp, or *H. influenzae*. Rare pathogens include *Neisseria* spp. and *Chlamydia*. For conjunctivitis of the newborn see page 572.

Symptoms Discharge with eyelids stuck together in the mornings, red eye, and ocular irritation. Usually starts in one eye then spreads to the other. Presentation may suggest the causative organism:

- Hyperacute (<12 hrs): *N. gonorrhoeae*, *N. kockii*, *N. meningitides* (rare).

- Acute: *S. pneumoniae*, *H. aegyptius*, Staphyloccal spp.

- Subacute: *H. influenzae* (thin watery discharge), *E. coli*, *Proteus* spp.

- Chronic: *Chlamydia*.

Signs The lids may be mildly oedematous with tear film debris (Fig. 4.8). There is conjunctival injection ± papillae, or rarely a pseudomembrane or true membrane. Exclude corneal epithelial defects or ulceration. Lymphadenopathy is usually absent except with *Chlamydia* or gonococcus. Gonococcus can produce a secondary iritis.

Differential diagnosis Consider viral conjunctivitis (systemic viral features, less discharge, follicles), allergic conjunctivitis (atopy, itch, papillae), blocked nasolacrimal duct (look for reflux with pressure on a mucocele), blepharitis, and acute ocular cicatricial pemphigoid.

Investigations Consider sending conjunctival swabs for culture and sensitivity. For hyperacute, severe, purulent discharge or (pseudo-) membranes send urgent conjunctival scrapings for Gram stain. Inoculate onto blood agar and chocolate agar.

Treatment Advise patients to clean away discharge, wash hands, and avoid spreading infection to family and colleagues via towels or direct contact. Topical antibiotics, e.g. G. chloramphenicol q.d.s., may speed resolution. Avoid prolonged or repeated treatment that may cause drop allergy. G. prednisolone 0.5% q.d.s. may reduce the scarring often seen following pseudomembranous conjunctivitis but generally avoid steroid use. If microscopy shows Gram-negative intracellular diplococci treat for *Neisseria* with hourly G. chloramphenicol and i.v. cefotaxime 500 mg q.d.s. once, but check latest protocols with a sexually

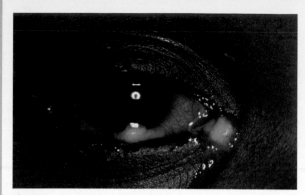

Fig. 4.8: Bacterial conjunctivitis.

transmitted disease service. Regularly irrigate the fornices with saline and refer to a sexual health clinic for contact tracing. Delay may lead to perforated cornea, endophthalmitis, septicaemia, or meningitis.

Follow-up Most cases are seen once and discharged. For hyperacute, severe, purulent discharge or (pseudo-) membranes examine daily until improving then every 2–3 days until resolved.

Adenoviral Keratoconjunctivitis

Background The most common acute viral infection of the external eye. Virus may spread systemically and shed via tears, resulting in secondary ocular infection. External spread may occur by aerosol or direct contact, e.g. hands and clinical instruments. Numerous viral serotypes can cause the disease.

History Incubation period is ≈8 days with three typical presentations:

- *Acute non-specific follicular conjunctivitis*: produces a red eye initially with mild irritation and tearing, but little photophobia. Lid swelling occurs after 48 hours. Usually bilateral, separated by 1–3 days. Usually resolves rapidly.

- *Pharyngoconjunctival fever (PCF)*: a follicular conjunctivitis with systemic viral features.

- *Epidemic keratoconjunctivitis (EKC)*: commonest in autumn and winter. Produces acute red eye, tearing, and irritation. There may be minimal systemic symptoms in adults but children may get fever, sore throat, and ear ache. Bilateral in ≈40% with onset usually separated by 4–5 days.

Ask about contact with conjunctivitis, and systemic viral features such as myalgia, sore throat, cough, fever, and gastrointestinal disturbance.

Examination

- Tender preauricular lymphadenopathy.

- Lids: mild to moderate swelling.

- Conjunctiva: there is typically diffuse injection with variable chemosis and serous discharge, ± ecchymoses, ± petechial haemorrhages. Look for follicles (p. 110, Fig. 4.1) on the lower tarsal conjunctiva and papillary hyperplasia of upper tarsal conjunctiva. Pseudomembranes with mucopurulent discharge may occur, or rarely, true membranes.

- Cornea: variable involvement (30% in PCF, ≈80% in EKC). In the first week there may be fine pin-point epithelial erosions on retroillumination that do not stain with fluorescein or rose bengal and often resolve. In the second week there may be focal or diffuse, fine or coarse punctate keratitis that stains with fluorescein and rose bengal. There may be pseudodendrites, fine epithelial or anterior stromal oedema, or filamentary keratitis. At 12–17 days there may be subepithelial

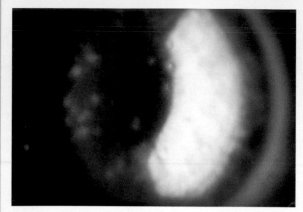

Fig. 4.9: Adenoviral keratoconjunctivitis with subepithelial infiltrates.

punctate keratitis. Subepithelial infiltrates (Fig. 4.9) may occur in the visual axis, causing blurred vision and glare.

■ Anterior chamber: may have a mild cellular reaction in the second week.

Wash hands and clean the slit-lamp after use. Do not routinely check IOP because of the risk of cross-infection.

Differential diagnosis Bacterial conjunctivitis (more discharge, fewer follicles, and no systemic viral features), acute haemorrhagic conjunctivitis caused by enterovirus 70, coxsackie A24, or *Streptococcus pneumoniae* (usually resolves within 2–4 days), and allergic conjunctivitis (more likely to have itch, atopy, and papillae). Papillae have a central vessel at their apex, whereas follicles have fine vessels around their base.

Investigations Swabs have a low yield but consider if the diagnosis is uncertain and onset within 12 days.

Treatment There is no effective antiviral. Suggest warm compresses and G. hypromellose 0.3% q.d.s. to relieve irritation. Explain that the disease is highly contagious for 2 weeks, so avoid work and close contact with family members (separate towels and face cloths), wash hands, and keep hands out of eyes. Use G. chloramphenicol q.d.s. if there is bacterial super infection and Oc. chloramphenicol q.d.s. for pseudomembranes. Corticosteroids are sometimes used for severe corneal involvement with symptomatic infiltrates in the visual axis or pseudomembranes (G. prednisolone 0.5% six times daily for 2 weeks, then taper over 10–12 weeks). Corticosteroids may increase the viral load if given in the first 2 weeks during active viral replication. After this period, steroids probably do not alter the basic pathogenesis, but merely suppress inflammation. Subepithelial infiltrates may reappear when steroids are tapered off. These usually resolve with a second course of steroids.

Follow-up Most cases spontaneously resolve within 8–10 weeks, often sooner. Review those with keratitis in clinic and beware emergence of a true dendritic ulcer and steroid-responsive IOP elevation. Permanent visual loss is very rare but corneal subepithelial infiltrates may rarely recur for several years.

Chlamydial Conjunctivitis

There are three species of chlamydiae: *C. trachomatis*, *C. psittaci*, and *C. pneumoniae*. Almost all ocular disease is caused by *C. trachomatis* with three distinct ocular syndromes: adult inclusion conjunctivitis (AIC), neonatal inclusion conjunctivitis (p. 572), and trachoma.

Adult inclusion conjunctivitis

Background Adult inclusion conjunctivitis (AIC) is a sexually transmitted infection (STI) caused by immunotypes D–K, producing urethritis, proctitis, epididymitis, and prostatitis in men; cystitis, cervicitis, salpingitis, and pelvic inflammatory disease in women. Spread is usually through direct contact with infected genital secretions, but also by direct eye-to-eye contact or by poorly chlorinated swimming pools.

Symptoms Acute or subacute onset of redness, irritation, mucopurulent discharge 2–19 days after inoculation. Initially unilateral, then bilateral.

History Assess the risk of a sexually transmitted infection.

Examination Look for conjunctival injection with well-developed follicles. Unlike trachoma, the inferior fornix is more affected than the superior fornix. There may be fine to coarse superficial punctate keratitis and a limited number of irregular subepithelial limbal infiltrates after several weeks. Check for preauricular lymphadenopathy.

Investigation Apply topical anaesthetic then scrape the tarsal conjunctiva with a spatula and apply to a glass slide for fluorescent monoclonal antibody testing (≈95% sensitivity, ≈85% specificity). Use tissue culture (70–90% sensitivity, 100% specificity) if legal ramifications are likely. Take bacterial and viral conjunctival swabs. Polymerase chain reaction (PCR)-based tests are replacing culture and antibody-based tests in many laboratories; samples must be taken before fluorescein is applied.

Management Approximately 50% of adults with AIC have concurrent *C. trachomatis* genital tract infection and 25% of men with chlamydial urethritis are asymptomatic, so refer to genitourinary medicine clinic for investigation, treatment, and contact tracing. Topical antibiotics suppress the ocular manifestations of AIC but do not eradicate the genital reservoir, so systemic treatment is required. Once all ocular and genital swabs have been taken, treat with a single dose of azithromycin 1 g p.o.

and await symptomatic improvement over 2–4 weeks. Conjunctival follicles may last for months and corneal infiltrates persist for months to years. Significant conjunctival scarring is rare.

Trachoma

Background Caused by immunotypes A–C. Rare in the developed world but endemic to North Africa, the Middle East, India, and Southeast Asia. Usually self-limiting but repeated infection leads to conjunctival cicatrization and corneal scarring.

Clinical features Acute infection begins 5 days after inoculation as a bilateral follicular, nonpurulent conjunctivitis. After 2–3 weeks follicles appear on the superior tarsal conjunctiva and superior limbus. The diagnosis of trachoma requires at least two of the following:

- ≥ 5 follicles on the superior tarsal conjunctiva
- Limbal follicles or their sequelae (Herbert's pits, Fig. 4.10)
- Tarsal conjunctival scarring
- Vascular pannus.

There may be tender preauricular lymphadenopathy.

Management Infection provides no immunity, so endemic areas require control with community health education and mass treatment. Surgery may be required for lid deformities such as entropion and aberrant lashes, or severe corneal opacity.

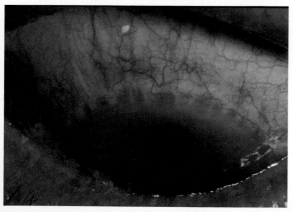

Fig. 4.10: Herbert's pits (Courtesy DH Verity).

Allergic Conjunctivitis

Allergic conjunctivitis includes acute allergic conjunctivitis, seasonal allergic conjunctivitis (SAC), perennial allergic conjunctivitis (PAC), vernal keratoconjunctivitis (VKC), atopic keratoconjunctivitis (AKC), drop hypersensitivity, and contact lens-associated papillary conjunctivitis (CLPC), of which giant papillary conjunctivitis (GPC) is the most severe and drop hypersensitivity.

Acute, seasonal, and perennial allergic conjunctivitis

Background Allergic conjunctivitis, often (70%) associated with atopy or a family history of atopy.

History Ask about major (hayfever, asthma, atopic dermatitis, eczema) and minor (idiopathic urticaria, nonhereditary angioedema, food allergies) atopies. Seasonal symptoms include ocular itch, tearing, often with allergic rhinitis (sneezing and nasal congestion). Acute reactions may occur, with marked conjunctival swelling as well as systemic reactions.

Examination Ocular inflammation is usually mild with lid erythema, conjunctival oedema, papillae, and increased tear film mucus. Acute allergic reactions may produce profound chemosis with pale, boggy conjunctiva ballooning over the eyelid margins.

Treatment Acute allergic swelling of the conjunctiva can be reduced with cool compresses and G. adrenaline 0.1% stat. For recurrent allergic conjunctivitis attempt to eliminate the allergens and advise cool compresses. During periods of antigen exposure, prescribe topical mast cell stabilizers (e.g. G. nedocromil b.d.), antihistamines (e.g. G. emedastine 0.05% b.d.), or a combined mast cell stabilizer and antihistamine (e.g. G. olapatidine 0.1% b.d.). Prescribe systemic antihistamines, e.g. loratidine (Clarityn) 10 mg o.d. p.o.

Follow-up Two weeks if necessary

Vernal keratoconjunctivitis (spring catarrh)

Background A rare but serious form of chronic allergic conjunctivitis. Most common in males, aged 5–15 years,

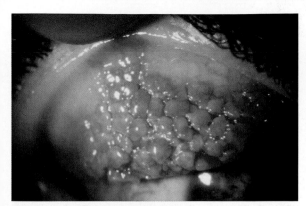

Fig. 4.11: Cobblestone papullae in severe vernal keratoconjunctivitis.

particularly Arabs and Afro-Caribbeans. Management can be challenging.

History There is frequently a family or personal history of atopy. Symptoms typically occur annually in spring or summer but may persist throughout the year. Itch is the main symptom but ropey discharge, photophobia, and pain occur.

Examination A mild mechanical ptosis may be present. Evert the lids and look for large pleomorphic, irregularly distributed cobblestone papillae (Fig. 4.11), more pronounced than in the lower tarsal conjunctiva. Follicles or scarring are rare. There may be Tranta's dots (chalk-white, raised, superficial infiltrates straddling the limbus) (Fig. 4.12). The conjunctiva may have a pinkish tinge and mild oedema. Mucous strands are thicker and more ropey than in SAC. Superficial punctate keratitis, epithelial macroerosions or 'shield' ulcers (Fig. 4.13), plaques or subepithelial scarring may occur.

Treatment Initial treatment includes cool compresses, lid hygiene for blepharitis, antigen avoidance, and artificial tears or saline for antigen dilution. For mild to moderate VKC consider: mast cell stabilizers (e.g. G. nedocromil sodium b.d. or lodoxamide b.d.); H_1 antihistamines, e.g. emedastine 0.05% b.d.; combined antihistamine/mast cell stabilizers, e.g. olopatadine 0.1% b.d. For more severe flare-ups use short-term G. fluorometholone 0.1% t.d.s., or dexamethasone 0.1%/prednisolone 1% titrated against the disease severity, with regular IOP assessment. Trials show that topical ciclosporin (various formulations) is very effective without

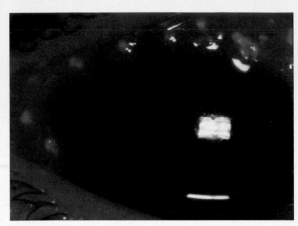

Fig. 4.12: Trantas dots (Courtesy of DH Verity).

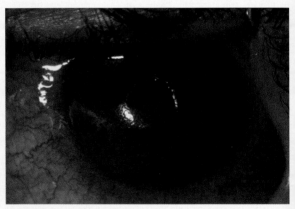

Fig. 4.13: Vernal shield ulcer (Courtesy of DH Verity).

the side effects of steroids, but tolerance is a problem with preparations dissolved in oils. Ciclosporin (and mast cell stabilizers) are poorly tolerated during disease exacerbations and can be introduced as soon as the disease has been partially controlled with steroids. Rarely, systemic therapy with steroids and sometimes ciclosporin is needed; aspirin may be helpful in older children. Shield ulcers (vernal plaques) may heal spontaneously once the conjunctival disease is controlled. If an associated epithelial defect persists, peel off the vernal plaque with a crescent blade and the control the disease to promote healing.

Follow-up Review every 1–2 weeks until inflammation is controlled, then 3 monthly. Corneal scars (from plaques), steroid-induced glaucoma, and cataracts are the causes of visual loss in VKC, which resolves after puberty in 90% of cases.

Atopic keratoconjunctivitis

Background Severe atopic conjunctivitis associated with keratitis.

History Ask about ocular itch, burning, foreign body sensation, tearing, and mucoid discharge.

Examination Look for eyelid dermatitis, chronic blepharitis, conjunctival oedema, papillae, and increased mucus in the tear film and inferior fornix. Cicatrizing conjunctivitis may develop with chronic inflammation, as may corneal scarring, vascularization, and visual loss.

Treatment Treat as for VKC. Care of periocular skin is also very important. Moisturize with E45 cream or aloe vera b.d. Use topical steroids (e.g. 1% hydrocortisone skin ointment o.d. b.d.), with care due to the risks of systemic absorption, depigmentation, and superinfection. Tacrolimus 0.03% ointment may be effective for severe atopic eyelid disease.

Follow-up Every 2 weeks until inflammation is controlled then 3 monthly, often long-term.

Contact lens-associated papillary conjunctivitis (including giant papillary conjunctivitis)

Background Most commonly seen in contact lens and prosthesis users where the papillae are often small. CLPC shares the conjunctival features of VKC and AKC but without corneal involvement. Giant papillary conjunctivitis (GPC) is the most severe form but is rarely seen since the widespread use of disposable and frequently replaced contact lenses (Fig. 4.14). GPC is more common in prosthesis users and as a result of broken or protruding sutures.

History Contact lens wearers may report decreasing lens tolerance and mucous discharge. Ocular itch may occur. Ask about contact lens wear and cleaning regimen (p. 207).

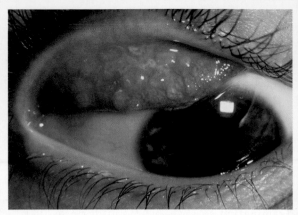

Fig. 4.14: Giant papillary conjunctivitis (Courtesy of DH Verity).

Examination Evert the eyelid and look for hyperaemia, infiltrate, and papillary response (best seen using 2% fluorescein drops). Giant papillae are those >1 mm. There may be epithelial erosion of the apices of the papillae and mucus trapped between the papillae. Examine contact lenses for damage.

Treatment Replace damaged lenses. If the patient must wear contact lenses, reduce the wearing time and optimize the lens cleaning regimen, including frequent (2–4 times weekly) protein removal. Daily disposable lenses, different lens material or edge design, and mast cell stabilizers may help. Remove broken sutures. Ocular prostheses can be repolished and coated. Treat any associated atopic conjunctivitis.

Follow up Review contact lens wearers in clinic only if symptoms persist. Ensure patients remain under regular review by their contact lens practitioner if they are not under medical review.

Drop toxicity (contact hypersensitivity)

Background A relatively common condition, particularly with certain drops including neomycin and atropine; however, prolonged treatment with any preserved (especially benzalkonium chloride) drop may result in a type IV contact hypersensitivity.

History Ask about itch and periocular rash. List all topical medications.

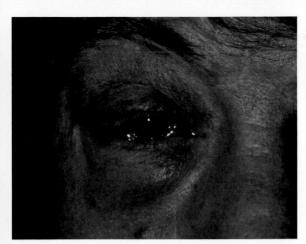

Fig. 4.15: Contact hypersensitivity secondary to eyedrops.

Examination Look for erythematous, dry, scaly dermatitis, particularly in the lower lid but often extending to the cheek (Fig. 4.15). There is diffuse conjunctival injection with follicles, especially in the lower fornix. The cornea is rarely involved.

Investigation Occasionally, patch testing is required.

Treatment Advise cool compresses, withdraw offending medication where possible, or replace with preservative-free drops. Rarely, dermal steroids (e.g. 0.5% hydrocortisone ointment b.d. for 5 days) are required.

Follow-up If the offending agent is withdrawn the dermatitis settles in a few days. Review any changes in long-term ocular medications as required.

Stevens-Johnson Syndrome (Erythema Multiforme)

Background A type III immune reaction most commonly affecting children, adolescents, and young adults. Circulating immune complexes trigger a skin reaction 7–14 days after stimulation. Although self-limiting, there is significant mortality and morbidity.

History Ask about fever, malaise headache, loss of appetite, nausea, vomiting, and skin rash. Try to identify the precipitating agent:

- Drugs: sulfonamides (dorzolamide, acetozolamide), sulfonylureas (chlorpropamide), antiepileptics (barbiturates, phenytoin, carbamazepine), chlorpromazine, thiazide diuretics, allopurinol, salicylates, codeine, antibiotics (tetracycline, penicillin, chloramphenicol).

- Infection: viral (herpes simplex, mumps, vaccinia), bacterial (streptococci, tuberculosis, yersinia, orf), and fungal (histoplasmosis).

- Connective tissue disease: rare.

- Malignancy: rare.

- Idiopathic: 50% of cases.

Examination Symmetrically distributed target lesions (papules with central pallor/erythematous surround or central erythema/pale surround) spread proximally along the limbs, with bullae on the back of hands, palms, forearms, feet and soles, or dependent parts in prostrated patients (Fig. 4.16). Nasal and oral mucosa is most commonly affected by ruptured bullae and haemorrhagic crusting (Fig. 4.17). The vagina and anus may be affected. Look for bilateral conjunctivitis ± bullae. There may be superficial punctate keratopathy, mild anterior uveitis, and occasionally panophthalmitis.

Treatment Remove known precipitating factors. Supportive treatment by physicians includes fluid management, systemic antibiotics, and skin care. Ophthalmic care includes G. atropine 1% o.d. and G. chloramphenicol q.d.s.; the value of topical steroids in the acute phase is uncertain and may promote infection. The use of oral prednisolone (80–100 mg o.d.) is controversial. Immunosuppression is contraindicated. Treat tear deficiency with tear substitutes, e.g. G. hypromellose 0.3%

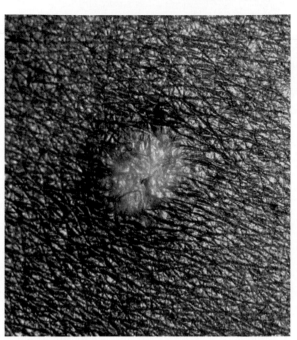

Fig. 4.16: Target lesion in Stevens-Johnson syndrome (Courtesy DH Verity).

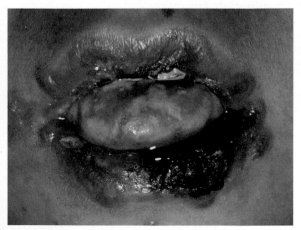

Fig. 4.17: Stevens-Johnson syndrome (Courtesy of DH Verity).

preservative free, 1–2 hourly, punctal occlusion, and moisture chambers as required.

Follow-up Review daily as an inpatient. Treat symblepharon formation (maintain the fornices by removing inflammatory debris and separating symblephara with glass rods and forceps). Exclude IOP rise and corneal ulceration. Taper any topical steroids and antibiotics after eye lesions have settled. Review weekly for 1 month, then as required. May fully resolve but possible sequelae include keratinized lid margins, dry eyes, eyelid deformities, conjunctival and corneal scarring. Late recurrences are probably infrequent but include recurrent conjunctival inflammation, late cicatrizing conjunctivitis, and late sclerokeratitis, all of which can exacerbate surface failure.

Ocular Mucous Membrane Pemphigoid

Background Ocular mucous membrane pemphigoid (OcMMP) is a type II hypersensitivity disease with antibodies to basement membrane and subsequent conjunctival scarring. There is a female preponderance with typical onset age 60–70 years. Previously termed ocular cicatricial pemphigoid.

History A chronic red eye is often misdiagnosed as infectious conjunctivitis. Ask about topical medications associated with OcMMP including pilocarpine, epinephrine, timolol, ecothiaphate iodine, and antivirals. There may be mucosal lesions of the nose, mouth, pharynx, trachea, oesophagus, anus, urethra, and vagina. If dysphasia and dyspnoea are present refer to an ENT specialist for endoscopic examination.

Examination

◾ Stage 1: chronic conjunctivitis with mild conjunctival and corneal epitheliopathy. Look for subtle subepithelial conjunctival fibrosis with a meshwork of fine white striae over the tarsus. The earliest sign is often a loss of the plica semilunaris as a result of subtle scarring.

◾ Stage 2: shortening of the fornices with abnormal surface wetting. Corneal keratinization may occur.

◾ Stage 3: Symblephara (Fig. 4.4, p. 112). Cicatrization deforms the lash follicles, lacrimal and meibomian gland ductules, with resultant aqueous and oil deficiencies, and also results in trichiasis due to cicatricial entropion. Mucin deficiency may exacerbate dry eye.

◾ Stage 4: ankyloblepharon, corneal keratinization, and totally dry eye.

Investigations Biopsy conjunctival and buccal mucosa for direct immunofluorescence. If skin lesions are present arrange a dermatology consultation and perilesional skin biopsy. Use specialist histology services, e.g. St John's Dermatology Unit, St Thomas' Hospital, London SE1 7EH; Tel: 020 7188 7188. False negatives are common in ocular disease (only 60–80% are positive) although not in buccal or skin disease. A positive biopsy or indirect immunofluorescence is not mandatory before treatment of typical disease.

Treatment This requires specialized knowledge. For mild to moderate disease use dapsone at an initial dose of 25 mg b.d., increasing up to 150 mg per day as required. Contraindications include sulfa allergy and glucose-6-phosphate dehydrogenase deficiency; anaemia is common. Sulfasalazine, an alternative sulfonamide, may be better tolerated at 1–2 g orally daily. If the response is incomplete, add methotrexate 7.5–15 mg p.o. weekly, azathioprine 2–3 mg/kg p.o. o.d., or mycophenolate 1 g b.d. If there is no response to a sulfonamide then discontinue this and use methotrexate, azathioprine, or mycophenolate alone. For severe disease or moderate disease unresponsive to these drugs use prednisolone 1 mg/kg/day p.o. with cyclophosphamide 1–2 mg/kg/day and taper off steroids once the inflammation is controlled; usually in 2–4 months. All these drugs require mandatory screening for side effects. Ciclosporin is not effective.

Local treatment is important. Remove any lashes abrading the cornea. Remove small numbers of lashes with electrolysis: for larger areas use a lid split and cryotherapy but beware reactivation of inflammation. Treat tear film deficiencies with punctal occlusion and preservative-free tear substitutes. Optimize meibomian gland function with warm compresses and lid massage. Bandage contact lenses may be used with caution. Keratinized tarsal conjunctiva may respond to topical retinoids. Oculoplastic surgery may be necessary to treat any lagophthalmos or reconstruct the fornices. Conjunctival or corneal surgery can trigger reactivation and patients should be effectively immunosupressed beforehand. Epithelial defects may fail to heal after surgery. Keratoprostheses are sometimes required.

Follow-up About 20% of patients have mild disease and can be reviewed annually to assess progression or more frequently if ongoing local therapy is require for surface disease. Patients on systemic drugs require blood tests to screen for toxicity, initially weekly. These can often be undertaken via the general practitioner, with 2–3 monthly ophthalmology review of treatment effect.

Subconjunctival Haemorrhage

History Most cases are idiopathic but ask about hypertension, Valsalva (coughing/constipation/heavy lifting), bleeding diathasis, anticoagulants, and trauma.

Examination Fresh haemorrhage appears as a bright red area, often over a large area (Fig. 4.18). Haemorrhage without a posterior margin may be associated with an intracranial bleed. Check BP and IOP.

Investigations Request coagulation screen and FBC only if recurrent.

Treatment None required. Reassure patients that the haemorrhage will fade over 2 weeks.

Follow-up Discharge with referral to a haematologist if a bleeding diathasis is detected, or general practitioner if hypertensive. Otherwise, no follow-up is required.

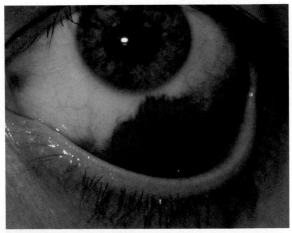

Fig. 4.18: Subconjunctival haemorrhage (Courtesy of Y Ramkissoon, K Mireskandari).

Superior Limbic Keratoconjunctivitis

Background A rare inflammatory conjunctivitis that tends to affect middle-aged women.

History Patients typically describe remissions and exacerbations of burning, foreign body sensation, mild photophobia, mucoid discharge, and tearing. Ask about contact lens wear, ocular surgery, and symptoms of thyroid dysfunction.

Examination Signs are usually bilateral but asymmetrical, and less severe than symptoms. Look for papillae (evert lids), conjunctival hyperaemia and thickening, most intense at the superior limbus, and fading towards the fornix, ± conjunctival keratinization. There is superior, superficial punctate keratitis (best seen with rose bengal) (Fig. 4.19) and micropannus, with filamentary keratopathy in 33% of cases. Tear deficiency may be present.

Investigations Thyroid function tests (50% have associated thyroid dysfunction).

Treatment Treat any thyroid dysfunction. G. acetyl cysteine 5% q.d.s. reduces filaments. Offer tear substitutes as required. Bandage contact lenses may help. In severe cases consider surgical resection of the superior limbal conjunctiva. Courses of topical corticosteroids can be useful for treatment of severe disease. The disease often remits after 2–4 years

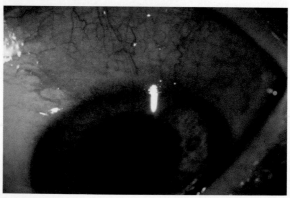

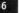

Fig. 4.19: Superior limbic keratoconjunctivitis.

Miscellaneous Conditions of the Conjunctiva

Pingueculum A yellowish raised area of bulbar conjunctiva in the palpebral aperture along the horizontal meridian (Fig. 4.20). May gradually thicken or become inflamed but often asymptomatic, and only noticed when the background conjunctiva becomes red, e.g. conjunctivitis. No treatment is usually required but if the area becomes inflamed consider topical lubricants or weak topical steroid, e.g. G. fluoromethalone (FML) t.d.s. reducing over 3 weeks. Excision biopsy is occasionally needed for symptomatic relief.

Oncocytoma (oxyphilic adenoma) Rare, 2–5 mm cystic yellow-tan caruncular mass presenting in older patients. Usually asymptomatic. May occur in the lacrimal gland, conjunctiva, and extraocular sites. No treatment is required for caruncular lesions but they can be excised if cosmetically embarrassing. Extracarunclar lesions may become malignant.

Kawasaki disease A rare condition occurring most commonly in girls aged 2 months to 9 years. Carries a 1–2% mortality rate. Produces conjunctivitis that does not require treatment, but this may be the presenting feature of the disease and hence requires urgent paediatric referral for management of extraocular features. These include cervical lymphadenopathy, dry

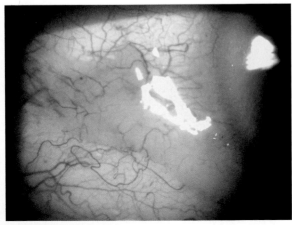

Fig. 4.20: Pingueculum.

lips, 'strawberry' tongue, arthralgia, arthritis, palmar erythema, and desquamation of fingertip skin.

Oculoglandular syndrome Also called cat-scratch fever and Parinaud's conjunctivits. Caused by a reaction to a cat scratch or more rarely pathogens such as *M. tuberculosis*, *T. pallidum*, and *C. trachomatis*. Produces grossly visible preauricular lymphadenopathy, low-grade fever, and unilateral conjunctival granulomata with focal necrosis ± ulceration. Consider cat-scratch disease skin test ± conjunctival biopsy. Resolves spontaneously over 2–3 months. Excision of solitary granulomata may be curative. A course of oral tetracyclines speeds resolution of cat-scratch disease.

Chemical Injury

Background Compounds include alkalis, acids, solvents, and detergents. Alkalis penetrate ocular tissue and are the most harmful, e.g. ammonia, lye in drain cleaner, caustic potash, $Mg(OH)_2$ from 'sparklers', lime in wet plaster, cement, and mortar. Acids usually produce more superficial damage but concentrated acids may produce effects that are indistinguishable from alkali injury.

Treat as an emergency, even before vision testing.

Immediate treatment Measure the pH of both eyes (normal: 7.3–7.6). Instil topical anaesthetic and eyelid speculum and irrigate the eye(s) copiously with saline or Ringer's lactate solution delivered via i.v. tubing for at least 30 minutes. Avoid acidic solutions to neutralize alkalis or vice versa. Pull down the lower lid and double-evert the upper lid to irrigate the fornices and remove any particulate matter. This may rarely require a general anaesthetic. Five minutes after ceasing irrigation, retest the pH. Continue irrigating until neutral. Persistently elevated pH suggests retained material.

History Document the chemical, time, nature of exposure, and any first aid measures. If available, examine the chemical container labels and test its pH. Contact a poisons centre for more information if required (p. 710).

Examination Record VA, facial injuries, and IOP. Apply fluorescein and systematically note:

- Lids: may be burned or oedematous.

- Conjunctiva: extent of epithelial loss, chemosis, and haemorrhage. Grade any limbal ischaemia:

  I = little or none.

  II = < 50% of the limbus (Fig. 4.21).

  III = 50–100% limbal ischaemia, but proximal conjunctiva preserved.

  IV = 50–100% limbal ischaemia and loss of proximal conjunctiva. Severe ischaemia may produce a deceptively white eye.

- Cornea: clarity, size and depth of any defects. Total epithelial defects may be easy to miss. Bowman's layer is slow to take up fluorescein compared with the stroma and basement membrane.

- Anterior chamber: depth and activity.

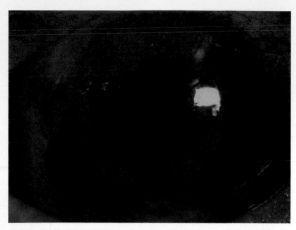

Fig. 4.21: Grade II limbal ischaemia with associated corneal damage (Courtesy of DH Verity).

- Lens: clarity.

- Retina: retinopathy may result from penetration of alkali through the sclera.

Subsequent treatment The majority of injuries are mild; if there is no limbal ischaemia or epithelial defect, give G. chloramphenicol q.d.s. for 1 week but review moderate to severe cases in 1–2 days as ischaemia may not be apparent immediately. If there is any ischaemia treat as follows:

1. *Acute phase (day 0–7)* Debride clearly necrotic corneal and conjunctival epithelium which may stimulate inflammation and contain residual chemicals. Use preservative-free eyedrops if available. Prevent melting with G. sodium ascorbate 10% 2 hourly and vitamin C 1 g p.o. q.d.s. For grade II–IV injuries add G. sodium citrate 10% 1 hourly and sodium citrate 2 g q.d.s. p.o. Control anterior uveitis with topical steroid, e.g. dexamethasone 0.1% 4–6 times daily; otherwise, avoid steroid use in the acute phase. Prescribe G. chloramphenicol q.d.s., cycloplegia, and analgesics. If IOP is raised or not measurable, add acetazolamide 250 mg q.d.s. p.o., and topical medication if further IOP reduction is required. Lyse conjunctival adhesions with a glass rod. A scleral shell may be required to prevent symblephara. Admit all grade II–IV injuries or see daily as outpatients.

2. *Early repair phase (day 7–21)* Monitor re-epithelialization. Epithelial defects should be closed in grade I and healing in

grade II. Grade III and IV epithelial defects persist. The degree of ischaemia may initially be under- or overestimated so reassess. Continue ascorbate and citrate until the epithelium has healed. Taper off corticosteroids to promote repair, replacing with progestational steroids (e.g. medroxyprogesterone 1% from i.v. preparation 4–6 times daily) or NSAIDs (e.g. G. diclofenac 0.1% t.d.s). Once the epithelium has closed, topical corticosteroid may be restarted if necessary. Doxycyclin 100 mg o.d. p.o. may be useful for its anticollaginase activity.

3. *Late repair phase (from day 21)* Grade II injuries may heal with conjunctival epithelium in the ischaemic sector. Grade III injuries may also re-epithelialize from the conjunctiva with associated superficial and deep stromal vascularization, persistence of goblet cells in the epithelium, and poor epithelial basement membrane adhesion. Grade IV injuries fail to re-epithelialize and require surgical intervention. In more severe chemical injuries corneal inflammation, collagen synthesis, and collagenase activity peak at this time. Continue treatment to minimize inflammation and collagenase activity. Correct any tear deficiency.

Surgical interventions An amniotic membrane patch sutured over the entire ocular surface, and secured to the skin and fornices, may aid healing in severe disease unresponsive to conservative measures in 10–14 days. Tissue glue is useful for impending or small (<1 mm) perforations (p. 156). Tectonic keratoplasty may be required for larger perforations. The success of future surgical interventions, e.g. penetrating keratoplasty, is dependent upon an adequate tear film and the population of limbal stem cells. These may be harvested from the contralateral eye in uniocular injuries, or as an allograft. Keratoprosthesis may be required for severe bilateral chemical injuries.

Optometry and General Practice Guidelines

General comments

The commonest external eye disease seen in primary care is conjunctivitis. The symptoms, pattern of redness, and type of discharge usually suggests the diagnosis. Diffuse conjunctival injection is typical, whereas perilimbal injection, intraocular pain, and photophobia suggest uveitis or corneal disease. Ask about contact with conjunctivitis. Purulent discharge and surface irritation is typical of bacterial infection. A watery discharge and systemic viral features suggests viral conjunctivitis. A personal or family history of atopy and ocular itch suggest allergic conjunctivitis. There is no specific treatment for adenoviral conjunctivitis but it spontaneously resolves in 2–3 weeks. Provide appropriate advice about cross-infection and offer topical hypromellose q.d.s. p.r.n. It is commonplace to prescribe antibiotics (e.g. G. chloramphenicol q.d.s.) for presumed bacterial conjunctivitis although it will often resolve without treatment. Avoid protracted (>7 days) antibiotics that commonly cause drop hypersensitivity (look for periocular skin redness, papillae, and itch.). Treat allergic conjunctivitis by mast cell stabilizers, e.g. G. nedocromil sodium b.d. for 1 month, and consider antigen avoidance (avoid house pets if possible and maintain a hypoallergenic bedroom and domestic environment as for asthma protocols). Most cases of conjunctivitis can be treated in primary care. Swabs are not necessary for typical cases but send viral, bacterial, and chlamydial swabs if there is no improvement in 5 days. Refer if there is no improvements in 2 weeks or if the vision changes at any time. The commonest findings on referral are adenoviral conjunctivitis, blepharitis, drop hypersensitivity, and dry eye.

General practice

Do not prescribe steroid eyedrops without specialist review. A single episode of subconjunctival haemorrhage does not routinely require investigation or referral but ask about bleeding/bruising/anticoagulants and check BP. Refer unexplained, recurrent subconjunctival haemorrhage.

Optometrists

For blepharitis, recommend lid hygiene b.d. (p. 113) for 1 month and refer if symptoms persist.

The following guide to referral urgency is not prescriptive, as clinical situations vary.

Immediate

- Chemical injury: instil anaesthetic eyedrops (if available) then rinse immediately with clean neutral liquid, e.g. sterile saline. Following copious irrigation transfer all serious injuries to an eye unit by ambulance.   p. 139

- Suspected gonococcal conjunctivitis   p. 117

Same day

- Suspected chlamydial conjunctivitis   p. 122

- Stevens-Johnson syndrome (systemic features may require more urgent referral to physicians)   p. 130

Urgent (within 1 week)

- Nonresolving conjunctivitis   p. 117

- Viral conjunctivitis with corneal involvement (keratoconjunctivitis)   p. 119

- Vernal keratoconjunctivitis   p. 124

- Ocular mucous membrane pemphigoid   p. 133

Soon (within 1 month)

- Pyogenic granuloma   p. 35

- Inflamed pingueculum   p. 137

Routine

- Blepharitis   p. 113

- Uninflamed pingueculum causing ocular discomfort   p. 137

- Superior limbic keratoconjunctivitis   p. 136

- Recurrent subconjunctival haemorrhage   p. 135

Chapter 5

CORNEA

Anatomy

The normal cornea

- The air–tear interface is the most powerful refracting interface of the eye.

- The cornea is aspheric, with the central cornea steeper than the periphery, i.e. prolate.

- The refractive power of the optical zone (central 4 mm) is ≈43 D.

- The average adult transverse corneal diameter is 11–12 mm, and 9–11 mm vertically.

- Corneal clarity depends upon an ordered lamellar collagen structure and relative dehydration, requiring a minimum endothelial cell density of ≈1000 cells/mm^2. The mean endothelial cell density falls by ≈0.6% per year.

- The central corneal thickness remains constant between the second and sixth decades but varies with the time of day (thickest in the morning) and race (Afro-Caribbeans and Chinese ≈530 μm, Caucasians ≈550 μm at 60 years).

- Normal corneal innervation is essential for the maintenance of an intact epithelial surface.

- The stem cells that generate the epithelium are located at the junction between the cornea and the sclera, probably in the palisades of Vogt.

- The normal cornea is avascular.

History and Examination

History

Ask about the presenting complaint, past ocular and medical history, medications, allergies, family, and social history. Document the presence or absence of the following key symptoms and determine their severity, nature, duration, and any relieving or exacerbating factors.

- Reduced vision.

- Abnormal sensation: direct stimulation of the corneal nerves usually gives rise to severe, sharp pain. Inflammation produces a duller, aching pain. Photophobia is a spasmodic pain on exposure to light caused by ciliary spasm. Irritation or grittiness is a symptom of epithelial disturbance. Itch usually indicates allergy. A diseased anaesthetic cornea may be asymptomatic.

- Tearing: multiple causes including corneal epithelial breakdown and stromal inflammation (see also p. 55).

- Red eye: ask if friends or family are affected, suggesting infection.

- Discharge: ask if this is purulent, mucoid, or ropey. Ask if friends or family are affected. Discharge is most often secondary to ocular surface infection or allergy.

- Contact lens: ask about contact lens wear including the type, cleaning routine, pattern of wear (i.e. daily or overnight), and duration of use (see also p. 207).

Examination

Corneal structure and function are dependent upon the lids, tears, conjunctiva, and sclera. Examine as follows, documenting relevant positive and negative findings.

- General habitus, hands and face: for example, rheumatoid hand changes may help diagnose the cause of peripheral corneal thinning.

- Vision: record uncorrected, best corrected, and pinhole VA. High-contrast Snellen VA may be maintained despite reduced contrast sensitivity from corneal opacity or astigmatism.

■ Eyelids: note inflammation, abnormal contour, incomplete closure, misdirected lashes, and lid margin disease (blepharitis, meibomian gland plugging).

■ Tears: note the quality (discharge, debris) and quantity (meniscus height). Measure tear break-up time (p. 158) if the tears appear abnormal, and tear volume with Shirmer I test (p. 147).

■ Bulbar conjunctiva: note scarring (location, extent) and subconjunctival haemorrhage. If inflamed, note depth (conjunctival, episleral, scleral) and location (perilimbal, sectoral, diffuse, localized).

■ Tarsal conjunctiva: evert the upper and lower lids to look for keratinization, scarring, foreign bodies (FBs), and the presence of membranes, papillae, and follicles.

■ Corneal epithelium: note any defects (size, location, pattern, e.g. superficial punctate keratitis, dendritic, geographic), FBs, infiltrates (pattern, size, location, depth), oedema (extent and severity, e.g. bullae), deposits (location, pattern, material, e.g. iron, calcium, filaments).

■ Corneal stroma: record the size, location, depth, and pattern of opacities. Infiltrates tend to have feathery margins. Scars have defined edges on retroillumination and often result in corneal thinning. Areas of oedema have soft, diffuse edges on retroillumination and increased corneal thickness. Note the depth, number of clock hours, and distance of corneal new vessels from the limbus. Ghost vessels carry no blood and appear grey. Inactive vessels may have blood flowing through them but appear to have sharp edges on retroillumination. Active vessels have a cuff of oedema producing a less-defined edge.

■ Corneal endothelium and Descemet's membrane: Note thickening, guttata, folds or breaks in Descemet's membrane, and the extent and distribution of deposits (KPs, pigment, blood).

■ Drawings: draw any corneal abnormities using a frontal and slit view. Baseline photographs may help quantify changes seen at subsequent examinations.

Further clinical tests may be indicated based on the history and examination (see next page).

Investigations

Consider the following tests and investigations, as indicated by the history and examination.

Corneal sensation Corneal anaesthesia may be due to corneal disease or predispose to it. Warn the patient, and then lightly touch the peripheral cornea with a cotton-tipped bud. Compare sides. Be aware; testing can affect vital staining and spread infection between eyes. For quantitative assessment use a Cochet and Bonnet aesthesiometer.

Vital dyes

1. *Fluorescein 2%* Viewed with a cobalt blue light this fluorophore has multiple uses including:

   ■ *Tear film assessment* Can be used to assess tear volume (meniscus height), quality (tear break-up time, p. 158), and drainage (Jones tests and fluorescein disappearance test, p. 58).

   ■ *Corneal disease* Raised areas have a thinner layer of fluorescein over them and appear bluer. Thinned cornea with an intact epithelium 'pools' fluorescein, appearing green. Dead epithelial cells and exposed basement membrane stain green, e.g. corneal abrasion. Bowman's layer stains slowly.

   ■ *Aqueous leakage* (Seidel's test) Fluorescein 2% is applied to areas of suspected leakage. The usually dark-orange 2% fluorescein is diluted by leaking aqueous, turning bright green under a blue light.

2. *Rose Bengal 1%* should only be applied after topical anaesthetics. Warn patients that it may sting. Desiccated, devitalised conjunctival or corneal epithelial cells stain pink. Wash out afterwards with normal saline.

Schirmer I test Bend a Schirmer strip at the preformed notch by 90° and place into the conjunctival sac at the junction of the mid and temporal thirds of the lower lid, without using topical anaesthetic. Conduct the test in ambient lighting, with the patient blinking normally, eyes open and looking slightly up, and away from bright lights. Allow the paper to wet by capillary action. Aqueous tear deficiency is diagnosed if the strip wets by ≤5 mm over 5 minutes. From 5 to 10 mm is borderline. The Schirmer II test uses topical anaesthetic before testing and has been used as a measure of 'baseline' tear production which is probably unphysiological, as all tear production is reflex.

Pachymetry Measuring the central corneal thickness (CCT) is useful for monitoring corneal grafts, prior to refractive surgery, and for normalizing IOP measurements. For normal values, see page 144. There are several devices that measure CCT.

- *Orbscan®* has the advantages of being noncontact and producing a thickness map. Standard deviation (SD) of CCT is $\approx 10\,\mu m$ centrally (greater in the periphery). It may not be possible to capture data with some corneal curvatures, the posterior corneal surface must be visible, it is time consuming, and requires good patient cooperation.

- *Ultrasound* requires topical anaesthesia. Any area of the cornea can be measured. Record which area was measured. Touch the probe gently on to the cornea, perpendicular to the surface, to avoid overestimating corneal thickness. The SD of CCT is $\approx 3\,\mu m$, taking seven measurements and averaging the middle five. Alternatively, take the smallest value that is consistent with the others, since this is most likely to indicate perpendicular placement of the probe on the cornea.

- *Partial coherence interferometry* is fast, noncontact, precise ($SD \approx 0.75\,\mu m$) with low interobserver variability. It requires a transparent cornea, and peripheral measurements are hard to obtain.

- *Optical slit lamp-based pachymetry* can be used with a contact lens in situ and to measure the depth of corneal scars. It is less accurate than the methods above.

Keratometry Dedicated instruments for measuring central corneal curvature, such as the Javel-Schiotz and Bausch and Lomb keratometers express the corneal curvature as a radius of curvature or in dioptric power. Automated devices such as the IOL Master®, Orbscan® and videokeratoscopes also provide measures of corneal curvature.

Corneal topography Several devices measure the corneal shape or curvature.

- *Placido-based videokeratoscopy* measures the corneal reflection of circles of light (mires) of known radius. Tear film abnormalities degrade the image. Videokeratoscopy does not measure beyond the surface and therefore the corneal power is derived mathematically. The reconstruction algorithms vary. Peripheral measurements are less accurate because the relationship between the corneal curvature and the refractive power varies, and fewer points are analyzed.

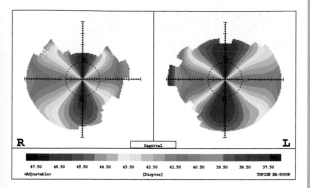

Fig. 5.1: Corneal topography showing with-the-rule astigmatism (Topcon videokeratoscope). Compare with Fig. 5.6 (p. 161).

■ *Scanning slit-beam systems* The computerized corneal mapping devices that use a calibrated video and slit beam system, e.g. Orbscan®. A mathematical representation of the true topographic anterior and posterior corneal surfaces is formed, from which the surface curvature is calculated. The image must be captured in 30 msec to prevent degradation from eye movement.

All methods produce similar results in the visually important, central 3 mm of the cornea. Data points taken along meridians from centre to periphery are converted into colour-coded contour maps. Yellows and greens represent normal corneal powers, cool colours represent lower power, and warm colours, higher power. Scales are not standardized and need to be selected carefully for meaningful interpretation. Topography of fellow eyes usually produces mirror images (enantiomorphs). Videokeratography of regular astigmatism results in a bow-tie pattern (Fig. 5.1).

Wavefront scanning technology can be used to measure the total ocular aberrations. Data acquisition and manipulation vary between manufacturers. Maps show the difference between the ideal planar wavefront and the wavefront distorted by the eye's aberrations, including lower-order aberrations (prism, sphere, and cylinder), higher-order aberrations (all the rest), and point spread function (light scatter).

Specular microscopy permits visualization and photography of the endothelium. Computer analysis produces quantitative and qualitative indices that can be used to monitor cell loss from contact lens wear and intraocular surgery.

Corneal Abrasions and Foreign Bodies

Background A shearing force or foreign body breaches the epithelium to expose the subepithelial nerve plexus.

Symptoms Pain, photophobia, foreign body (FB) sensation, and tearing.

History Ask about the material (organic, metallic, or other) and mechanism of injury. Could a high-velocity FB have entered the eye from metal striking metal? Would safety goggles have been appropriate?

Examination Instil proxymetacaine 0.5% prior to examination then evert both lids to exclude subtarsal FBs (Fig. 5.2). Use 2% fluorescein to show conjunctival defects. If these coexist with subconjunctival haemorrhage that obscures the sclera, dilate the pupil to exclude an intraocular FB. Subconjunctival pigment may indicate uveal prolapse from scleral penetration. Note the pattern of corneal fluorescein staining such as a geographic abrasion, superficial punctate keratitis or linear scratches. Draw the abrasion location, size (in millimetres), and depth (percentage of corneal thickness). Iron FBs may be surrounded by a rust ring or sterile infiltrate, especially if present >24 hr (Fig. 5.3). The base of uninfected abrasions should be clear. Mild anterior uveitis may be present but iris or lens defects suggest an intraocular FB.

Differential diagnosis Treat expanding or new infiltrates associated with purulent discharge, severe redness, or pain as

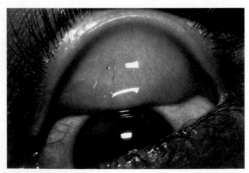

Fig. 5.2: Subtarsal foreign body with associated corneal fluorescein uptake.

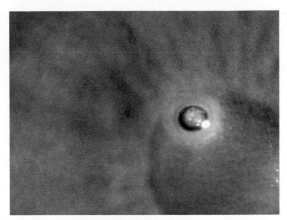

Fig. 5.3: Corneal FB with rust ring.

bacterial keratitis (p. 171). For apparently spontaneous epithelial defects consider corneal dystrophy and recurrent erosion syndrome. Exclude chemical and penetrating injury.

Management Remove foreign bodies (Box 5.1). Stat G. homatropine 1% or cyclopentolate 1% relieve pain from ciliary spasm. Offer oral analgesics as required.

Box 5.1: Removal of superficial corneal foreign body

1. Explain the procedure and warn that discomfort may increase when the anaesthetic wears off.

2. Instil topical anaesthesia, e.g. 3 drops of proxymetacaine 0.5%.

3. Multiple superficial FBs are sometimes more easily removed by irrigation.

4. Remove embedded FBs at the slit lamp using a 20-gauge needle with a bent tip. Remove any rust ring with a needle or dental burr. Deep rust rings in the visual axis that cannot easily be removed should be left to resolve spontaneously. Mild iron staining is not visually significant.

5. Document the epithelial defect size (post-removal).

6. Apply Oc. chloramphenicol and paraffin embedded mesh, e.g. Jellonet, and pressure pad unless there is a risk of infection, e.g. organic matter, finger nail scratch, or contact lens wearer.

Follow-up

1. Contact lens wearers

   ■ In contact lens wearers, without a clear history of a fingernail injury, an 'abrasion' is often the first sign of bacterial keratitis. If in doubt about the diagnosis, treat as bacterial keratitis. Otherwise, prescribe G. ofloxacin four times daily until the eye is comfortable, indicating epithelialization. Ask the patient to return as an emergency if symptoms deteriorate, suggesting infection.

   ■ Re-start contact lens wearing 1 week after the epithelium has healed.

2. Non-contact lens wearers

   ■ Small abrasion at low risk of infection: remove the pad after 24 hours. Use Oc. chloramphenicol q.d.s. for five days then stop. Review only if symptoms persist.

   ■ Larger abrasions or high risk of infection: use Oc. chloramphenicol q.d.s. and review at 24 hr. If the abrasion is healing well and the patient is comfortable, continue ointment for five days then stop. If not, instil G. homatropine 1%, continue Oc. chloramphenicol q.d.s. and review in 24 hr.

Recurrent Corneal Erosion

Background Traumatic, dystrophic, or degenerative damage interferes with corneal epithelium–basement membrane adhesion, resulting in recurrent epithelial breakdown (recurrent erosion syndrome). Determining the causative mechanism is important in selecting appropriate therapy. See also persistent corneal epithelial defects (p. 155).

Symptoms Recurrent attacks of pain, tearing, and redness, typically during sleep or at awakening.

History Ask about prior corneal abrasions, especially those from organic material such as a tree branch or finger nail. Ask if there is a family history of recurrent erosions or corneal disease.

Examination Epithelial defects vary from focal superficial punctate keratopathy (SPKs) or immature epithelium (Fig. 5.4), to full-thickness defects. The anterior chamber may have scanty cells. Examine the other eye with fluorescein and retroillumination for signs of a corneal dystrophy.

Differential diagnosis Epithelial basement membrane dystrophy (syn. Cogan's, or map-dot-fingerprint dystrophy) is the most common cause and often presents with recurrent erosion. Recurrent erosion is also frequent in Thiel-Behnke, Reis-Bücklers, lattice, granular, and Meesman's dystrophies.

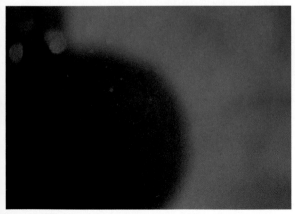

Fig. 5.4: Recurrent corneal erosion with subsequent subepithelial cysts in the affected area in a patient with map-dot-finger print dystrophy.

Management Most cases respond to conservative management with stat G. homatropine 1%, Oc. chloramphenicol and pressure pad, with review in 24 hours if not settled. Repeat if the epithelium has not healed. If not healed in 3 days insert a bandage contact lens (BCL), e.g. 'Night and Day', to relieve discomfort and promote healing. Inflamed eyes may better tolerate a BCL if treated with topical NSAID (G. diclofenac 0.1% b.d.) and cylcoplegic (G. homatropine 1% b.d.) for 2 days. Use the BCL for 2–3 months. Cases not responding to padding and BCL may benefit from focal debridement of loose epithelium using a cellulose sponge under topical anaesthesia. Remove any residual strands with plain forceps. Avoid sharp instruments. Focal abnormalities occurring off the visual axis may respond to anterior stromal puncture using the needle on an insulin syringe (bend the tip at 90° to the shaft with tying forceps, leaving a point shorter than the corneal thickness to avoid a corneal perforation): make multiple fine punctures through Bowman layer in the affected area. Use surgical superficial keratectomy or phototherapeutic keratectomy (PTK) for recalcitrant cases, particularly if there is excessive aberrant epithelial basement membrane and subepithelial collageneous pannus (commonest in map-dot-fingerprint dystrophy).

Once healed, prescribe a lubricant ointment at night until asymptomatic for at least 3 months.

Follow-up Review daily until the epithelial defect has closed (see comments above). Those with ocular surface disease, BCLs or on topical steroids are at increased risk of microbial superinfection and require close follow-up.

Persistent Epithelial Defect

Background Persistent corneal epithelial defects (PCEDs) occur in association with a large and heterogeneous group of ocular and systemic diseases. Detection and treatment of any underlying autoimmune diseases may facilitate corneal healing and avoid potentially lethal vasculitis.

History and examination Look for facial, eyelid, and tear film abnormalities. Test corneal sensation and note the location and size of epithelial defects (usually oval with slightly heaped edges, in the palpebral aperture), the percentage of stromal thinning, and presence of any infiltrate. Exclude the following potential causes:

- *Local*: eyelid or eyelid margin disease; neurotrophic keratitis; neuroparalytic keratitis (e.g. Bell's palsy); following corneal infections, burns, and surgery (including keratorefractive procedures); diabetes; skin disease (e.g. acne rosacea; psoriasis); atopic or vernal keratoconjunctivitis; Mooren's ulcer; staphylococcal marginal ulcer; herpetic keratitis; allograft rejection.

- *Systemic*: nutritional disorders (e.g. keratomalacia); leukaemia, Sjögren's syndrome; graft-versus-host disease; collagen vascular disorders (rheumatoid arthritis, ocular mucous membrane pemphigoid, Stevens-Johnson syndrome, relapsing polychondritis, systemic lupus erythematosus, polyarteritis nodosa, Wegener's granulomatosis).

Treatment Treatment is directed at the underlying cause.

- Discontinue unnecessary topical medications and use ointment that may reduce the shearing forces of the eyelids on the corneal epithelium.

- A low-toxicity unpreserved antibiotic drop or ointment such as chloramphenicol is usually used as prophylaxis against bacterial infection.

- Use preservative-free drops if possible, especially if the patient requires more than six drops daily.

- Manage infiltrates as microbial keratitis (p. 171). Patients on topical steroids may have infection without an infiltrate.

- Treat dry eye with tear substitutes, serum tears, or punctal occlusion. Avoid continuous use of hydrogel bandage contact lenses if there is aqueous tear deficiency. The risk of superinfection is high.

Box 5.2: Applying corneal glue

1. Apply topical anaesthetic, e.g. proxymetacaine 0.5%.

2. Trephine a circular patch of clear plastic from a sterile drape using a 4 mm skin punch. To one side apply a drop of KY jelly. This allows the patch to be picked up using an applicator, such as a cotton-tipped stick.

3. Lift the patch and turn it over. To the other side apply a small drop of cyanoacrylate (e.g. Histacryl) tissue glue.

4. Dry the corneal defect with a cellulose (e.g. Weccel) sponge.

5. Place the patch over the defect, glue-side down. Leave the polythene patch in place.

6. Use a cellulose sponge to confirm that the defect is sealed.

7. Apply a bandage contact lens.

Complications include early loss of glue, neovascularization, and infection. Advise patients not to rub the eye and use preservative-free drops while the contact lens remains in situ. Review within 24 hours. Tectonic corneal grafting may be required if the leak continues.

- If treatment of the underlying disorder and the use of lubricants fails, then consider lid closure with Botox injection (p. 24) or a temporary central tarsorrhaphy with a 4/0 mattress suture and bolster. Human amniotic membrane grafting is an alternative for refractory PCED or if rapid stromal thinning threatens perforation.

- Treat small perforations (<1 mm) with tissue glue (Box 5.2), a contact lens and prophylactic topical antibiotics. For larger perforations, a therapeutic lamellar or penetrating keratoplasty is necessary.

- If all these treatments fail, a conjunctival flap will sacrifice vision but reduces discomfort and ocular inflammation, and promotes healing. If no conjunctiva is available due to scarring, a free buccal mucous membrane graft will usually result in a stable epithelium.

Follow-up Weekly until healed.

Dry Eye (Keratoconjunctivitis Sicca)

Background Tear dysfunction occurs in 15–33% of the population with a female preponderance. It may be idiopathic or result from a variety of causes:

■ *Abnormal wetting (mucin deficiency)*: e.g. conjunctival cicatricial disease, trachoma, chemical burns and lid margin disease.

■ *Aqueous tear deficiency (reduced lacrimal gland function)*: postmenopause, autoimmune disease (e.g. Sjögren's syndrome, rheumatoid arthritis, SLE, sarcoidosis), drug induced (diuretics, topical or systemic beta blockers, antimuscarinics, antihistamines, sedatives, nasal decongestants, opiate based medicines, e.g. some antitussives, analgesics and antidiarrhoeals), corneal anaesthesia, Riley Day syndrome, lacrimal gland disease, lymphoma, HIV, amyloidosis, and irradiation.

■ *Abnormal spreading and lagophthalmos*: reduced blink frequency when concentrating on tasks such as driving, facial nerve palsy, parkinsonism, lid malposition, proptosis, pingeculae, pterygia, and contact lenses.

Symptoms Complex symptomatology may include surface discomfort, photophobia, redness, itch, ropey discharge, eyelid fatigue, and blurred or fluctuating vision. Paradoxically, tear deficiency can cause excessive compensatory lacrimation. Symptom severity may correlate poorly with the signs.

History Enquire about the exact nature of symptoms, relieving and exacerbating factors including the effect of blinking. Take a full medical and drug history, noting the potential causes listed above.

Examination

1. Lids: blink, contour, and lid margin disease.

2. Tears.

   ■ *Quantity*: The inferior marginal tear strip is usually 0.5–1 mm high, if <0.5 mm suspect dry eye. Perform the Schirmer I test (p. 147).

   ■ *Quality*: Look for excessive foam, oils or mucous debris (best seen by gently pushing up the lower lid so they can be viewed against the pupil). Measure the *tear film break up time* (TBUT).

a. Prior to lid manipulation or any eyedrops, instil a small volume of fluorescien on an applicator strip with unpreserved saline.

b. Ask the patient to blink a few times then stare straight ahead.

c. Use a slit lamp with a broad, tangential, blue beam.

d. The time between a complete blink and the appearance of a corneal tear film defect (dark blue spot) is the TBUT.

e. A normal TBUT is >10 seconds, a TBUT more than the blink interval lacks significance, <1–2 seconds is usually abnormal, suggesting mucin deficiency.

3. Conjunctiva: note any injection, scarring, keratinisation, and symblephara. Fluorescein or rose bengal staining suggest mucin deficiency. Eyes with disturbed tear function quickly become red during examination.

4. Cornea: note the pattern and extent of rose bengal and fluorescein staining, focal abnormal wetting, thinning (dellen), infection, keratinization, scarring, and filaments (strands of mucous and degenerated corneal epithelial cells).

Treatment There is no panacea for dry eye.

■ *Eliminate underlying causes*: Treat meibomian gland dysfunction with warm compresses, lid hygiene, and doxycycline (p. 114). Treat ocular surface inflammation with a weak preservative-free steroid (e.g. prednisolone 0.1–0.5% 2–4 times daily) for 2 weeks. Treat excess mucus with G. N acetyl cysteine 5% q.d.s. Discontinue unnecessary eyedrops, especially those with preservative. If available, use vitamin A for conjuctival keratinization, e.g. G. retinoic acid 0.01–0.1% q.d.s.

■ *Tear substitutes*: Many products are available. Inappropriate, excessive, or long-term treatment may cause intolerance, especially with drops containing preservative, e.g. benzalkonium or cetrimide, that is not diluted by normal tear flow. Limit preservative-containing drops if possible, but if unavoidable use no more than 6 times daily in severe aqueous tear deficiency. For refractory cases autologous serum may be beneficial but is expensive, time-consuming to manufacture, and can become contaminated.

- *Punctal occlusion*: This prevents tear drainage and prolongs the effect of tear substitutes. Treat any blepharitis beforehand as occlusion may exacerbate symptoms. Options include temporary collagen or silicone plugs, and permanent surgical occlusion. Try plugs first to assess the therapeutic effect and the risk of epiphora, but note that not all temporary plugs fully occlude the canaliculi and may fail to predict epiphora. Permanent occlusion is achieved by cautery: anaesthetise, insert the tip of a hand-held cautery fully into the canaliculus, activate, then withdraw, denuding the adherent epithelial lining.

- *Contact lenses*: Rigid gas permeable scleral contact lenses cover the cornea and most of the conjunctiva, preventing tear evaporation. They also protect from abnormal lids.

Treatment options also depend on disease severity:

- *Mild*: G. preserved tear substitutes 3–4 times daily (e.g. G. hypromellose 0.3% or G. polyvinyl alcohol).

- *Moderate*: Unpreserved tear substitute (e.g. G Hypromellose 0.3% unpreserved up to 2 hourly). Use spectacles to reduce evaporation from the surface (about 30% reduction); wrap around spectacles or side shields increase effectiveness.

- *Severe*: If there is some lacrimation (see Schirmer I Test, p. 147), occlude the lower punctum with temporary plugs, if not, plug the upper and lower puncti. Consider permanent occlusion depending on the effect. Use hourly unpreserved tear substitute.

- *Very Severe*: Use hourly unpreserved tear substitutes, such as:

  a. Low viscosity: unpreserved hypromellose 0.3%.

  b. Gel: unpreserved carbomer, hyaluronic acid.

  c. Viscous: carboxymethylcellulose sodium 0.5% solution or ointments.

Consider punctal occlusion (plugs initially), lacrimal stimulation with oral pilocarpine, limbal-fit or scleral gas-permeable contact lenses, autologous serum drops, and tarsorrhaphy.

Keratoconus

Background Keratoconus (KC) is the commonest primary corneal ectasia. It is characterized by noninflammatory, central corneal thinning, typically presenting in the second and third decades.

History Ask about blurred vision, rapidly changing spectacle prescription, eye rubbing, and contact lens (CL) wear. Review past refractions if available. Family history exists in ≈8%. Sudden onset of pain, redness, loss of vision, and photophobia suggests hydrops (see below). Many conditions are associated with KC, including atopic dermatitis, vernal keratoconjunctivitis, Down's syndrome, Ehlers Danlos syndrome, and Laurence-Moon-Bardet-Biedel syndrome, among others.

Examination Corneal changes are nearly always bilateral, but may be asymmetrical. The cornea has a variably shaped cone (Fig. 5.5), that is thinned at the apex. This produces a focal lid convexity in downgaze (Munson's sign, Fig. 5.5B). The corneal substrate may appear normal but several signs may be present including: a rust-coloured Fleischer ring at the base of the cone (best seen using oblique cobalt blue illumination); Vogt's striae (deep stromal vertical stress lines); fine subepithelial scarring at the cone apex; a scissor reflex on retinoscopy; an oil drop red reflex; and prominent corneal nerves. Acute rips in Descemet's membrane occur in ≈5% (higher in Down's syndrome or allergic eye disease), resulting in a sudden onset of profound stromal hydration (*hydrops*).

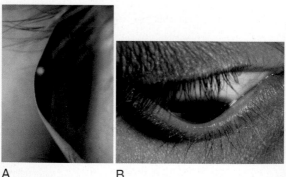

A   B

Fig. 5.5: **(A)** Keratoconus. **(B)** Munson's sign (Courtesy of DH Verity).

Investigation Subtle irregular astigmatism is the first finding. Corneal topography is the most sensitive investigation and may show keratoconus minus (a.k.a. *forme fruste*) with asymmetric localized steepening of the inferior cornea (Fig. 5.6). Keratoconus plus (anterior keratoconus) is the same plus one or more classic signs.

Treatment

■ *Astigmatism*: Progression is variable but slows with age. When spectacles no longer correct the astigmatism, try rigid gas permeable CLs. Advanced cases with CL instability require keratoplasty or scleral CLs. Keratoconus may rarely recur in the graft. Penetrating or deep anterior lamellar keratoplasty (PK or DALK) are currently the procedures of choice. Epikeratophakia (onlay lamellar keratoplasty) is only rarely used as the quality of vision is poor.

■ *Scarring*: Consider PK or lamellar keratoplasty if scarring limits the corrected VA. DALK avoids the risk of rejection, but the extra interface may degrade the VA. Previous hydrops usually results in a posterior split during lamellar dissection and is an indication for PK.

■ *Hydrops*: Usually resolves in 8–10 weeks but may take 6 months. Offer G. hypertonic sodium chloride 5% q.d.s. and G. homatropine 1% b.d. Examine every 2–4 weeks until resolved. PK may be required if there are no signs of improvement at 3 months, or earlier in corneas that start vascularizing.

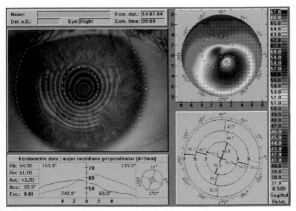

Fig. 5.6: Corneal topography showing keratoconus. Normal astigmatism is shown in Fig. 5.1.

Other corneal ectasias

Pellucid marginal degeneration Onset age 20–40. A characteristic arcuate band of thinning 1–2 mm wide is seen from 4–8 o'clock, located 1–2 mm central to the limbus. There may be marked central corneal flattening along the vertical meridian before inferior thinning is detectible.

Keratoglobus Stromal thinning extends to the peripheral cornea resulting in a globular corneal profile (Fig. 5.7).

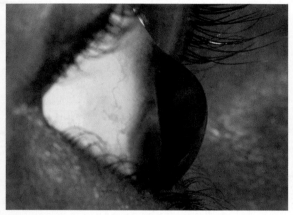

Fig. 5.7: Keratoglobus (Courtesy of DH Verity).

Peripheral Corneal Thinning

Background Peripheral ulcerative keratitis (PUK) is often idiopathic (Mooren's ulcer) or may be associated with rheumatoid arthritis (RA) and type III autoimmune diseases (polyarteritis nodosa, relapsing polychondritis, Wegener's granulomatosis).

Examination Scleritis is absent in Mooren's ulcer, variably present in RA, and severe, usually necrotizing, in autoimmune diseases. PUK is destructive, beginning peripherally and progressing centrally, circumferentially, and posteriorly, leaving thinned neovascularized cornea.

Differential diagnosis See table 5.1.

Investigations PUK may be the presenting feature of potentially fatal systemic, vasculitic disease. Check cANCA, pANCA, RhF, ANA, ENA, ESR, CRP, sACE, CXR, and urine for protein and casts.

Treatment Involve senior clinicians. Unilateral Mooren's ulcer may resolve with surgery (conjunctival resection/tissue glue), bandage contact lenses, topical treatment (steroids, acetylcysteine, antibiotic), and oral doxycyline. Severe or bilateral Mooren's ulcer and PUK associated with type III autoimmune disease requires systemic immunosuppression.

Follow-up Aim for 1 year of remission (and ANCA normalization in Wegener's granulomatosis) then taper immunosuppressants. Monitor for side effects of systemic treatment (p. 343). 'Burnt-out' Mooren's ulcer may reactivate with cataract or corneal graft surgery, so immunosuppress beforehand.

Table 5.1: Differential diagnosis of peripheral corneal thinning

Condition	Sex	Pain	Epithelium intact?	Age	Most common site	Laterality	Progression	Perforation	Comments
Terrien's marginal degeneration (Fig. 5.8)	M = F	No	Yes	3–4th decade	Superior nasal	Bilateral	Yes, slowly	No, unless trauma	Variable and intermittent limbal inflammation, anterior chamber (AC) uninflamed. Lipid in vascularized, superficial cornea. Topical steroid rapidly controls inflammation.
Herpes zoster ophthalmicus (HZO) Herpes Simplex Virus (HSV)	M = F	No	No	Elderly	Any quadrant	Unilateral	Yes	Yes	Reduced corneal sensation, mild uveitis. For treatment see p. 182 (HZO) or p. 178 (HSV)

Pellucid margin degeneration	M = F	No	Yes	2–3rd decade	Inferior	Bilateral	Yes, slowly	No, unless trauma	Conjunctiva and AC uninflamed. No lipid deposition. Abnormal topography. No treatment.
Marginal keratitis and ocular rosacea	M = F	No	Yes	Any	Multifocal	Uni- or bilateral	Yes, with recurrent episodes	No	For treatment see p. 116 and p. 170
Furrow degeneration	F = M	No	Yes	Elderly	Peripheral to arcus senilis	Bilateral	Very slowly	No	Conjunctiva and AC uninflamed. Associated with rheumatoid arthritis. No treatment
Dellen (Fig. 5.9)	M = F	No	Yes	Any	Adjacent to limbal or corneal elevation	Unilateral	Very slowly	No	Conjunctiva and AC uninflamed. Eliminate elevation if possible Topical lubricants.

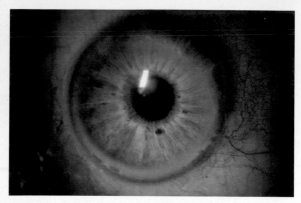

Fig. 5.8: Terriens marginal degeneration.

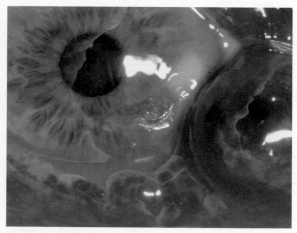

Fig. 5.9: Dellen from an adjacent, elevated subconjunctival haemorrhage (Courtesy of DH Verity).

Interstitial Keratitis

Background A corneal stromal inflammation without epithelial loss, usually caused by an immune reaction to trapped antigens. Interstitial keratitis (IK) is a sign rather than a diagnosis. It may be necrotising or non-necrotising. Causes are listed in Table 5.2.

Symptoms Red eye, irritation, tearing, photophobia, and reduced VA if the visual axis is involved.

History Ask about previous episodes (especially herpetic eye disease), sarcoidosis, maternal syphilis (congenital syphilis may present age 5–20), previous sexually transmitted infection (syphilis, chlamydia), reduced hearing (syphilis, Cogan's syndrome), foreign travel (parasites), rashes (measles, mumps, syphilis).

Examination

Face Look for features of congenital syphilis (saddle nose; frontal bossing; Hutchinson's triad of IK, notched upper central incisors and sensorineural deafness), or leprosy (loss of temporal eyebrow; hypopigmented/anaesthetic skin patches). Herpes zoster ophthalmicus (HZO) may have frontal scarring.

Conjunctiva Exclude follicular conjunctivitis (chlamydia).

Cornea Bilateral or unilateral? (*Mycobacteria* spp, mumps, HSV, HZV, acquired syphilis, congenital syphilis may initially have unilateral onset). Focal (HSV disciform lesions), multifocal (HZO nummular keratitis) or diffuse (greyish pink 'salmon patch' of syphilitic IK) distribution. Check IOP. Long-standing IK results in stromal scarring with deep neovascularisation or ghost vessels.

Anterior chamber Granulomatous uveitis may occur.

Table 5.2: Causes of interstitial keratitis

Necrotizing	Non necrotizing		
	Focal	Multifocal	Diffuse
Herpes simplex virus (HSV)	HSV	Adenovirus	HSV
Herpes zoster ophthalmicus (HZO)	HZO	Chlamydia	Syphilis
	Epstein Barr virus	Epstein Barr virus	Cogan's syndrome
Non virulent bacteria (*Mycobacteria*, *Strep. viridans*, Brucella)	Sarcoidosis	Mumps (rare)	Measles (rare)
	Cogan's syndrome	Parasites (oncocerciasis, malaria, trypanosomiasis, cystercicosis)	

Pupil/iris Nodules (leprosy, sarcoidosis), miosis (syphilis, secondary to uveitis).

Fundus Salt and pepper chorioretinopathy of syphilis. Optic atrophy.

Differential diagnosis Acanthamoeba, fungi, or low virulence microbial keratitis with epithelial healing e.g. *Nocardia*.

Investigations Check syphilis serology; sACE (sarcoid); CXR (TB, sarcoid); tuberculin skin test; hearing (Cogan's syndrome, congenital syphilis, leprosy). Other tests as indicated.

Treatment Prescribe topical steroids (e.g. prednisolone 0.5% q.d.s.) and cycloplegia as required. Treat the underlying cause and any elevated IOP. Treatment of syphilis does not affect the course of IK.

Follow-up Depends upon underlying cause e.g. IK of congenital syphilis lasts 3–4 weeks. Residual scarring may necessitate corneal grafting. Beware recurrence in the graft.

Phlyctenulosis

A type IV hypersensitivity reaction historically associated with tuberculosis, but now with staphylococcus, herpes simplex virus (HSV), and varicella-zoster virus (Fig. 5.10). Granulomatous lesions form at the limbus and ulcers develop within a few days. Treatment with topical steroids causes involution in 2–4 days e.g. prednisolone 1% b.d., then taper. Treat associated staphylococcal lid disease with topical antibiotic and lid hygiene, and add oral aciclovir for HSV.

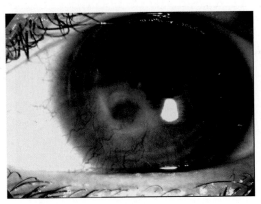

Fig. 5.10: Phlycten.

Marginal Keratitis

Patients with staphyloccal disease of the eyelids or conjunctiva may present with small superficial round infiltrates as an immunological response to the organism or its toxins (Fig. 5.11). Initially, the epithelium is intact, but may later break down. No culture is required. The infiltrates resolve with topical steroids (e.g. G. prednisolone 0.5% q.d.s.) and lid hygiene, followed by topical antibiotic ointment to the lid margin (e.g. Oc. fucithalmic b.d.). Taper treatment according to response.

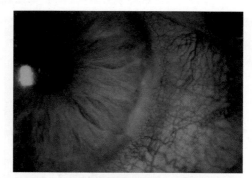

Fig. 5.11: Marginal keratitis.

Bacterial Keratitis

Symptoms Unilateral red eye, discharge, tearing, and blurred vision.

History Ask about onset, progression, treatment, level of discomfort, trauma, contact lens wear, and ocular or systemic disease.

Examination Examine adnexae, eyelids, conjunctiva, and cornea of both eyes for predisposing factors, e.g. dry eyes. Draw the size, location, depth, shape and colour of corneal infiltrate. Test corneal sensation. Perform Seidel's test (p. 147) if perforation is suspected. Document anterior chamber cellular activity, including the size of any hypopyon. These are usually sterile unless Descemet's membrane has been breached (Fig. 5.12).

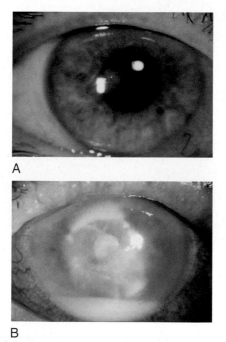

A

B

Fig. 5.12: Bacterial keratitis. **(A)** Small pneumococcal infiltrate. **(B)** Severe pseudomonal keratitis with hypopyon.

Differential diagnosis Consider herpes simplex, acanthamoeba keratitis, or fungal keratitis, sterile peripheral infiltrates from contact lenses, and phlyctenular keratitis. Rarer causes of progressive infection include anaerobic bacteria (propionobacterium, capnocytophaga), *Nocardia*, mycobacterium (particularly post-LASIK), and microsporidia.

Management Perform a corneal scrape (Box 5.3) to guide therapy, remove debris, and improve antibiotic penetration. Prescribe regular cycloplegia (e.g. G. homatropine 0.5% b.d.). If the cornea is thinned, apply a shield, without padding. Start empiric therapy with G. cefuroxime 5% and gentamicin 1% hourly, 30 mins apart, or alternatively G. ofloxacin 0.3% hourly in

---

Box 5.3: Taking a corneal scrape

1. Liaise with microbiology staff. Request an urgent Gram stain.

2. Warm refrigerated media to room temperature.

3. Instil G. proxymetacaine 0.5% then G. amethocaine 1%.

4. Explain the procedure.

5. At the slit lamp, use a Kimura spatula, No. 15 Bard Parker blade, or 20-gauge needle to remove superficial debris from the ulcer, and then scrape the edges and base.

6. Streak material onto two glass slides for Gram and Giemsa staining (or other preferred stain). Air dry and label with pencil.

7. Take additional scrapes, one for each culture medium. Streak material onto agar plates without breaking the surface. Flame the blade and cool for 20 seconds between scrapes, or select a fresh needle.

8. Plate onto blood agar, chocolate agar, and Sabouraud's agar.

9. If acanthamoeba is suspected, streak onto the centre of a non-nutrient agar plate.

10. Tape covers onto the plates to prevent evaporation.

11. Inoculate brain–heart infusion and cooked meat broth by agitating the blade or needle in the media, (or by dropping a sterile cotton swab into the media).

12. Culture contact lenses, cases, and solutions. Document that the patient understands these will be destroyed in the process.

13. Label all material, and transport immediately to the laboratory.

14. Cultures may be positive in 24 hours, but can take up to 3 weeks for fungi, acanthamoeba, or anaerobes.

countries such as the UK, where quinolone resistance is rare. Some streptococcal species are less sensitive to fluoroquinolones. Treat day and night for 2 days then day only. Admit if rapid onset, only eye, risk of perforation, or poor compliance. Otherwise, review with microbiology results in 2 days. If responding, continue treatment unaltered and review in a corneal clinic in 5 days. If improving at that visit, reduce antibiotics to q.d.s. and consider adding G. prednisolone 0.5% q.d.s. to reduce inflammation. Address any precipitating factors. If not responding, consider early review, admission, re-scraping, and altering antibiotics based on sensitivities.

Fungal Keratitis

History Ask about ocular or systemic disease: candida keratitis is commonest in debilitated patients or those with preexisting corneal disease. Ocular trauma is associated with filamentous fungi, e.g. *Aspergillus* or *Fusarium* spp.

Symptoms Unilateral red eye, tearing, and blurred vision. Pain and photophobia are initially mild, but become severe relative to the clinical signs.

Signs The corneal surface typically appears grey with a dry rough texture. Filamentous fungi classically grow in a feathery branching pattern, but may be very rapidly progressive and indistinguishable from bacterial keratitis (Fig. 5.13). Candida produces a small ulcer with expanding infiltrate in a collar-stud configuration, often superimposed on a debilitating corneal condition. There may be an endothelial plaque under the lesion and satellite lesions at the edges. Suppurative keratitis, fibrinoid uveitis, hypopyon, and elevated IOP may occur.

Differential diagnosis Herpes simplex virus, acanthamoeba, and atypical bacterial keratitis, e.g. *Nocardia*, *Mycobacterium*, *Propionibacterium*.

Investigations Take a corneal scrape for smear and culture (p. 172). The diagnosis can often be made with the smear. Liaise with the microbiologist. If culture negative after 7 days and the patient is not responding, perform a partial-thickness corneal biopsy. This must be large (3 mm) and deep enough to include the affected areas. Send half to microbiology, half in formalin to histology. If available, in vivo confocal microscopy may be diagnostic.

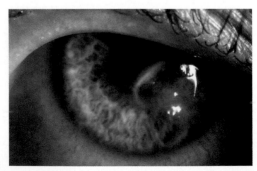

Fig. 5.13: Fungal keratitis (*Aspergillus fumigatus*) (Courtesy SJ Tuft).

Treatment

- Discontinue any steroid treatment immediately.

- Candida keratitis: G. amphotericin 0.15% (from i.v. preparation) hourly for 5 days then reducing to 4–6 times daily until the disease resolves. Use systemic treatment for peripheral or deep corneal ulceration (e.g. fluconazole 400 mg p.o. stat then 200 mg daily p.o. or i.v.). The frequency of topical therapy is as for candida keratitis above.

- Filamentary fungal keratitis: G. amphotericin (as above) or G. econazole 1%, and itraconazole 100 mg b.d. for deep or peripheral lesions.

- Shield without pad if the cornea is thinned.

- Treat raised IOP.

- Provide cycloplegia and analgesia as required.

Follow-up Initially 1–2 times weekly until there are signs of improvement or deterioration halts. This may take days or weeks. A minimum of 12 weeks' therapy is required for deep infection. Topical steroids are contraindicated in filamentary fungal infection as they promote fungal growth. Consider keratoplasty if the disease progresses after 2 weeks of optimal therapy; persisting with conservative treatment in this situation will lead to intraocular invasion (without perforation). A therapeutic penetrating keratoplasty is required in ≈25%, enucleation in 3%. Steroids should not be introduced after keratoplasty for 1–3 months because of the risk of recurrence in the host corneal ring. Continue antifungals 4 times daily for several weeks after therapeutic keratoplasty.

Acanthamoeba Keratitis

Background Most (85%) cases occur in contact lens wearers. Protozoa may be isolated from contact lenses, water (fresh, salt, tap, swimming pools, hot tubs), dust, soil, or sewage.

History Ask about contact lens cleaning regimen, swimming and showering in lenses, and the use of tapwater to clean lenses. Initially, pain and photophobia are mild; later they are often, but not always, severe relative to the clinical signs.

Examination Signs are usually unilateral and highly variable. The cornea may show superficial punctate keratitis, reduced sensation, and dendritiform lesions. Perineural infiltrates may be peripheral or central. Stromal infiltrates are initially minimal, patchy, and widespread. Focal lesions are uncommon. Paracentral infiltrates may coalesce to form characteristic ring infiltrates (Fig. 5.14). Other features include disciform oedema, scleritis, and mild uveitis. Hypopyon suggests bacterial superinfection.

Differential diagnosis Herpes simplex, fungal, or bacterial keratitis (e.g. *Nocardia*).

Investigations A corneal scrape must be taken (p. 172). Culture contact lenses, cases, and solutions. Explain that these will be destroyed in the process. A corneal trephine biopsy may be necessary in culture-negative cases that progress. Confocal microscopy, if available, can be diagnostic.

Treatment *Acanthamoeba* cysts are highly resistant and in vitro susceptibility correlates poorly with in vivo activity.

- First line: G. PHMB 0.02% or G. chlorhexidine 0.02% hourly, as signs of resolution appear reduce to q.d.s.

- Second line: add G. propamidine 0.1%, G. hexamidine 0.1% or G. metronidazole 0.5% (from i.v. preparation) hourly.

- First and second line drugs are often combined (G. PHMB 0.02% with G. hexamidine 0.1%).

Provide NSAID analgesia. Consider oral steroids and ciclosporin for painful scleritis resistant to treatment with NSAIDs.

Follow-up 1–2 weekly until signs of resolution occur, then monthly as treatment is tapered off. Delay topical steroid use for at least 2 weeks as this may interfere with macrophage activity required to clear cysts. Do not use steroids if the inflammation is subsiding spontaneously.

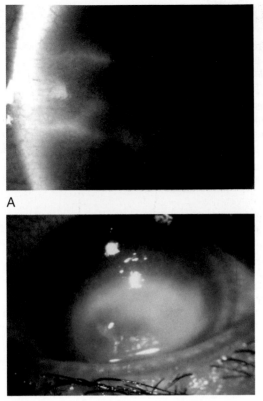

A

B

Fig. 5.14: Acanthamoeba keratitis. **(A)** Perineural infiltrates. **(B)** Ring infiltrate.

Herpes Simplex Keratitis

Background Herpes simplex virus keratitis (HSVK) may occur as a primary infection in adults and children, but is more commonly due to reactivation of latent viral infection. Nonocular primary infection may be asymptomatic.

History Ask about potential triggers for recurrence such as UV light, trauma, cold, menstruation, psychological stress, systemic illness, and immunosuppression. Ask about previous labial, genital, or ocular HSV.

Examination Test corneal sensation: hypoaesthesia occurs early. Examine the eye fully, as multiple sites may be involved.

- Primary HSV
  Common signs include eyelid rash (clear vesicles on erythematous eyelids and later crusting), conjunctival follicles (± pseudomembrane), punctate keratitis, subepithelial corneal infiltration or ulceration, dendritic ulcers, and disciform lesions.

- Recurrent HSV keratitis

  1. *Epithelial HSV*: Blotchy, stellate, or a filamentary keratitis usually progresses in 1–2 days to a classic dendritic pattern (branching lesions with feathery edges, and bulbs at the end) (Fig. 5.15). Fluorescein stains the ulcer and rose bengal stains the swollen epithelial cells at the ulcer's

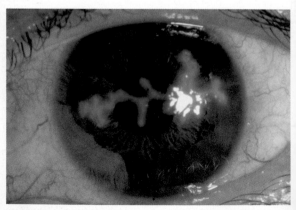

Fig. 5.15: Dendritic corneal ulcer (Courtesy of DH Verity).

edge. There may be underlying, slightly larger subepithelial ghost infiltrates. With prolonged infection or steroid use, a geographic or amoeboid ulcer may occur. There may be a mild anterior chamber cellular reaction.

2. *Stromal HSV*: Three main patterns of disease exist:

   a. Disciform ± endotheliitis: A circular area of oedema with minimal infiltrate or vascularization (except in recurrent disease) (Fig. 5.16). Fluorescein staining shows an intact epithelium, pushed forward by the underlying oedema. Oedema also produces folds in Descemet's membrane. Granulomatous KPs occur under the disciform or elsewhere. There may be anterior chamber cells and the IOP is often raised.

   b. Necrotizing interstitial keratitis: typically shows intact epithelium, greyish-white stromal patches, corneal thinning, and neovascularization.

   c. Necrotising interstitial keratitis with loss of the epithelium: beware rapid corneal melting. A hypopyon may occur with stromal necrosis or secondary to bacterial superinfection.

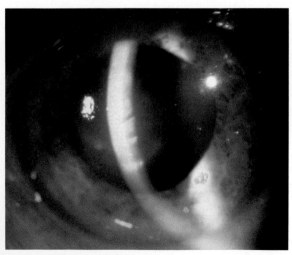

Fig. 5.16: Disciform lesion.

Differential diagnosis

■ Epithelial disease: varicella-zoster keratitis, recurrent corneal erosion, healing abrasion, and contact lens pseudodendrite.

■ Stromal disease: other causes of interstitial keratitis, acanthamoeba, and bacterial keratitis.

Investigations Viral cultures have an approximate 70% recovery rate if taken within 2–3 days and prior to antiviral therapy (only 4% after treatment).

Treatment

■ Lid involvement

In the immunocompetent host, HSV is usually self-limiting. Lid lesions can be treated with warm compresses and Oc. aciclovir 3% t.d.s., or aciclovir 400 mg t.d.s. p.o.

■ Epithelial HSV

1. Debride loose epithelium using topical anaesthetic and a cotton wool swab. Instil G. homatropine 1%, Oc. chloramphenicol and pad overnight. Avoid if there is stromal involvement.

2. Oc. aciclovir 3% five times daily for 14 days or for 7–10 days after healing. Treatment may initially aggravate subepithelial ghosting. This usually fades within a year and does not require steroid therapy.

3. Treat mild uveitis with G. homatropine 1% b.d.

4. While ulceration persists use G. chloramphenicol q.d.s. as prophylaxis against bacterial superinfection.

5. Do not use topical steroids.

■ Stromal HSV

1. Steroids may be unnecessary for disciform HSVK as some episodes resolve spontaneously. Epithelial breakdown during steroid use can lead to rapidly progressive corneal thinning.

2. If steroids are necessary (e.g. failure of antiviral therapy, moderate to severe involvement, raised IOP) use G. prednisolone 1.0% q.d.s. or G. dexamethasone 0.1% q.d.s.

3. Prescribe Oc. aciclovir 5 times daily or aciclovir 400 mg t.d.s.p.o.

4. Prescribe G. chloramphenicol q.d.s. if there is an epithelial defect.

5. Systemic steroids are not useful.

6. If epithelial healing has not occurred within 3 weeks, consider toxic or trophic epithelial defects. Change topical aciclovir to oral, and preserved topical steroids to unpreserved.

7. Infection may be prolonged and damaging in immunocompromised patients.

8. Threatened or actual corneal perforation requires glue or tectonic keratoplasty. Penetrating keratoplasty has a high risk of HSV recurrence and rejection, so defer until the eye is uninflamed and steroid free.

For recurrent corneal epithelial or stromal disease use aciclovir 400 mg b.d. p.o. for 1–2 years as prophylaxis. This reduces recurrences by 50%.

Herpes Zoster Ophthalmicus (Ophthalmic Shingles)

Background Years to decades after primary varicella infection (chickenpox), latent virus in the trigeminal ganglion may reactivate. This produces eye disease and frontal/eyelid/nasal rash (ophthalmic division, V_1).

Symptoms Headache, fever, malaise, chills, and neuralgia. Ask about precipitating factors such as physical trauma, surgery, immunosuppression, and systemic illness.

Signs Multiple sites may be involved.

- Skin/lids: crops of clear vesicles on inflamed hyperaesthetic skin with V_1 distribution, typically occurring 2 days after neuralgia. Vesicular fluid becomes turbid and remains contagious until scabbed (Fig. 5.17). Occasionally dermatitis does not develop.

- Conjunctiva: a follicular or papillary conjunctivitis is extremely common.

- Episclera/sclera: focal inflammation.

- Cornea: keratitis develops in ≈65% of patients, often with a marked decrease in corneal sensation and a varied appearance. Fine or coarse punctate epithelial keratitis occurs. 'Dendrites' differ from those of herpes simplex virus (p. 178) in that they are fine, greyish, nonulcerated, elevated, linear

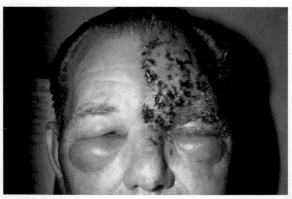

Fig. 5.17: Herpes zoster ophthalmicus (HZO).

lesions that appear painted on (Fig. 5.18). They stain poorly with fluorescein and lack terminal bulbs. Gentle debridement does not produce a fluorescein-staining ulcer, unlike HSV. Coarse, nummular, anterior stromal infiltrates may occur subsequent to epithelial disease. Neurotrophic keratitis occurs in ≈50%. Disciform, necrotic, interstitial or peripheral ulcerative keratitis, or sclerokeratitis may occur.

- Anterior chamber: 40% have cells and flare.

- IOP: may be low, normal, or elevated. Marked elevation occurs in 10% (33% if keratouveitis).

- Fundus: optic neuritis, central retinal vein occlusion, central retinal artery occlusion, necrotizing retinitis (acute retinal necrosis, ARN), thrombophlebitis, localized arteritis ± exudates may occur.

- Cranial nerves: palsies are not uncommon.

Investigations HZO is a clinical diagnosis, but virus may be cultured from vesicles for 3–5 days. Take a careful history to exclude immunocompromise and investigate if suspected.

Acute treatment

- Aciclovir 800 mg 5 times daily p.o. for 7–10 days or famciclovir 500 mg t.d.s. p.o. for 7 days, ideally starting within 72 hours of onset.

- Use skin toilet with or without topical disinfectants to prevent bacterial superinfection.

- For epithelial defects prescribe Oc. chloramphenicol 1% q.d.s.

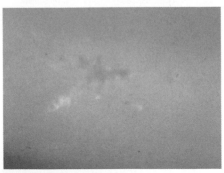

Fig. 5.18: Microdendrites.

- For iritis or moderate to severe disciform disease with intact epithelium use topical steroids commensurate with the severity.

- If HSV is suspected, prescribe Oc. aciclovir 3% five times daily.

- For unstable tear film or exposure keratitis add tear substitutes, e.g. unpreserved hypromellose 0.3% 2-hourly.

- Offer appropriate analgesia and cylcoplegia as required.

- For neurotrophic ulcers consider botulinum toxin protective ptosis or central tarsorrhaphy.

The use of systemic steroids, bandage contact lenses, tissue glue, tarsorrhaphy, and corneal grafts all require senior input, as do immunocompromised patients.

Treatment and follow-up of chronic disease

Corneal anaesthesia recovers fully in 60% in 2–3 months, but 25% develop permanent anaesthesia and neurotrophic keratitis. Disciform immune keratitis responds slowly and may require long-term, low-dose steroids to prevent recurrence. Skin lesions may take weeks to heal, and leave scars.

Post-herpetic neuralgia (neuralgia lasting >6 months or >1 month after the skin heals) may be severe. Consider capsaicin cream 0.025% or 0.075% q.d.s. to affected skin. Burning sensation or erythema occurs in 30%. Capsaicin takes 2–3 weeks for onset of action. Taper frequency when pain relief begins: age <55 years with pain for <3 months, stop 3–5 months after pain relief; age >70 with pain >6 months, continue for 3 years. Restart if pain recurs on cessation. Amitriptyline may help (initially 25–50 mg p.o. nocte, increasing in 25 mg increments every 3–4 days until taking 75–100 mg). If the pain is uncontrolled with these treatments refer to a pain clinic.

Thygeson's Keratitis

Background An uncommon superficial punctate keratitis of unknown aetiology.

Symptoms Intermittent episodes of irritation/foreign body sensation/pain ≈50%, photophobia ≈50%, blurred vision ≈50%, redness ≈15%, and tearing ≈15%. May rarely be asymptomatic

Signs VA is only mildly affected (6/9 or better in ≈80%), and rarely worse than 6/18. Usually bilateral but may be very asymmetrical. The cornea has discrete, elevated, whitish, crumblike epithelial opacities that stain with fluorescein. Subepithelial ghosts may be present. Opacities are mainly in the pupillary area (Fig. 5.19).

Differential diagnosis Viral keratoconjunctivitis, granular dystrophy, and superficial punctate keratopathy.

Treatment Fluorometholone (FML) 0.1% q.d.s. Unresponsive cases may require a stronger steroid, e.g. dexamethasone 0.1% q.d.s. Bandage contact lenses give symptomatic relief as an alternative to steroids.

Follow-up Review at 1 week; if settling, taper steroid slowly. Control of symptoms may require long-term treatment used as necessary. The clinical course is characterized by exacerbations and remissions with a good visual prognosis (corneal scarring and vascularization do not occur). Monitor for complications of long-term steroid use.

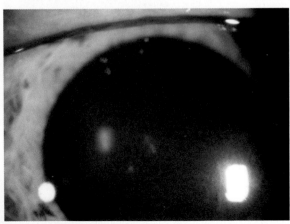

Fig. 5.19: Thygeson's keratitis (Courtesy of SJ Tuft).

Corneal Dystrophies

Predominantly epithelial corneal dystrophies

■ *Epithelial basement membrane dystrophy* (map-dot-fingerprint dystrophy, Cogan's dystrophy): not a true dystrophy. Abnormal attachment between the epithelium and Bowman's layer causes recurrent erosions and persistent epithelial defects. These result in subepithelial 'maps' (geographic opacities), 'dots' (intraepithelial microcysts) and 'fingerprints' (subepithelial ridges) (Fig. 5.20). Any condition with repeated epithelial breakdown may produce a similar clinical picture, e.g. chronic epithelial oedema. Symptoms are usually nocturnal or on waking, varying from mild to severe depending on the size of the erosion. Minor trauma can trigger major epithelial breakdown. The severity of clinical symptoms may not parallel slit lamp findings. Fluorescein may show localized epithelial irregularity and epithelial defects. High-magnification examination of the other eye against the red reflex of a dilated pupil may uncover subtle abnormalities when the affected eye is too uncomfortable to examine in detail. Treat as recurrent

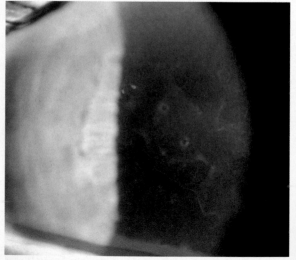

Fig. 5.20: Epithelial basement membrane dystrophy (Courtesy of SJ Tuft).

corneal erosion syndrome with ointment at night to reduce the frequency of exacerbations, bandage contact lenses to stabilize the epithelium, anterior stromal puncture, or excimer laser phototherapeutic keratectomy (PTK) to create focal debridement just into Bowman layer.

▪ *Meesmann's dystrophy* (juvenile familial epithelial dystrophy): rare, autosomal dominant (AD), bilateral epithelial dystrophy that becomes evident in the first few months of life. Small, clear/grey-white bubble-like epithelial opacities occur in both eyes (Fig. 5.21). Bowman's layer is unaffected and there are no associated systemic disorders. The central cornea is more affected than the periphery. Initially asymptomatic, as it slowly progresses symptoms of mild ocular irritation, photophobia, and blurred vision may occur. Basement membrane thickening may cause irregular astigmatism. PTK may be effective initially, but the cysts recur.

Corneal dystrophies of Bowman's layer

▪ *Thiel-Behnke corneal dystrophy* (curly fibre corneal dystrophy, corneal dystrophy of Bowman's layer type II, honeycomb corneal dystrophy, Waardenburg-Jonkers dystrophy): often confused with granular corneal dystrophy (GCD) type III and commonly called Reis-Bückler's dystrophy. AD inheritance. Painful corneal erosions start during childhood. Subepithelial corneal opacities with honeycomb pattern are seen centrally with a clear zone at the corneoscleral junction. Recurrent erosions

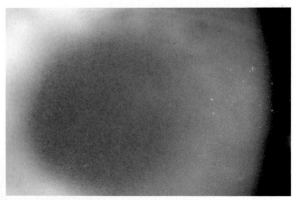

Fig. 5.21: Meesmann's dystrophy (Courtesy of SJ Tuft).

result in subepithelial scarring, irregular astigmatism, and reduced acuity by the second decade. The pathognomonic subepithelial 'curly' fibres can only be identified by transmission electron microscopy of biopsy material. PTK may be effective initially, but deep anterior lamellar keratoplasty (DALK) may be required later. Disease may recur in the graft.

■ For 'true' Reis-Bückler's dystrophy see GCD type III below.

Predominantly stromal corneal dystrophies

■ *Lattice corneal dystrophy* (LCD): Characterized by radially orientated, interdigitating or branching filamentous opacities within the corneal stroma (Fig. 5.22). The lattice lines do not coincide with corneal nerves but relate to linear deposits of amyloid.

  a. LCD type I: recurrent epithelial erosions are common and usually begin during the first decade of life. Inheritance is AD. Although asymmetrical, both corneas contain foci of amyloid scattered throughout the central corneal stroma and sometimes immediately beneath the epithelium. The peripheral cornea remains relatively transparent. Corneal sensation is diminished. The endothelium and Descemet's membrane are spared. LCD I is slowly progressive and usually leads to substantial discomfort and visual impairment before the sixth decade.

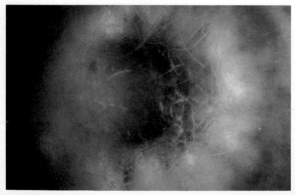

Fig. 5.22: Lattice corneal dystrophy (type I).

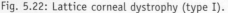

Contact lenses and PTK are often helpful. Results of penetrating keratoplasty (PK) are good, but there may be recurrence in the graft.

b. LCD type II (familial amyloid polyneuropathy type IV – Finnish or Meretoja type; Meretoja syndrome): both corneas contain randomly scattered short, fine, glassy lines that are less numerous, more delicate, and more radially orientated than LCD I. The peripheral cornea is chiefly affected and the central cornea is almost spared. Corneal sensitivity is reduced. Epithelial erosions are not a feature. Inheritance is AD with changes from the second decade, but earlier in homozygous patients. Vision is usually not significantly impaired before age 65 years. Grafts are rarely required. The corneal abnormalities are accompanied by a progressive bilateral neuropathy involving the cranial and peripheral nerves, dysarthria, a dry and lax itchy skin with amyloid deposits in the arteries and sclera. A characteristic masklike expression with protruding lips, pendulous ears and blepharochalasis are also features.

■ *Granular corneal dystrophy* (GCD)

a. GCD type I (classic granular dystrophy, Groenouw type I dystrophy): small white sharply demarcated spots that resemble breadcrumbs or snowflakes become apparent in the central cornea beneath Bowman's layer within the first decade of life (Fig. 5.23). Inheritance is AD. VA gradually decreases and painful RES is common (≈60%). The

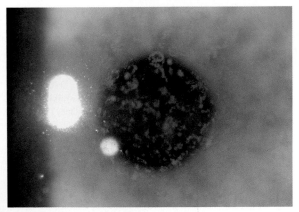

Fig. 5.23: Granular dystrophy (type I).

peripheral 2–3 mm remains clear, as does tissue between the opacities. RES or reduced VA may necessitate excimer PTK. Occasionally DALK or PK is required for deep stromal opacities.

b. GCD type II (GCD with amyloid, Avellino dystrophy, combined lattice–granular dystrophy): less common and severe than GCD I, with onset during the second decade. Inheritance is AD. Corneal opacities are typically shaped like disc, rings, stars and snowflakes. Painful RES (≈15%) occurs especially in women. Contact lenses and PTK are helpful.

c. GCD type III (superficial GCD, 'true' Reis-Bückler's dystrophy, corneal dystrophy of Bowman's layer type I, geographic corneal dystrophy): usually presents in the second and third decades with bilateral painful RES with AD inheritance. Subepithelial deposits typical of GCD type I progress to anterior corneal scarring with an irregular and roughened surface. Visual loss is more pronounced than Thiel-Behnke dystrophy. Corneal sensitivity is reduced or absent. The deep stroma, Descemet's membrane, and endothelium are unaffected.

d. GCD type IV (French GCD): phenotype intermediate between GCD I and GCD III. RES begins in early childhood. Inheritance is AD.

■ *Central crystalline dystrophy* (Schnyder's dystrophy): classically presents early in life with yellow/white ring of needle-shaped, polychromatic crystals in Bowman layer and anterior third of the stroma. The epithelium, Descemet's membrane, and endothelium are normal. Usually stabilizes after childhood, but gradual corneal opacification may reduce the VA to the point where corneal grafting is required. The dystrophy may recur in the graft. May have associated hypercholesterolaemia, xanthelasmata and genu valgum. Inheritance is AD.

■ *Macular corneal dystrophy* (Groenouw type II dystrophy): autosomal recessive disease that usually begins in the first decade of life. Irregular greyish-white opacities with indistinct edges appear within a hazy corneal stroma. Initially central and superficial, the opacities gradually merge causing progressive clouding of the peripheral and deep stroma. There is primary involvement of Descemet's membrane with corneal thinning and endothelial guttata (fine wartlike endothelial excrescences). Visual impairment occurs by the fifth decade. Three immunotypes (I, IA, and II) appear similar clinically. PK may become necessary. Rarely there is subclinical recurrence in the graft.

Posterior corneal dystrophies

■ *Congenital hereditary endothelial dystrophy (CHED)* (hereditary corneal oedema): diffuse, bilateral, symmetrical corneal oedema varies from milky ground glass opacification to mild haze (Fig. 5.24). May have epithelial microbullae and thickening of Descemet's membrane. There are no guttata, interstitial inflammation, or neovascularization. Check IOP. If the cornea doesn't clear when raised IOP is normalized, suspect concomitant CHED. Type I (AD) progresses slowly to manifest during the first 2 years of life with photophobia and tearing and no associated ocular or systemic abnormalities. Type II (infantile hereditary endothelial dystrophy) is autosomal recessive and becomes manifest at, or shortly after, birth and is associated with nystagmus.

■ *Posterior polymorphous corneal dystrophy*: Asymmetric, vesicular or annular opacities with surrounding halos are seen at the level of Descemet's membrane. There is no stromal oedema or vascularization (Fig. 5.25). May have peripheral anterior synechiae. Usually asymptomatic with preserved VA but sometimes progresses slowly from teens. AD inheritance. If grafting is required, disease may recur in graft.

■ *Fuchs' endothelial dystrophy* (late hereditary endothelial dystrophy): although AD, there is poor penetrance and most

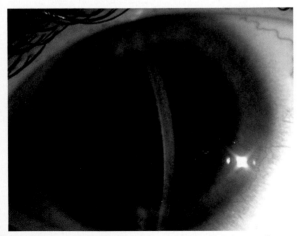

Fig. 5.24: Congenital hereditary endothelial dystrophy (Courtesy of SJ Tuft).

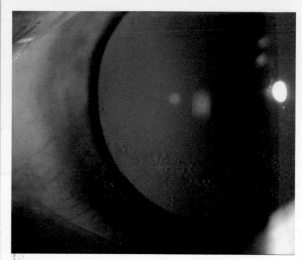

Fig. 5.25: Posterior polymorphous corneal dystrophy (Courtesy of SJ Tuft).

patients lack a family history. Patients present in their fifth to sixth decades with irritation or blurred vision, often worse on waking. Females predominate, 3:1. Endothelial dysfunction produces stromal oedema that starts axially and spreads peripherally (Fig. 5.26). Subsequent epithelial involvement causes painful ruptured bullae with fibrovascular pannus. The endothelium typically has a beaten-metal appearance with pigmented guttata. Nonpigmented guttata may also occur with degenerative corneal disease, trauma, or inflammation. Nonprogressive guttata in the peripheral cornea of young patients (Hassall Henle bodies) may be AD inherited and are of no clinical significance. Pachymetry in Fuchs' dystrophy shows corneal thickening; specular microscopy shows increasing polymegethism and polymorphism. Treatment includes G. hypertonic sodium chloride 5% q.d.s. to dehydrate the epithelium, and tear substitutes for surface irritation. Intraocular surgery may accelerate disease progression, so take precautions (p. 259). Bandage contact lenses may relieve discomfort but should be used with caution, due to the high risk of microbial keratitis. Ruptured bullae can be treated as corneal erosions (p. 153). Ultimately, PK or endothelial keratoplasty (posterior lamellar keratoplasty) are required for vision and comfort. The dystrophy does not recur in the graft.

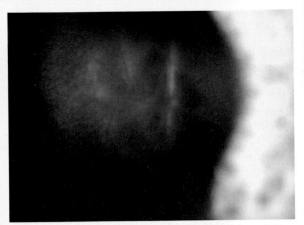

Fig. 5.26: Fuchs' endothelial dystrophy (Courtesy of SJ Tuft).

Pterygium

Background Conjunctival overgrowth onto the cornea, typically in young to middle-aged patients, with a male preponderance. There may be history of exposure to high ultraviolet levels, wind, and low humidity, e.g. outdoor work in hot dry climates.

Signs A fleshy triangular growth encroaches a variable distance onto the cornea, with the base arising from the conjunctiva (Fig. 5.27). The lesion is usually on the horizontal meridian, particularly the nasal side, and may be inflamed. There may be subepithelial scarring or iron deposition at the apex (Stocker's line), and dellen with elevated pterygia. Measure the distance onto the cornea.

Differential diagnosis

- *Goldenhar's syndrome* (oculoauriculovertebral dysplasia): page 79.

- *Inflammatory pannus*: usually less bulky, often not on the horizontal meridian, and often associated with ocular rosacea and underlying corneal thinning.

- *Dysplasia*: abnormal epithelium arising from the limbus does not have a triangular shape.

Treatment Use sunglasses to reduce exposure to sunlight. Treat ocular irritation with tear substitutes. If inflamed, try G. fluorometholone 0.1% q.d.s. for 1 month. Excise, or avulse, with

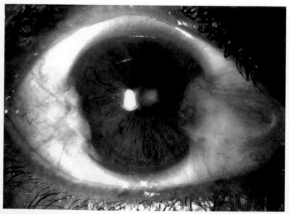

Fig. 5.27: Pterygium.

conjunctival autografting if symptoms are uncontrolled by conservative therapy or when there is encroachment into the visual axis. Send specimens for histology.

Follow-up If asymptomatic, review as necessary. If on topical steroids, check IOP in 4–6 weeks. Taper by one drop per fortnight when inflammation settles, then see as required.

Band Keratopathy

Background Calcium deposits in the basement membrane, Bowman's layer, and anterior corneal stroma. Associated with various ocular diseases including chronic low-grade uveitis (10–50% of juvenile chronic arthritis), corneal dystrophies (posterior polymorphous and CHED), phthisis, silicone oil keratopathy, prolonged glaucoma, and longstanding corneal oedema. Metabolic causes include hypercalcaemia and hyperphosphataemia (Fig. 5.28). Band keratopathy (BK) may also be inherited (juvenile and mature type) or idiopathic.

History and examination BK is a sign not a diagnosis. Take a full ocular and systemic history and examine for underlying causes. The amorphous pale grey deposits are seen peripherally in the anterior cornea, mainly in the palpebral aperture. With time, the central cornea becomes affected. There is a transparent limbal zone.

Investigations Consider serum calium phosphate if there is no obvious ocular disease to account for BK.

Treatment

▪ Manage the underlying condition.

▪ *Mild irritation*: topical lubricants.

▪ *Moderate irritation:* bandage contact lens and preservative-free topical lubricants.

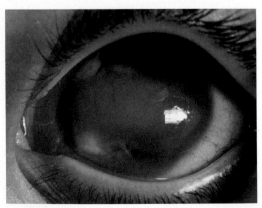

Fig. 5.28: Band keratopathy in an eye with buphthalmos (Courtesy of DH Verity).

■ *Severe irritation and reduced VA*: superficial keratectomy ± ethylene diamino tetra acetic acid chelation (EDTA), or excimer phototherapeutic keratectomy (PTK).

Follow-up Review 3–12 months, depending on the symptoms and underlying cause.

Corneal Degenerations and Deposits

Climatic droplet keratopathy (spheroid degeneration of the cornea, Labrador keratopathy, Bietti's keratopathy, pearl diver keratopathy) (Fig. 5.29). Occurs mainly in men who work outdoors due to exposure to ultraviolet light. Early on, fine subepithelial yellow droplets form superficially in the peripheral cornea. Later, droplets become central with subsequent corneal clouding and reduced vision. Excimer phototherapeutic keratectomy (PTK) may be necessary.

Terrien's marginal degeneration See page 164.

Band keratopathy See page 196.

Lipid keratopathy Extracellular lipid deposition from corneal vessels (Fig. 5.30). May be idiopathic or associated with previous keratitis or disordered lipid metabolism (e.g. fish-eye syndrome).

Saltzmann's nodular degeneration Degeneration of the superficial cornea involving the epithelium, Bowman's layer, and stroma preceded by chronic corneal inflammation. Patients may complain of red eyes, irritation, and blurred vision. Bluish-white nodules of amyloid result in irregular astigmatism (Fig. 5.31). Treat

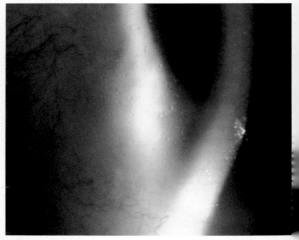

Fig. 5.29: Climatic droplet keratopathy (Courtesy of SJ Tuft).

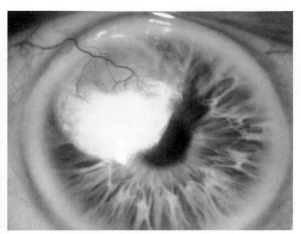

Fig. 5.30: Lipid keratopathy from herpes keratitis (Courtesy of SJ Tuft).

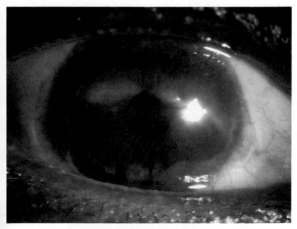

Fig. 5.31: Salzmann's nodular degeneration (Courtesy of SJ Tuft).

the underlying cause. Consider superficial keratectomy ± PTK. A lamellar graft is rarely required. The disease may recur.

Corneal degenerations and deposits not requiring treatment

Arcus senilis (corneal annulus, anterior embryotoxon) Extremely common, bilateral, benign, peripheral corneal degeneration. Appears as a hazy grey ring ≈2 mm in diameter with a lucent zone between it and the limbus (Fig. 5.32). Caused by lipid droplets in all layers of the cornea, especially the anterior and deep stroma. Check lipids in those under the age of 50; otherwise, no treatment is required.

Kayser-Fleischer ring Copper deposition immediately superficial to Descemet's membrane, 1–3 mm inside the limbus – usually only visible with gonioscopy. Variable colour: brown, ruby red, bright green, blue, or yellow. Associated with hepatolenticular degeneration (Wilson's disease) and chronic hepatobiliary disease. Disappears with penicillamine treatment used to treat the systemic disease.

Fleischer ring Accumulation of ferritin within and between basal epithelial cells at the base of a keratoconus cone.

Vortex keratopathy (vortex corneal dystrophy, corneal verticillata of Fleischer, hurricane keratopathy, striate melanokeratosis). Pigmented whorl-shaped lines in the epithelium (Fig. 5.33). Associated with chloroquine, indomethacin, amiodarone, phenothiazine (e.g. chlorpromazine), tamoxifen use and clofazimine toxicity. Seen in Fabry's disease (X-linked recessive) and asymptomatic female carriers, so examine family members if there is no drug cause.

Hudson-Stähli line Horizontal iron deposition line at the junction of the lower and middle thirds of the cornea

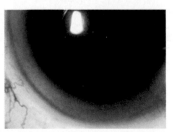

Fig. 5.32: Arcus senilis.

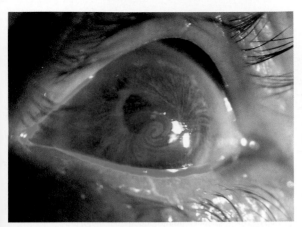

Fig. 5.33: Vortex keratopathy.

corresponding to the line of lid closure. A normal occurrence in the elderly.

Ferry's line Iron deposition line adjacent to limbal filtering blebs.

Stocker's line Iron line at the apex of a pterygium.

Phototherapeutic keratectomy An iron deposition line may occur at the perimeter of treatment.

Haemosiderin Golden-brown stromal deposits following large hyphaema with prolonged raised IOP. Tends to resolve with time.

Corneal farinata Small grey punctate opacities seen pre-Descemet's membrane in the elderly. Does not affect VA. May be associated with ichthyosis and keratoconus. Sometimes larger, more polymorphous types of comma, circular and dotlike opacities are seen.

Limbal girdle of Vogt Involves the interpalpebral, superficial stroma. Type I has no clear zone at the limbus with chalky-white deposits due to actinic damage. Type II has a clear zone at the limbus with lucent areas in superficial opacity. May be indistinguishable from early band keratopathy.

Corneal Graft Rejection

Background Immunologically mediated graft rejection may occur at any time but most often within 2 years of penetrating keratoplasty (PK). It may affect any part of the graft. Monitor corneal thickness and carefully document all keratic precipitates (KPs). If the cornea thickens, new KPs appear (with or without uveitis), then start treatment as per endothelial rejection (see below). Treat stromal and endothelial rejection as an emergency.

Epithelial rejection A slightly raised linear opacity, confined to the epithelium, starts peripherally and migrates centrally over several days (Fig. 5.34). Mild perilimbal injection may be present but there are usually few symptoms. Complete by 3 weeks postgrafting. No change in treatment or review schedule is required as it seldom leads to endothelial rejection.

Subepithelial rejection May occur up to 1 year following PK. Small, round, subepithelial infiltrates in Bowman's layer are confined to the graft (Krachmer spots). There may be mild irritation and photophobia, KPs, flare and AC cells, and mild perilimbal injection. Although unlikely to induce endothelial rejection, treat with topical steroids to speed resolution of the infiltrates, e.g. G. prednisolone 0.5% q.d.s., until inflammation is resolved, then taper gradually.

Stromal rejection Only 1–2% of rejections. Rapidly spreading, dense, even infiltrate affecting all stromal layers, but confined to the graft. Vascularization occurs late. Treat as per endothelial rejection.

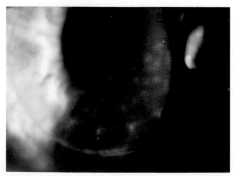

Fig. 5.34: Epithelial graft rejection.

Endothelial rejection Carries potential for irreversible damage to the endothelium and subsequent corneal decompensation (Fig. 5.35). Two patterns occur:

■ *Focally progressive* (25–45% of rejections): begins at the graft host junction. Cytotoxic lymphocytes from marginal vessels then form an advancing demarcation line (Khodadoust line) with clear cornea centrally and stromal oedema behind it. KPs, cells and flare are present. The differential diagnosis includes diffuse rejection, suture abscess, and epithelial ingrowth (usually occurs later and without uveitis or stromal swelling behind the line).

■ *Diffuse* (25–45% of rejections): tends to occur later than focally progressive cases. Variable severity. Cytotoxic lymphocytes from the uvea result in AC cells and flare. KPs are confined to the graft endothelium. The graft may be oedematous or remain clear if there is only mild rejection. The differential diagnosis includes anterior uveitis (KPs not confined to graft, more AC cells), herpes simplex keratitis, raised IOP (no new KPs, AC quiet). Treat as follows:

1. Admit if compliance with treatment is likely to be poor.

2. Intensive topical steroids (e.g. G. prednisolone 1.0% hourly 0600 to 2400 hours, then Oc. dexamethasone 0.1% nocte, or hourly day and night for severe cases).

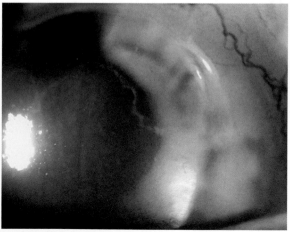

Fig. 5.35: Endothelial corneal graft rejection.

3. Cycloplegia (e.g. G. homatropine 1.0% b.d.)

4. Systemic steroids if not responding within 24–48 hours, or if recurrent episode (e.g. prednisolone 40–80 mg o.d. p.o. with ranitidine 150 mg b.d. p.o.)

5. Control IOP if raised (e.g. acetazolamide SR 250 mg b.d. p.o).

6. Review every 3–7 days until there are signs of improvement, then taper steroids.

Anterior Segment Trauma

Background Common traumatic ocular injuries described elsewhere include corneal abrasion (p. 150), angle recession (p. 313), uveitis (p. 335), retinal commotio, tears and ruptured globe (p. 551), and optic neuropathy (p. 661). If an injury results from an alleged assault or workplace injury, carefully document the timing and circumstances of the injury and measure or preferably photograph all wounds. Consider tetanus prophylaxis.

Conjunctival laceration

Look for a laceration with rolled or retracted edges and foreign bodies (FBs). Prolapsed Tenon's capsule appears white and oedematous. Brown pigment suggests a scleral laceration and prolapse of uveal tissue. Be aware of the potential for involvement of the extraocular muscles or of a scleral perforation obscured by subconjunctival haemorrhage. Remove FBs and prolapsed Tenon's capsule. Small, clean conjunctival lacerations require no suturing. Prescribe Oc. chloramphenicol q.d.s. 1 week. Larger (>15 mm,) more complex lacerations may require suturing with interrupted 8/0 Vicryl. Avoid suturing the plica or caruncle. Be careful to appose the conjunctiva rather than Tenon's capsule. If sutured, review at 1 week.

Corneal laceration

History Pain, red eye, foreign body sensation, watering eye, and reduced vision.

Examination If the globe is ruptured, pressure on the globe may risk further ocular injury, so avoid tonometry, gonioscopy, and indented fundoscopy. Note the site, location, extent, and depth of the corneal wound. Siedel testing (p. 147) may be negative with full-thickness shelving wounds that self-seal. Note the anterior chamber depth, cellular activity, and any hyphaema. Look for pupil irregularity or iris prolapse through the wound. Traumatic mydriasis is common. Test for an RAPD due to traumatic optic neuropathy or retinal detachment. The IOP may be low, normal, or elevated. Dilate and examine the posterior pole and periphery.

Management

- *Partial thickness*: anaesthetize e.g. G. proxymetacaine 0.5%, and remove any debris. Only suture gaping wounds, in theatre, with 10/0 Nylon.

■ *Full thickness*: apply a protective shield and prescribe antiemetic if required. Treat clean, self-sealing, full-thickness lacerations with prophylactic oral antibiotics (ciprofloxacin 750 mg b.d. p.o. for adults; co-amoxiclav t.d.s. for children) and topical G. chloramphenicol 0.5% q.d.s. for five days. Treat minimally leaking lacerations with a bandage contact lens and G. unpreserved chloramphenicol 0.5% q.d.s. Leaking full-thickness lacerations require debridement and suturing (10/0 Nylon) in theatre. Admit, nil by mouth, except for prophylactic oral antibiotics. For more extensive damage, treat as a ruptured globe (p. 553).

Follow-up Review daily until the epithelium heals. Stop topical and oral antibiotics at 1 week if settled. Explain the symptoms of retinal detachment, endophthalmitis, and sympathetic ophthalmia, with advice to attend promptly if these develop.

Contact Lenses

Background The fitting and review of contact lenses for low refractive errors is predominantly carried out by community optometrists. In the UK, hospitals generally review contact lens problems or fit lenses for more complex indications such as:

- Refractive: high myopia (>10D); aphakia; postcorneal graft; anisometropia; anisekonia; high hypermetropia (>5.00D); irregular astigmatism (keratoconus); postinfective keratitis; postrefractive surgery.

- Therapeutic: 'bandage lenses' are used for pain relief by covering rough or unstable epithelium, to mechanically protect the ocular surface, maintain corneal hydration, or tamponade leaking wounds. Common examples include recurrent erosion syndrome, bullous keratopathy, keratinized lids, misdirected eye lashes, and corneal exposure.

- Cosmetic: aniridia; scars; albinism; iris coloboma; unable to wear glasses due to facial deformity.

Abbreviations

- RGP rigid gas permeable (hard) contact lens.
- BVD back vertex distance.
- BVP back vertex power.
- BOZR back optical zone radius (back radius).
- TD total diameter (diameter).

History Ask about:

1. Lens type:

   - *Material*: RGP or soft. Soft lenses are usually hydrogel but silicone hydrogel (SiH) and silicone rubber (SiR) are sometimes used.

   - *Size*: corneal or scleral.

   - *Mode of wear*: daily disposable, frequent replacement (e.g. weekly, monthly or 3 monthly) or longer use.

2. Pattern of wear: average wearing time per day (in hours) and number of days per week, any overnight wear and if so the number of nights, maximum wearing time per day, contact lens wearing time on the day of consultation and/or if the lens was removed before the consultation, how many hours previously.

3. Cleaning regimen: typical routine is: remove the contact lens from the eye, 'rub' (clean), rinse, overnight disinfection and storage, rinse, then replace on the eye. All-In-one solutions are widely used but for patients who react to them recommend separate solutions for each step. Common cleaning solutions include surfactant cleaners, e.g. Miraflow (Ciba) or LC65 (Allergan), and, for rigid lenses, polymeric beads (Boston cleaner by Bausch & Lomb). Saline is often used for rinsing. Disinfecting may involve unpreserved cold chemicals, e.g. hydrogen peroxide with neutralization in the morning (2-step, the 'gold standard'), or 1-step peroxide systems. Storage cases should be rinsed daily and air dried, scrubbed with a brush and boiled weekly, and replaced at least 3 monthly. Protein deposits can be removed with enzyme tablets. Always wash and dry hands before handling lenses. Never use tap water (risk of acanthamoeba keratitis).

4. Use of topical medications: preservatives may lead to ocular surface toxicity.

5. Any adverse symptoms (Table 5.3).

Examination Note the contact lens fit (see below), the presence of scratches and deposits, and wetting. Remove the lens and examine the eye for the common contact lens-related problems shown in Table 5.3. Evert the eyelid to check for papillae.

Investigations Arrange corneal topography if there is suspected corneal warpage or early keratoconus.

Fitting a contact lens The aim is to fit a lens that optimizes VA, is stable on the cornea, produces minimal ocular surface disruption, and is comfortable. A good fit depends upon the lens diameter, back radius, and design. Begin by measuring refraction, keratometry (K), ± topography (p. 148). Choose the lens type (RGP, soft, combination, scleral). If the cylinder is ≤1.0 D it is appropriate to use soft lenses, but if >1.0 D use a rigid lens, toric soft lens, or rarely a soft lens with spectacle astigmatic correction. Trial diagnostic contact lenses are used to find the best fit.

■ Soft lens

1. Select a trial lens with a TD slightly larger than the corneal diameter, e.g. 14.0 mm.

2. Select the BOZR, typically 8.7.

3. Select the power, as close to refraction as possible, correcting for BVD.

Table 5.3: Adverse symptoms

Diagnosis	Symptoms	Corneal signs	Other signs	Treatment
Microbial keratitis	Pain, watering, photophobia, red eye, purulent discharge	Ulceration Cellular infiltrate	Severe injection Limbal > diffuse ± AC activity ± hypopyon	See p. 171
Sterile marginal keratitis	Pain, watering, photophobia, red eye	Small, peripheral, superficial, round infiltrate(s). Epithelium may break down later	Variable – moderate injection adjacent to infiltrate	Remove lens Topical steroid e.g. G. prednisolone 0.5% q.d.s. for 2 weeks. See p. 170
Corneal abrasion	Sudden onset pain, watering, red eye, photophobia	Linear or geographic epithelial break No infiltrate	Variable – moderate injection Limbal > diffuse	See p. 150
Papillary conjunctivitis	Irritation / itching, clear mucus discharge. May be asymptomatic.	None / mild superficial punctuate keratopathy	Variable – moderate, diffuse injection Mild to 'giant' tarsal papillae	Review CL hygiene, frequency of lens replacement, the lens material and fit. See p. 124
Toxic epitheliopathy /hypersensitivity	Irritation, maximal immediately after lens insertion	Diffuse punctate epithelial erosions	Variable – moderate injection Limbal > diffuse	Stop lens wear or change lens and solution(s)

209

Limbal metaplasia	Irritation, lens intolerance	Opaque limbal epithelium may extend onto cornea ± superficial neovascularization	Mild limbal injection	Stop lens wear if possible. Change to unpreserved solutions and drops.
Chronic epithelial microcystic epitheliopathy	None/ mild irritation	Epithelial microcysts. Normal stroma and no infiltrate	Normal conjunctiva	None or preservative free topical lubricants
Surface irritation	None/ mild irritation	Superficial neovascularization	Normal conjunctiva	Review lens fit and cleaning regimen. Increase lens DK (oxygen transmission).
Acute hypoxic epitheliopathy	Pain, watering, photophobia, red eye (several hours after lens removal). May progressively worsen after lens insertion	Central punctate epithelial erosions ± epithelial loss ± oedema	Variable – moderate injection Limbal > diffuse	Omit lens, reduce wearing time, choose lens with increased DK
Hypoxic stromal oedema	None / blurred vision	Stromal oedema ± Descemet's folds	Normal conjunctiva	Stop lens wear if possible Increase lens DK
Hypoxic neovascularization	None / blurred vision	Deep neovascularization ± corneal oedema ± lipid deposition	Variable – moderate injection Limbal injection	Stop lens wear if possible Increase lens DK
Corneal warpage	Good contact lens vision, poor vision with glasses	Irregular topography	Normal conjunctiva	Refit lenses Topography usually normalises

4. Fit the lens, wait 20 minutes, then assess fit without fluorescein.

   a. *Satisfactory fit*: well centred, lens moves freely on digital displacement but not more than 0.5 mm on blinking.

   b. *Tight/steep fit*: lens indents conjunctiva, poor movement on blink or upgaze, poor tear exchange, or bubbles under the lens.

   c. *Loose/flat fit*: moves >0.5 mm on blinking, poor centration, or unstable vision. Try increasing the TD in 0.5 mm steps if the lens does not centre well.

5. Specify (prescribe) the material or lens manufacturer, lens type, side (L/R), BOZR, TD, power, any tint (e.g. Coopervision; Proclear Biocompatibles; L; 8.60 : 14.20 : +15.50. tint: blue).

■ Hard lens

1. Start with a TD of 9.5–10 mm.

2. Select a BOZR equal to the flatter K reading for most aspheric lens designs.

3. Select power as close to refraction as possible, correcting for BVD.

4. Insert the lens, wait until reflex lacrimation has abated, then instil fluorescein 2% and assess the fit. Ask the patient to blink normally a few times to spread the dye.

   a. Satisfactory fit: the lens lies within the limbus in all directions of gaze with ≈0.5 mm of movement on blinking. At the periphery there should be a 0.5 mm halo of fluorescein clearance with the tear meniscus. On a regular cornea there should be an even spread, or slight pooling of fluorescein centrally (Fig. 5.36). Fluorescein should circulate under the lens within a few blinks.

   b. Astigmatic fit: steep fit in one meridian, flat fit in the orthogonal meridian.

5. Specify: lens manufacturer, lens model, material, side (R/L), BOZR, TD, power, any marks, or tint (e.g. CIBA, Aspheric, Boston XO, R 7.70: 9.70: +14.00, engrave R, tint blue).

When the correct fit is achieved with a hard or soft lens, perform subjective over-refraction using a spectacle trial frame and

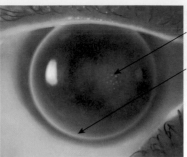

Central alignment
with slight pooling

Edge clearance with
tear meniscus

Fig. 5.36: Rigid contact lens fitting example.

document the VA. The final contact lens power will be the sum of contact lens power + spectacle power. If the latter is ≥4.0D, correct for BVD using standard tables.

Special situations

- *High myopia*: patients usually have large flat corneas; use lenses with a high oxygen transmissibility (e.g. Boston XO) or high water content. Silicone hydrogels are currently not available in high powers.

- *Adult aphakia*: negative RGP lenses may drop so negative edge carriers, high axial edge lift designs, larger diameters, etc. are frequently needed. Use lenses with high oxygen transmissibility (e.g. Boston XO) or high water content. Silicone hydrogels are currently not available in high positive powers.

- *Keratoconus*: consider corneal topography, degree of corneal toricity, and degree of ametropia. The corrected VA must be balanced with lens tolerance and effect on corneal integrity. Start with an RGP designed for keratoconus (e.g. Woodward KC3 or Rose K). Look for a good fit with fluorescein but some apical touch is likely. With highly protrusive or markedly decentred cones, some compromise is likely, but look for a lens that offers good VA, stays in on most gaze excursions, avoids indenting the cornea, and minimizes corneal contact. Figures 5.37–5.40 show examples of lens fits and management options in keratoconus.

- *Following penetrating keratoplasty*: use the flatter K for initial estimate of base curve. Bespoke multi-curve RGP lenses frequently 10 mm to 12 mm in diameter are usually used. 'Reverse-geometry' RGP lenses are sometimes required for flat central corneal shapes.

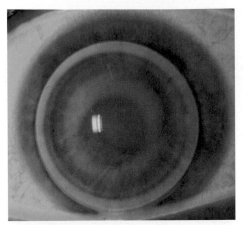

Fig. 5.37: Contact lens fitting example. *Fit*: Acceptable fit (regular three-point touch) with apical contact (blue), deep mid-peripheral pool (green), and peripheral contact zone (blue) (Courtesy KW Pullum). *Management*: No change, but apical contact could be eased with a steeper BOZR and using a lens design with a smaller BOZD could ease the annular peripheral contact.

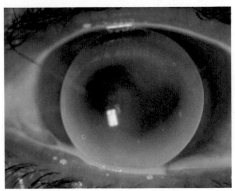

Fig. 5.38: Contact lens fitting example. *Fit*: Flat fit with heavy apical contact, excessive edge clearance and 'stand off' inferiorly (Courtesy KW Pullum). *Management*: Needs a steeper BOZR, larger BOZD.

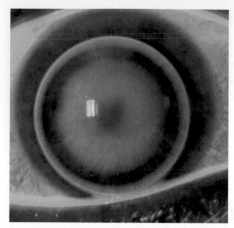

Fig. 5.39: Contact lens fitting example. *Fit*: Ideal edge clearance with ≈0.5 mm bandwidth, glancing contact apically, but excessive peripheral contact zone. *Management*: Flatten central BOZR, or reduce BOZD, smaller TD.

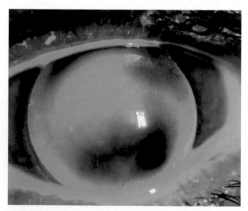

Fig. 5.40: Contact lens fitting example. *Fit*: Decentred apex with hard touch, irregular excessive edge clearance. Bottom edge of lens resting on the lower eye lid. *Management*: Difficult to improve corneal fit, if unstable try a scleral lens.

■ *Presbyopia*: For those aged ≥40, single vision lenses seldom provide adequate depth of focus. The usual solution is a contact lens distance correction and reading spectacles, varifocal, or bifocal over-correction. Alternatives include monovision (dominant eye focused for distance, other for near – but this can interfere with binocular vision) and multifocal contact lens (these tend to reduce low contrast vision).

Choosing a therapeutic contact lens

■ Choice: First → Last

Pain relief: Hydrogel → SiH → Limbal RGP → Scleral

Epithelial healing: SiH → Hydrogel → Limbal RGP → Scleral

Perforation: SiH → Hydrogel → Limbal RGP → Scleral

Sensitive eye: Hydrogel → SiH → Limbal RGP → Scleral

Ease of fit: Hydrogel → SiH → Limbal RGP → Scleral

■ Severity: Mild → Severe

Hydrogel → SiH → Limbal RGP → Scleral

(Suitable for exposure, dry eye, corneal protection, irregular astigmatism)

Useful lenses First choice contacts lenses include:

■ Irregular corneas, mild to moderate dry eye: Proclear Biocompatables (Coopervison) 8.60:14.20

■ Steep corneas (Proclear too loose): D75 (e.g. Cantor & Nissel) 8.00:15.00 or 7.80:13.50

■ Large corneas, unstable lens fit, limbal or scleral defects: D75 9.50:16.50, M&L 75 (e.g. Cantor & Nissel) 8.60:18.00 or 8.80:20.00

■ Persistent epithelial defect, leaking wounds: Purevision (Bausch & Lomb) 8.60:14.00 or Night & Day (CIBA Vision) 8.40 & 8.60:13.80

Laser Refractive Surgery

Background Excimer laser refractive surgery procedures are commonly used to correct myopia, hypermetropia and astigmatism. In the UK, this is predominantly undertaken in the private sector, but treatment can influence the management of conditions seen in the NHS, e.g. cataract and glaucoma. Some post operative complications may present acutely to the accident and emergency department e.g. dislocated LASIK flaps or deep lamellar keratitis. A basic understanding is therefore worthwhile.

Basic principles Excimer (excited dimer) laser photoablation can be used to remove corneal tissue with submicron accuracy without thermal build up or adjacent tissue damage. Myopia can be corrected by removing tissue from the central cornea resulting in central flattening and reduced refractive power. In hyperopia tissue is removed from the peripheral cornea resulting in steepening of the central cornea and increased refractive power.

Contraindications Relative ocular contraindications include severe dry eyes, severe atopy, keratoconus, previous herpetic keratitis, neurotrophic corneas and nystagmus.

Relative systemic contraindications include collagen vascular diseases, pregnancy, hormone replacement therapy, and immunocompromise e.g. HIV infection.

Surgical techniques There are three main procedures (Table 5.4): Photorefractive keratectomy (PRK), laser assisted in situ keratomileusis (LASIK) and laser subepthelial keratomileusis (LASEK). All three are performed under topical anaestheasia.

■ PRK

PRK involves removal of the corneal epithelium followed by photoablation of Bowman's layer and the anterior stroma. After treatment a bandage contact lens (BCL) is inserted. Mild to severe foreign body (FB) sensation is normal for 3–4 days post operatively until the corneal surface has re-epithelialised. PRK is safe and effective for correcting low myopic refractive errors. The use of PRK is limited by the corneal wound healing response causing corneal haze, with subsequent reduced contrast sensitivity and Snellen acuity, and unpredictable refractive regression.

■ LASIK

A hinged flap is cut in the anterior stroma with a mechanical microkeratome attached to the eye with a suction ring. The

Table 5.4: Efficacy and safety of excimer laser refractive procedures

Parameters	PRK	LASIK	LASEK
Technique	Surface ablation	Intrastromal ablation	Surface ablation
Refractive predictability (± 1 D)	91%	98%	98%
Refractive stability	1–3 months	2–3 weeks	3–4 weeks
Visual recovery	3–7 days	24 hours	3–7 days
Postoperative pain	Moderate, 24–48 hours	Very mild, 12 hours	Mild, 24–48 hours
Postoperative topical steroids	3 weeks to 3 months	1–2 weeks	3 weeks to 3 months
Significant intraoperative complications	Rare	Flap related problems (0.3 %)	Rare
Postoperative complications	Corneal haze (1–2%)	Flap and interface problems (4%), infectious keratitis (1:7500), epithelial ingrowth (<1%), diffuse lamellar keratitis (<1%), dry eyes, keratectasia	Corneal haze
Recovery from dry eyes	4 weeks to 6 months	Up to 12 months	4 weeks to 6 months

flap is usually 120–180 μm thick and 8–9 mm in diameter. The hinge may be superior or nasal. The flap is lifted and the excimer laser treatment applied to the exposed stromal bed. The flap is then repositioned. Visual recovery is rapid and stable. There is minimal damage to the epithelium so post operative FB sensation is mild and short lived. Haze is only seen at the periphery of the flap where Bowman's layer has been cut. However, the procedure is technically more challenging with the risk of intraoperative and post operative flap related complications and post operative ectasia if a residual stromal bed of ≤250 μm has not been left, or the patient had *forme fruste* keratoconus pre operatively.

■ LASEK (epi LASIK)

LASEK/epiLASIK are modifications of PRK that preserve the epithelial sheet. The epithelium is peeled back with a modified mechanical keratome (epiLASIK) or manually after application of 20% ethanol (LASEK). The excimer laser treatment is applied to the stromal bed. The epithelium is then repositioned and a bandage lens applied to protect the epithelium while it heals. The retention of the epithelium is said to reduce post operative pain and increase the rate of visual recovery. The problem of haze formation with surface ablations is thought to be reduced, at least in the short term, by the intraoperative application of Mitomycin C.

Outcomes

■ Results obtained with different lasers and microkeratomes are not directly comparable

■ Excimer laser refractive procedures are safe and effective for the correction of mild to moderate myopia. The predictablility decreses in high myopia (>8D), hypermetropia >4D, astigmatism >3D, and therapeutic treatments e.g. correction of post peretrating keratoplasty astigmatism.

■ Better understanding and treatment of corneal wound healing, the use of wavefront guided treatments and iris recognition are leading to improved clinical outcomes.

■ Dislocated or wrinkled flaps of short duration can be floated back into position in the operating theatre. If this is not possible referral to a corneal surgeon for suturing is advised. Amputation of the flap may be necessary.

■ Following LASIK the interface between the flap and the stroma may become inflamed (deep lamellar keratitis, DLK). DLK may occur in the immediate post operative period or later in response to epithelial abrasion or superficial infection. The triggering event should be treated and frequent topical steroids applied unless otherwise contraindicated e.g. G prednisolone 1.0% 6 times daily. As the inflammation settles, steroids can be tapered off.

- Interface infection is rare and often caused by low virulence organisms e.g. *Mycobacteria*. Emergency treatment is required. It may be necessary to lift the flap to obtain material for culture and sensitivity testing (p. 172). Frequent, fortified broad spectrum topical antibiotics should be applied. Amikacin is particularly useful for its activity against low virulence organisms e.g. *Nocardia*, *Mycobacteria*. Amputation of the flap may be necessary.

- Epithelial ingrowth is unusual unless the flap has been lifted for retreatment. Refer back to the treating surgeon.

- Most keratometers and topography systems assume that the cornea has a spherical profile with a constant relationship between the anterior and posterior corneal surfaces. Following excimer refractive surgery these assumptions no longer hold true. As a consequence conventional biometry is inaccurate. Following treatment for myopia biometry tends to underestimate IOL power required, resulting in post operative hypermetropia. Following refractive surgery advanced biometric calculations are required.

Optometry and General Practice Guidelines

General comments

The most urgent corneal referral is microbial keratitis. A lesion close to the centre of the cornea is especially dangerous. Compared to conjunctivitis, there is less likely to be a history of contact with eye infection or systemic viral features such as a sore throat, and more likely to be history of pain, reduced vision, contact lens wear, or preexisting corneal disease. Look for a white infiltrate and focal fluorescein staining. Corneal scrapes taken prior to antibiotic therapy have a higher yield, so if microbial keratitis is suspected refer without starting treatment. Conjunctival swabs have a low yield in corneal infection. Advise contact lens wearers to bring their lenses, solutions, and cases for testing.

Immediately refer patients with corneal grafts if they notice blurred vision, inflammation, or pain, as the risk of rejection lasts for life.

Optometrists

Patients with corneal diseases and poor spectacle-corrected acuity may have irregular astigmatism. A marked improvement may be achieved by fitting a contact lens but also consider early keratoconus. Tear film abnormalities may cause visual changes when the patient concentrates and the blink rate reduces, such as when driving or reading. Tear substitutes such as hypromellose are available over the counter but treat any accompanying blepharitis. Compared to bacterial keratitis, the sterile corneal infiltrates associated with contact lenses tend to be smaller, more discrete, with less inflammation and little or no discharge. This distinction can, however, be difficult, so most patients require urgent hospital review. Marginal keratitis is another common cause of corneal infiltrates in patients with blepharitis. Urgent referral may be required to rule out bacterial keratitis.

General practice

If a slit lamp is not available, consider using other magnifiers to visualize small corneal abnormalities such as foreign bodies, ulcers, and abrasions: try using the ophthalmoscope (dial up a plus lens) or an auroscope with the earpiece removed. Fluorescein is extremely helpful in this setting – one drop of proxymetacaine in both eyes may also make the examination easier. Many corneal

...nditions such as herpes simplex keratitis, Thygeson's keratitis, ...nd recurrent erosion syndrome run a relapsing and remitting course, with recurrence even while the patient is being treated. It is preferable to refer back urgently rather than to alter medication. The use of topical steroids should be supervised by the treating ophthalmologist.

The following guide to referral urgency is not prescriptive as clinical situations vary.

Immediate

Same day

Urgent (within 1 week)

Routine

Chapter 6

CATARACT SURGERY

Preoperative Assessment

Background Cataract is the most common cause of treatable blindness worldwide. Most cataracts are age-related. An estimated 30% of those aged over 65 have visually significant (<6/12) cataract and 70% of those over 85 years. Whilst age is the predominant risk factor for cataract formation, the process is multifactorial and remains to be fully elucidated. To date, surgery is the only effective treatment. Modern, small incision cataract extraction by phakoemulsification with foldable intraocular lens implantation allows rapid visual rehabilitation with low complication rates.

For congenital cataract, see page 562.

Indications for cataract surgery

◼ Reduced visual function due to cataract.

◼ Cataract limiting assessment or treatment of posterior segment disease.

◼ Lens-induced disease (phakolysis, phakoanaphylaxis, phakomorphic angle closure).

◼ Second eye cataract surgery to improve stereopsis and reduce anisometropia.

◼ Refractive lens extraction ('clear lens' or 'pre-cataract'), particularly in high ametropia.

History

◼ *Symptoms*: ask about the duration and character of any visual loss (reduced VA, contrast sensitivity, or glare), and the impact on daily activities. Validated symptom questionnaires may help determine the need for surgery.

◼ *Past ocular history*: spectacle or contact lens (CL) use, amblyopia, strabismus, previous anisometropia, glaucoma, surgery including refractive procedures, trauma, uveitis or scleritis, and blepharospasm. In patients with a preexisting squint it is generally better to operate on the fixing eye first to avoid fixation switch and possible diplopia.

- *Past medical and surgical history*: especially deafness, confusion, neck disease, orthopnoea, difficulty lying flat, and seizures.

- *Drug history*: especially anticoagulants, tamsulosin (flomax), and allergies to iodine or antibiotics (some surgeons avoid subconjunctival cephalosporins in those with penicillin allergy due to the risk of cross-sensitivity).

- *Social history*: identify pre- and postoperative social support and any occupational visual requirements.

Examination

- *Best corrected VA* (BCVA): for near and distance and pinhole VA (PHVA, may indicate potential postoperative vision better than BCVA). Contrast sensitivity and glare disability are useful if symptoms are disproportionate to the VA loss, or the degree of cataract.

- *Binocular balance*: cover test and ocular motility.

- *Lids and adnexae*: blepharitis, ectropion, entropion, orbital, or lacrimal disease may need treatment prior to cataract surgery.

- *RAPD*: Check RAPD before dilating pupils.

- *Slit lamp examination*: assess the anterior segment including corneal clarity, guttatae, anterior chamber (AC) depth, pupil size, evidence of previous intraocular inflammation or trauma, pseudoexfoliation, irido- or phakodonesis, IOP, and gonioscopy if angle disease is suspected.

- *Cataract*: note the type (nuclear, cortical, posterior subcapsular, mixed) and grade (1+ to 5+) of cataract. Cortical cataracts are characterized by spokes, water clefts and vacuoles due to osmotic imbalances in lens epithelial cells. Nuclear cataracts result from accumulation of protein aggregates in the centre of the lens, becoming progressively harder and more brunescent with time. Posterior subcapsular cataracts occur at the posterior pole immediately beneath the lens capsule and are associated with the highest rates of cataract surgery.

- *Fundoscopy*: note posterior vitreous detachment (reduced risk of postoperative retinal detachment) or vitreous pigment cells, and exclude optic nerve or macula disease, retinopathy and peripheral retinal breaks or degenerations (especially in high myopes).

Investigations

- *Blood pressure*: should be controlled preoperatively – there is an increased risk of suprachoroidal haemorrhage with systolic BP ≥180 mmHg or a diastolic >100 mmHg.

- *BM*: diabetics may present with cataracts.

- *Other blood tests and ECG*: only if clinically indicated – routine testing does not reduce morbidity and mortality.
  If taking warfarin ensure the INR is in the therapeutic range (discontinuing warfarin increases the risk of stroke 1:100).

- *Special investigations*: as indicated, including B-scan ultrasound to exclude retinal detachment or mass lesion if there is no fundal view; corneal topography (particularly if high or irregular astigmatism) to plan astigmatic surgery; specular microscopy and pachymetry to assess endothelial compromise.

Consent

- *Benefits*: These may include

  1. Improved quality of vision.

  2. Improved fundal view to monitor or treat posterior segment disease.

  3. Reduced spectacle dependence (a reading correction is usually required)

  More than 90% of patients (without coexisting ocular disease) achieve a BCVA of 6/12 or better.

- *Risks*: Complications are infrequent and most can be treated. The overall risk of blindness is 1 in 1000, with 1:10000 chance of losing the eye as a result of surgery. There is almost no risk to the fellow eye. Potentially sight-threatening complications include: infectious endophthalmitis (0.1%), retinal detachment (<1%), suprachoroidal haemorrhage (0.1%), cystoid macular oedema (1–2%), and corneal decompensation (<0.3%). Other specific complications include: ecchymosis (common), posterior capsule rupture and/or vitreous loss (<5%), dropped nucleus (<1%), postoperative IOP rise (common), subluxation of intraocular lens implant, iris prolapse/wound leak, uveitis, refractive surprise, spectacle correction for best vision, drop allergy, diplopia, ptosis, further surgery, and posterior capsule opacification. There may be a guarded prognosis if there is coexisting ocular disease. Patients with a longstanding unilateral cataract and a divergent eye are at risk of intractable postoperative diplopia.

■ Also discuss:

1. The diagnosis and natural history of cataract.

2. Alternative nonsurgical options such as spectacles.

3. The patient's preferred refractive target and the risk of refractive surprise.

4. The surgical procedure, what to expect, and postoperative care.

5. Anaesthetic options: topical, LA or GA.

6. Admission: day case or inpatient.

7. Provide written information. (e.g. http://www.rcophth. ac.uk/public/booklets/UnderstandingCataracts.pdf) and give time to consider the options.

Biometry

Selecting the correct power of intraocular lens (IOL) for the desired refractive outcome relies on careful biometry. Measure the corneal curvature, axial length (AL), focimetry (or refraction) and, if keratometry is impossible, corneal topography.

Keratometry, K (Dioptres) Central corneal curvature is measured by manual or automated keratometry with paired readings taken in two orthogonal meridia. Take the average of 3 pairs of readings including axes. Corneal power in dioptres (D)=337.5/keratometry in mm, (where 337.5 is the hypothetical refractive index of the cornea).

Axial length of the eye (mm) Usually measured using either optical interferometery (e.g. IOLMASTER, Carl Zeiss) or A-Mode ultrasound. Ideally, contact lenses should be removed for as long as possible before measurements are taken. Tightly fitting contact lenses can induce a reversible corneal flattening which can lead to a postoperative gradual myopic shift.

- *Optical interferometery*: noncontact and measures AL to the RPE (rather than the vitreo-retinal interface as in ultrasound). A trace with a signal-to-noise ratio (SNR) of ≥2.0 is acceptable; however, the higher the SNR, the more accurate the reading. AL readings are typically 0.1 mm longer with the IOLMASTER compared to A-scan. As formulae for IOL power calculations have been tested with A-scan AL measurements, targets of −0.3 D to −0.5 D are recommended to achieve emmetropia when using optical biometry. Improved refractive targeting can be achieved by optimising IOL A-constants for optical biometry. The IOLMASTER has a built-in keratometer, facilities to measure preoperative 'anterior chamber depth' (ACD, the distance from the anterior corneal vertex to the anterior lens along the visual axis), horizontal white-to-white measurement (HWTW), optional settings, e.g. 'pseudophakia' (PMMA, silicone, and acrylic) or 'silicone oil filled vitreous', and software to calculate IOL implant powers using a selection of formulae.

- *A-Mode ultrasound*: essential if cataract is dense or other ocular opacity prevents optical measurement of AL, but more user-dependent. Immersion A-scan methods offer a reduced chance of foreshortening of eye by indentation (small potential error of 0.1 mm) but a much greater chance of misaligning the probe with respect to visual axis, which can lead to very high errors (≈mms). A small, high-frequency (typically 10 MHz) transducer is placed on the anaesthetized cornea (usually supported in spring-loaded assembly such as a tonometer holder). Between pulses, echoes are received from the ocular tissues and plotted as spikes on a display (Fig. 6.1). The height of the spike indicates the amplitude of the echo and the position along x-axis indicates time delay (converted to distance using assumed velocities in ocular tissue). A major source of error is poor alignment of the ultrasound probe; ensure central fixation with a perpendicular incidence (indicated by strongest echo with steepest rise time from baseline). The AL of silicone oil filled eye=anterior cornea to posterior lens plus [measured vitreal length × 0.64]. The length of the vitreous must be scaled to allow for the reduced velocity of sound in oil (both A & B-scan).

- *B-Mode ultrasound*: invaluable in babies, poorly cooperative patients, and to exclude staphylomata. Provides a cross-sectional image of the eye (Fig. 6.2) and orbit through closed eyelid (with a good system the anterior cornea and foveal pit can be imaged). Assumes a single velocity in ocular tissues. A skilled operator is required for accurate AL measurement; care must be taken not to indent globe as the probe is hand-held and considerably heavier than the A-scan probe.

Focimetry of old (pre-cataract) spectacles (or refraction) Assess spherical and astigmatic error in each eye and ensure this is consistent with other biometry data. Aim to minimize anisometropia to 2D or less, unless mono vision is desired (e.g. one eye focussed for distance; one for near). However, if the patient is adapted to longstanding anisometropia,

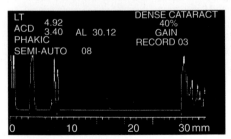

Fig. 6.1: A-scan: axial length (AL) 30.12 mm; anterior chamber length (ACD) 3.40 mm; lens thickness (LT) 4.92 mm: cursors at base of trace mark (from left to right) the anterior lens interface, posterior lens interface and vitreo-retinal interface, respectively.

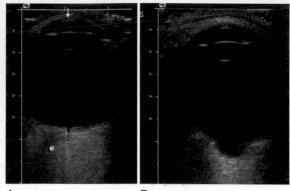

A   B

Fig. 6.2: Transverse (horizontal) central B-scan sections.
(A) Average length eye, anterior cornea (white arrow)
and foveal pit (black arrow). **(B)** Highly myopic eye with
gross posterior pole staphyloma.

correcting this can cause problems with image size disparity and
diplopia.

Corneal topography Keratometry rather than topography
readings should be used in IOL calculation. Topography can be
used to quantify significant keratometric astigmatism and exclude
irregular astigmatism or keratoconus prior to surgery and to assist
in planning incision placement, limbal relaxing incisions, or toric
IOL use.

IOL power calculation formulae IOL power is
calculated by entering keratometry and AL data into an
appropriate formula. Some formulae also require preoperative ACD
(Holladay 2, Haigis, and Catefract). Holladay 2 formula also
requires refraction, lens thickness, and HWTW measurements.
Any theoretical third-generation formula can be used (Hoffer Q,
SRKT, Holladay 1, Holladay 2, Haigis, and Catefract). Never use
obsolete formulae such as SRK II. Select a formulae based on
the axial length (Table 6.1). Highlight any special lens order
required.

An interocular difference in AL of >0.3 mm or K >1 D should be
checked with multiple readings and ideally with the patient's
refractive history or focimetry of old spectacles, i.e. before
cataract development. If the axial lengths differ by >0.6 mm
between fellow eyes and the history or focimetry are not
consistent, use A-scan to cross-check the readings obtained by

optical interferometery IOLMASTER. Do not target Plano '0' but choose −0.3 D as 'emmetropic correction'.

IOL power calculation after refractive surgery

Standard biometry will be inaccurate in patients who have undergone previous corneal refractive surgery. IOL power can be determined using three alternative methods:

- 1. *Refractive history technique*: Must have prerefractive surgery K values and refraction. Effective corneal power, K (D) for use in IOL power calculations is derived as follows:

  a. Calculate pre- and postprocedure refraction spherical equivalent at the corneal plane using:

  $$R_C = Rs / (1 - BVD \times Rs)$$

  where R_C = Refraction at corneal plane (D), Rs = Refraction at spectacle plane (D) and BVD = Back vertex distance (m).

  b. Determine change in refraction at the corneal plane by subtracting adjusted postprocedure refraction from adjusted preprocedure refraction. Take care with plus and minus signs.

  c. Effective corneal power,

  K(D) = Prerefractive surgery average K-value (D) + (Change in refraction at corneal plane).

  Take care with signs.

- 2. *Contact lens technique*: Useful when no pretreatment data exist. Spectacle refraction is performed followed by over-refraction with a hard CL of known base curve and plano (or low) power in situ:

  a. Calculate pre- and post-contact lens refraction spherical equivalent at corneal plane, as above for refractive history technique.

Table 6.1: IOL power calculation formulae	
Axial length	**Formula**
>22.0 mm	SRK/T
<22.0 mm	Hoffer Q when IOL ≤34 D Holladay 2 when IOL >34 D, piggy-back calculations or deep ACD

b. Effective corneal power:

K (D) = (Base curve of CL) + (Contact lens power) +
(Spherical equivalent at corneal plane with CL in situ) −
(Spherical equivalent at corneal plane without CL).

■ 3. *Nomograms*: See Table 6.2 (Vahid Feiz, et al. 2001).

Unexpected postoperative refractive outcome In
the event of a confirmed refractive surprise:

■ Re-check IOL choice, A-constant, formula used, and target
   refraction.

■ Re-measure AL and keratometry optically to exclude a
   biometry error.

■ Measure distance from anterior cornea to anterior surface of
   the IOL with either A- or B-scan (be careful not to measure to
   the posterior implant surface): too shallow or too deep will
   lead to myopic or hyperopic surprises, respectively (usually
   due to excess anterior or posterior vaulting of implant, often
   due to crimping of haptics).

■ In cases of myopic surprise, also consider retained visco
   elastic behind the implant – a distended bag may be visible on
   examination or with B-scan.

■ Beware manufacturing/pack errors with mislabelled implant
   power (implant thickness can be measured in situ on B-scan
   and compared to a correctly labelled implant of the same
   model).

Table 6.2: Nomogram for IOL power adjustment according to degree of previous refractive error correction	
Corrected myopia (D)	**Increase IOL power by (to nearest 0.25 D)**
1	0.5 D
3	1.5 D
5	2.75 D
Corrected hyperopia (D)	**Decrease IOL power by (to nearest 0.25 D)**
1	0 D
3	1.75 D
5	3.5 D

- Discuss treatment options with the patient.

- If the refractive outcome is tolerated, leave the IOL in situ and/or offer spectacle or CL correction.

- If not tolerated and no obvious biometry error, consider, IOL exchange, piggyback IOL *or* corneal refractive surgery.

- If the refractive outcome is not tolerated and if there is obvious biometry error, offer IOL exchange based on refraction *or* offer corneal refractive surgery. If the fellow eye has cataract consider equalizing refraction with second eye surgery or electing for anisometropic mono vision.

Management of Astigmatism

Background Visually significant keratometric astigmatism of ≥2.0 Dioptres (D) is present in up to 15% of patients undergoing cataract surgery. Cylindrical targeting using incision placement, limbal relaxing incisions, toric intraocular lenses (IOLs) or a combination of techniques can reduce or eliminate preexisting astigmatism and improve unaided distance vision (Fig. 6.3).

Incision placement Placing clear corneal incisions (CCI) on the steep meridian causes wound-induced flattening sufficient to control 0.75–1.50 D. Temporal CCIs are almost (0.25 D) astigmatically neutral if ≤3.4 mm in size and are recommended if there is negligible corneal astigmatism. Superior CCIs induce up to 1.50 D flattening. It is not always possible to operate on the steep meridian (e.g. if superonasal in the right eye or inferotemporal in the left eye, unless left handed or ambidextrous).

Limbal relaxing incisions (LRI) Safe, rapid, and reliably corrects up to 3.00 D keratometric astigmatism (Box 6.1). Paired arcuate limbal incisions centred on the steep meridian flattens the central cornea, and is usually combined with neutral

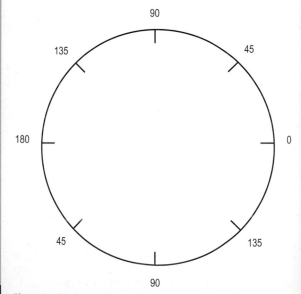

Fig. 6.3: Corneal axis.

Box 6.1: Limbal relaxing incision

1. Mark the limbus at the 90° position preoperatively, with the patient sitting upright at the slit lamp (avoids alignment error from cyclotorsion when supine after orbital block). Perform LRI at the start of surgery when the eye is firm and there is less risk of 'dragging' the corneal epithelium (if a large LRI is required at the site of the main wound, extend the LRI at the end of surgery).

2. Align a degree gauge (e.g. Mendez ring) on the cornea using the limbal reference marks (Fig. 6.4). Locate and mark the steep meridian. Confirm with intraoperative keratoscopy (reflected mires appear closer on the steep axis).

3. Define the required arc length centred on the steep meridian using either ink marks or a fixation ring with increment markers (e.g. Fine-Thornton-Nichamin).

4. Use a guarded diamond knife-style blade set at a depth of 600 microns (according to nomogram). Make accurate incisions at the most peripheral clear cornea (irrespective of vessels), keep the blade perpendicular and pull towards you. Wait 4–6 weeks for stable refraction.

temporal CCI. Measure the axis and amount of corneal astigmatism by keratometry or topography. Identify requisite LRI length (degrees of arc) from preferred nomogram, e.g. modified Gills or Nichamin (Table 6.3A, 6.3B). Complications include: wrong axis, perforation (rare), infection, misalignment, induced irregular astigmatism, decreased corneal sensation, and weakened globe.

Toric intraocular lenses Toric IOLs incorporate a cylindrical correction on a spherical optic for correction of preexisting regular keratometric astigmatism. They are useful when an LRI is inadequate or less predictable, e.g. astigmatism >3.00–3.75 D or in young patients (beware a forme fruste of keratoconus). Successful outcome relies on careful lens power calculation and selection, minimizing surgically induced astigmatism, meticulous cortical clean-up/capsule polish, and precise alignment of IOL cylindrical correction axis with the steep corneal meridian. Corneal reference marks should be made preoperatively as described above for LRIs. The greatest clinical experience exists with the STAAR single-piece silicone plate haptic toric IOL; available in astigmatic powers of 2 and 3.5 D (correcting approximately 1.5 and 2.25 D of astigmatism, respectively) and 2 lengths (TF 10.8 mm and TL 11.2 mm). However, significant IOL

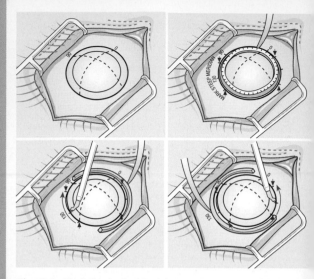

Fig. 6.4: Limbal relaxing incision.

rotation/axis shift occurs in more than 10% of eyes, reducing astigmatism correction (two-thirds of effect is lost with 20° deviation) and requiring repositioning within 1 week. Residual postoperative astigmatism is pseudophakic and cannot be corrected with a rigid contact lens (only with spectacles or soft toric contact lens). In addition, an increased capsular fibrosis rate is associated with silicone-plate haptic IOLs and risks decentration or dislocation into the vitreous following posterior capsulotomy. Second-generation toric IOLs include the HumanOptics Microsil® 3-piece silicone toric IOL (with Z-design haptics providing greater rotational stability) and the Alcon AcrySof single-piece SA60AT toric.

'Bi-optics' Refers to serial combined procedures to refine refractive and astigmatic outcomes from cataract surgery, e.g. using postoperative solid-state or excimer laser ablation or thermokeratoplasty.

Table 6.3A: Nichamin nomogram for clear corneal phako surgery

Astigmatic status='**spherical**': (+0.75×90; +0.50×180)
Incision design='Neutral' temporal clear corneal incision
(3.5mm. or less, single plane, just anterior to vascular arcade)

Astigmatic status='**against-the-rule**': (Steep Axis 0–30°/150–180°):
Intraoperative keratoscopy determines exact incision location
Incision design='Neutral' temporal clear corneal along with the following peripheral arcuate incisions:

Pre-op cylinder	30–40yo	41–50yo	51–60yo	61–70yo	71–80yo	81–90yo	>90
Nasal limbal arc only on steep axis							
+0.75→+1.25							
*Paired limbal arcs on steep axis	55°	50°	45°	40°	35°	35°	
+1.50→+2.00 on steep axis							
*Paired limbal arcs on steep axis	70°	65°	60°	55°	45°	40°	35°
+2.25→+2.75 on steep axis							
*Paired limbal arcs on steep axis	90° ↓ o.z. to 8 mm	80° ↓ o.z. to 9 mm	70°	60°	50°	45°	40°
+3.00→+3.75							
*Paired limbal arcs on steep axis	90°	90°	85°	70°	60°	50°	45°

Degrees of arc to be incised

* The temporal incision is made by first creating a two-plane, grooved phaco incision (600µ depth), which is then extended to the appropriate arc length at the conclusion of surgery. o.z., optic zone.

Table 6.3B: Nichamin nomogram for clear corneal phako surgery

Astigmatic status = 'with-the-rule': (Steep axis 45–145°):

Intraoperative keratoscopy determines exact incision location

Incision design = 'Neutral' temporal clear corneal (3.5 mm. or less, single plane, just anterior to vascular arcade) along with the following peripheral arcuate incisions:

Pre-op cylinder	30–40yo	41–50yo	51–60yo	61–70yo	71–80yo	81–90yo	>90
+1.00 → +1.50 Paired limbal arcs on steep axis	50°	45°	40°	35°	30°		
+1.75 → +2.25 Paired limbal arcs on steep axis	60°	55°	50°	45°	40°	35°	30°
+2.50 → +3.00 Paired limbal arcs on steep axis	70°	65°	60°	55°	50°	45°	40°
+3.25 → +3.75 Paired limbal arcs on steep axis	80°	75°	70°	65°	60°	55°	45°
Degrees of arc to be incised							

Reproduced with kind permission from Louis D. 'Skip' Nichamin, M.D., Laurel Eye Clinic, Brookville, PA, USA.

Local Anaesthesia

Background Most modern cataract surgery is performed under local anaesthesia (LA) with the advantage of reduced morbidity and mortality, reduced hospital stays, and increased patient satisfaction compared to general anaesthesia (GA). Anaesthesia can be achieved by topical means alone, but akinesia (paralysis of ocular movements) requires regional orbital block (sub-Tenon's, peribulbar, or retrobulbar). The choice of LA technique must be tailored to surgery, the patient's expectations, and the comfort of both patient and surgeon.

- *Patient selection*: Good communication before and during surgery reduces anxiety and improves cooperation. The patient should be able to lie still and relatively flat for the duration of surgery.

- *Monitoring*: all patients must be monitored (pulse oximetry, BP, ECG) by suitably trained personnel; if using sharp needle technique, an anaesthetist must be available and i.v. access in place.

- *Sedation*: Useful in certain patients (e.g. anxious or claustrophobic, may improve mild head tremor, but *not* for pain relief). Risks include inducing confusion, restlessness, and airway compromise. Requires postoperative monitoring and appropriate escort/transport arrangements.

- *General anesthesia*: preferred if the patient is unable to comply with instructions (e.g. confusion, learning difficulties), very severe claustrophobia, history of panic attacks, significant psychiatric disease, marked resting head tremor, young patient, previous adverse reaction, allergy or complication associated with LA, or if the patient declines LA.

Topical anaesthesia Increasingly popular, although regional block remains the standard in cataract surgery. Select well-motivated patients, routine cases, and an experienced surgeon. Avoid if there is a language barrier, hearing impairment, 'lid squeezers', extreme anxiety, dementia/confusion, nystagmus, combined or long surgical procedures. Warn the patient of pressure sensation and preservation of vision during surgery. Avoid unnecessarily bright illumination.

- *Advantages*: Noninvasive and quick, rapid visual recovery, avoids complications of orbital blocks/GA, inexpensive, useful if anticoagulated or long axial length.

- *Disadvantages*: Not suitable for all, limited to short procedures, drops can cause superficial punctate keratitis, epithelial haze/impaired view, without akinesia surgery may be challenging if the patient is uncooperative or if complications arise.

■ *Technique*: Apply G. proxymetacaine 0.5% (or G. benoxinate 0.4%) initially (less stinging than amethocaine) then 2–3 drops G. amethocaine 1% (better anaesthesia during surgery than proxymetacaine or benoxinate) 5 minutes preoperatively. Ensure application to the cornea, bulbar conjunctiva, inferior and superior fornices (to reduce speculum discomfort). Also instill G. proxymetacaine 0.5% once to the fellow eye. Instill a further three drops during surgery: before the first corneal incision, before intraocular lens insertion, and before subconjunctival antibiotic/steroid injection. Give additional drops at any stage as required, remembering that amethocaine can cause epithelial haze.

Adjunctive intracameral anaesthesia is not used routinely but is useful in eliminating the pressure sensation/pain sometimes experienced under topical alone: irrigate the AC with 0.5 mL preservative-free 1% lidocaine in BSS (without epinephrine) after the first incision.

Sub-Tenon's block

■ *Technique*: see Box 6.2 and Figure 6.5.

■ *Agents*: Use shorter-acting lidocaine 1 or 2% (without epinephrine), or longer-acting bupivacaine 0.5%, or a mixture

---

Box 6.2: Sub-Tenon's block

1. Position the patient supine, apply G. benoxinate 0.4% then one drop 5% povidone iodine, and insert the lid speculum. Button-hole the conjunctiva and Tenon's capsule 4 mm from the limbus in the inferonasal quadrant using spring scissors and forceps. Apply conjunctival cautery if required (Fig. 6.5A).

2. Blunt dissect to open sub-Tenon's space (Fig. 6.5B) then insert a curved blunt sub-Tenon's cannula between Tenon's and sclera. Gentle hydrodissection assists passage (Fig. 6.5C).

3. Keep the tip adjacent to the globe and pass posteriorly; there is usually some resistance at the equator (Fig. 6.5D).

4. Push beyond equator and inject 3–5 mL of LA to spread around globe and into the intraconal space. This often causes proptosis. If there is resistance to injection, reflux, or subconjunctival swelling, reposition the cannula or dissect more posteriorly before re-injecting.

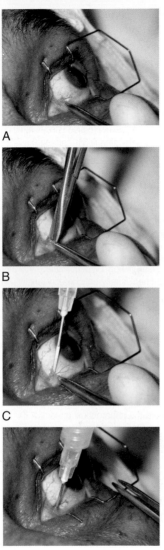

A

B

C

D

Fig. 6.5: How to perform a sub-Tenon's block. See Box 6.2.

of both, with or without hyaluronidase diluted to 15 i.u./mL (Hyalase® may prevent loculation of fluid behind the globe, reducing the risk of increased posterior pressure and its complications). The maximum safe dose of lidocaine without epinephrine is 3 mg/kg and bupivacaine 2 mg/kg (0.5%=5 mg/mL, 1%=10 mg/mL, 2%=20 mg/mL) e.g. maximum safe dose of 2% lidocaine for a 70 kg patient is $(3 \times 70)/20 = 10.5$ mL.

■ *Advantages*: safest orbital block (avoids sharp needle), relatively rapid action.

■ *Disadvantages*: less effective akinesia if poorly administered, subconjunctival chemosis or haemorrhage, and difficult to perform if previous buckle/conjunctival surgery.

Peribulbar block A sharp needle technique, but safer than retrobulbar. Check axial length, as long eyes are at higher risk of inadvertent perforation (use topical or sub-Tenon's instead).

■ *Technique*: Position the patient supine with gaze in the primary position. Apply G. benoxinate 0.4% then one drop 5% povidone-iodine. Usually only one conjunctival injection in the inferotemporal quadrant is required (Fig. 6.6A). Use a short 25-gauge needle (25–31 mm length), and carefully advance posteriorly to the hilt of the needle. Gentle side-to-side movement of the needle should not displace the globe, else suspect scleral puncture. Withdraw the plunger to ensure there is no reflux of blood before injecting 3–8 mL of LA into the extraconal space. Wait 10–15 minutes with digital massage or Honan's balloon to aid dispersion. An additional medial canthal injection via the caruncle may be given if needed (avoid the superonasal quadrant).

Retrobulbar block Avoid if inexperienced. Apply G. benoxinate 0.4% then one drop of 5% povidone-iodine. Give a single inferotemporal injection via the conjunctiva or lower lid skin at the junction of the outer and middle thirds of the inferior orbital rim. Use a short 25-gauge needle directed toward the occiput, then angle upwards when past the equator of the globe up to the needle hilt (Fig. 6.6B). Use manoeuvres as described for peribulbar block to check needle tip position before injecting a small volume (<3 mL) of LA into the intraconal space.

Complications of sharp needle blocks Retrobulbar haemorrhage, globe penetration/perforation (<0.1%, longer eyes at increased risk), optic nerve sheath haemorrhage, extraocular muscle trauma/toxicity causing diplopia, ptosis, rarely subarachnoid injection with brainstem anaesthesia (confusion, seizures, paralysis, respiratory arrest, circulatory collapse),

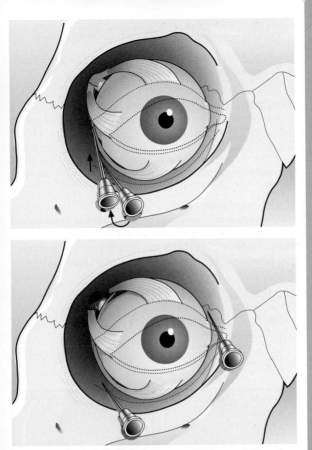

Fig. 6.6: Sharp needle orbital blocks. **(A)** Peribulbar.
(B) Retrobulbar.

intravascular injection of LA (seizures, resistant ventricular
fibrillation).

Websites The Royal College of Anaesthetists and The Royal
College of Ophthalmologists. Local anaesthesia for intraocular
surgery. 2001. http://www.rcophth.ac.uk/scientific/publications.
html.

The Royal College of Ophthalmologists. Cataract Surgery
Guidelines 2004. http://www.rcophth.ac.uk/scientific/publications.
html.

Basic Surgical Techniques

A 'standard' method of phako surgery is described, recognizing that surgeons will evolve their own techniques.

Preparation and draping

Antiseptic preparation of the surgical field (ocular surface, lids, lashes, cheek, and forehead) with aqueous povidone-iodine 5% (or chlorhexidine) and draping of the eyelashes reduces the risk of postoperative endophthalmitis.

Main incision

Construct small self-sealing clear (or near-clear) corneal incision as either a single plane stab or two or three step incisions (three step is more secure). Stabilize the globe using Thornton-Fine 'C-ring' or micro-grooved forceps (Fig. 6.7):

Step 1: Groove the cornea anterior to the limbus using a diamond or steel keratome (avoid incising the conjunctiva to prevent chemosis during phako).

Step 2: Create a stromal tunnel about 1 mm long using a 2.8 mm keratome (a longer tunnel is less likely to leak and essential if the AC is shallow).

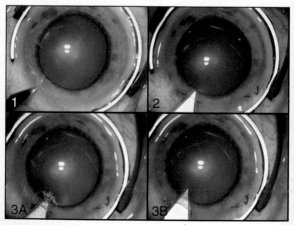

Fig. 6.7: Three-step corneal incision. Step 1, groove. Step 2, stromal tunnel. Step 3a, tilt keratome posteriorly. 3b, enter anterior chamber.

Step 3: Deliberately tilt the keratome posteriorly before advancing
the blade to enter the AC (note corneal striae on entry). A
temporal incision is preferred as it is astigmatically neutral
(if <3.4 mm) and allows better access. The site of incision
may be tailored to reduce preexisting corneal astigmatism
(p. 232).

Side port incision

Inject viscoelastic to stabilize the AC. Create a second, limbal
side-port incision (paracentesis) 45–90° from the main wound
using a diamond keratome or 15° blade; do not make this too
wide to avoid leaking or iris prolapse.

Continuous circular capsulorrhexis

Use a cystatome (preformed or bent insulin syringe needle) and/or
rhexis forceps (Figs. 6.8, 6.9). Puncture the capsule at the centre
and extend radially, ending with a 'J'-turn to create a curvilinear
fold in the favoured direction (clockwise or anticlockwise). Grasp
the capsular flap just in front of the tearing point, then pull

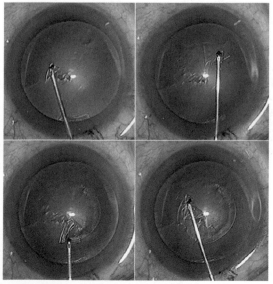

Fig. 6.8: Needle capsulorrhexis. Clockwise capsulorrhexis
with a bent insulin syringe needle.

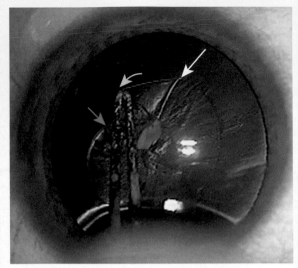

Fig. 6.9: Forceps capsulorrhexis. Start point (white arrowhead), tearing point (green arrowhead) and direction of pull (yellow curved arrow) are shown. Note anterior polar lens opacity adherent to anterior capsule.

circumferentially to create a continuous circular capsulorrhexis (CCC) of 5–6 mm diameter. To reduce the risk of losing control, re-grip the outer flap edge near the tearing point, ensure the AC depth is maintained with viscoelastic, and avoid pressure on the posterior lip of the wound. If the capsulorrhexis needs enlarging or if an irregular edge must be stabilized, cut the rhexis margin tangentially with Ong scissors to create a new flap to grip and extend with forceps (safest after IOL insertion). If the red reflex is poor/absent, inject filtered air into the AC then stain the anterior capsule with trypan blue 0.06% (Vision Blue™). Wash out after 30 seconds. In young patients, beware anterior insertion of the zonular fibres (identifiable by staining with trypan blue) and the more elastic capsule as both increase the risk of the capsulorrhexis tearing out. For management of capsule tears see page 260.

Hydrodissection

Separates the cortex from the capsule to mobilize the lens in the bag. Use a Rycroft or 27-gauge hydrodissection cannula (Pierce or J-cannula) on a syringe of balanced salt solution (BSS). Place tip of the cannula under the rhexis margin, immediately adjacent to the capsule, advance slightly, then gently inject BSS. A 'fluid wave' behind the lens confirms the correct cleavage plane (Fig. 6.10). Gently depress the nucleus to help move fluid around the lens. A single injection is preferred, but repeat the hydrodissection if necessary at a different site until the lens is freely mobile. *Hydrodelineation* cleaves the adult nucleus from the epinucleus: inject BSS into the lens matter and watch for 'golden ring' sign – epinuclear shell may not be easy to remove later but provides useful protection to the posterior capsule for phako-chop techniques.

Phakoemulsification

Know your machine! Piezoelectric crystal in the hand-piece oscillates the titanium phako needle at 35–45 KHz, generating ultrasonic energy in front of the tip. Emulsified lens matter is removed via a central aspiration port. The AC is maintained by fluid entering via the irrigation sleeve, also serving to cool the phako needle (ensure the holes of the sleeve are positioned horizontally so flow is not impeded and is away from the corneal endothelium). Phako machines are flow-based (usually a peristaltic

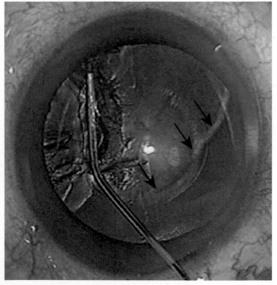

Fig. 6.10: Hydrodissection. Wavefront of fluid between lens and posterior capsule is shown by arrows.

pump) or vacuum-based (usually Venturi). Standard linear foot pedal control positions are:

- Position 1: off.

- Position 2: irrigation on (set by the infusion bottle height) with aspiration (set by flow rate and vacuum) increasing with pedal depression.

- Position 3: phakoemulsification increasing to maximum energy set.

Phako techniques A variety of methods are possible according to the type of cataract and surgical skill. Aim to develop an adaptable technique, minimize phako energy and fluid flow, and maintain a stable AC. AC stability is determined by irrigation (height of infusion bottle), vacuum setting, and wound integrity.

- *Divide and conquer*

   1. Aims to split the nucleus into quadrants for emulsification. The easiest technique to master. Set 60–70% phako power and 30–50 mmHg vacuum for the first stage. Make a central groove 1.5 times the width of phako tip (Fig. 6.11), sculpting deeper centrally than peripherally;

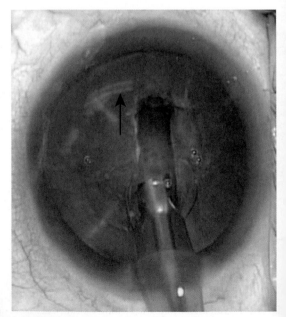

Fig. 6.11: Sculpting.

beware the rhexis margin. Advance the tip at same speed as emulsification (increase power as required) to avoid pushing the lens. Rotate the nucleus 180° to complete a long groove before sculpting a second long groove at right angles to the first. Alternatively, rotate the nucleus 90° at a time dividing into quadrants with four short grooves. Bimanual rotation minimizes zonular stress; if there is resistance to rotation repeat the hydrodissection. The depth of the groove for successful cracking varies with nucleus density; when the red reflex becomes apparent through the base of the groove, the depth is usually sufficient (Fig. 6.12).

2. To crack the nucleus (Fig. 6.13) make certain the second instrument and phako tip are at the base of the groove. Separate the instruments using an upward pivoting motion (rather than pure lateral movement); this is mechanically more efficient and reduces zonular stress. Ensure the crack extends along the full length. If unsuccessful, the groove is usually not deep enough. For quadrant removal, use 40–60% phako power but increase the vacuum to 140–350 mmHg (flow rate 25–35 mL/min). Position the quadrant to be removed opposite the phako tip. Use

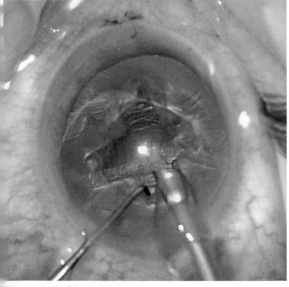

Fig. 6.12: Divide and conquer.

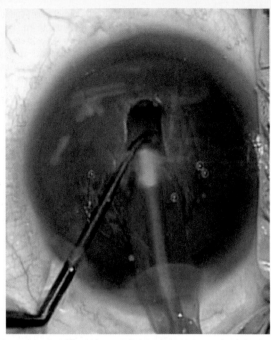

Fig. 6.13: Cracking the nucleus.

vacuum and phako to impale the centre of the fragment (tilting the apex of the quadrant forward aids this manoeuvre). Maintain occlusion without phako energy (foot position 2) and pull the quadrant to the centre of bag for emulsification. Pulse, burst, or cool-phako modes reduce the total phako energy required, especially in harder cataracts. Protect the capsule during quadrant removal by keeping the second instrument below the phako tip at all times.

■ *Stop and chop*: Stop and chop shortens phako time, is useful for hard nuclei, and reduces the stress on the capsule if the zonules are weak or the rhexis incomplete. Sculpt a single long groove, crack the nucleus into two halves, then 'stop' and 'chop' each heminucleus. Rotate the nucleus so that the groove is at 30° to the phako needle, then align the bevel of the tip parallel to the heminucleus to optimize tip occlusion. Increase vacuum (250–350 mmHg) to embed the phako tip into the heminucleus. To perform a horizontal chop, pass the chopper flat under the capsulorrhexis edge, engage opposite the equator of the nucleus, then pull the chopper toward the phako tip to split the nucleus (Fig. 6.14). Just before the instruments meet, move the chopper at right angles to release the wedge of nucleus for emulsification. For a vertical chop technique, use sharp tipped chopper to vertically incise the heminucleus (within the capsulorrhexis) toward the embedded phako tip. Lift the engaged nucleus slightly to facilitate cleavage before lateral separation of the chopper and phako tip to complete fracture. Rotate the nucleus clockwise and repeat the chopping action until the nucleus is completely removed.

■ '*Primary chop*': no sculpting required for this technique. Impale the nucleus with the phako tip just proximal to the centre and immobilize with high vacuum (phako power 40–60% on burst and vacuum 250–350 mmHg). Follow with either horizontal or vertical chop (as above).

■ '*Taco*' *technique*: useful for soft nuclei that are too soft to crack after sculpting a central groove. Fold the nucleus into the groove using aspiration and second instrument manipulation to 'tyre iron' the heminucleus into the phako tip (minimal or no phako energy is required).

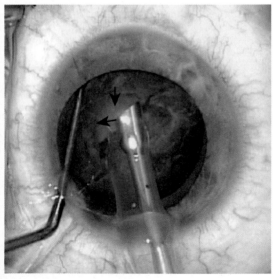

Fig. 6.14: Horizontal chop. Arrows indicate direction of pull of the chopper.

Cortical clean up

Residual cortical or soft lens matter (SLM) is removed using manual (Simcoe) or automated irrigation and aspiration (I&A) systems (Fig. 6.15). The authors favour the Simcoe. Engage SLM beneath the anterior capsule with the tip of the cannula and use aspiration to strip from the periphery to the centre. Excessive pulling (c.f. aspiration) risks PC rupture if the capsule is inadvertently engaged (indicated by star-shaped capsular striae). If the capsule is engaged, keep the instrument still and reflux immediately (if using automated I&A check the correct pedal action beforehand). Proceed circumferentially until all SLM is cleared. Difficult-to-remove subincisional SLM can be tackled with the Simcoe via the second instrument port or a second side port placed opposite the main incision. Ninety degree angled tips for the automated I&A are also available. Alternatively, remove the remaining SLM after IOL insertion – dialling the IOL can loosen material with the optic protecting the PC. Residual SLM may prolong postoperative inflammation and cause early PCO, but better to leave small amounts than risk PC tear.

Capsule polishing: The PC can be polished with automated I&A or a dedicated polisher with a roughened surface under viscoelastic. Manual focal irrigation after filling the bag with hypromellose is also effective at stripping residual cortex/plaque ('jetwash' technique). If there is a resistant plaque, try viscodissection to raise the edge then peel with rhexis forceps (very risky). Routine removal of residual lens epithelium from the equator (and anterior capsule) may reduce the risk of capsular fibrosis/PCO.

Insertion of folding posterior chamber IOL

Fill the capsular bag with viscoelastic and deepen the AC to protect the endothelium. Enlarge the section to 3.4 mm if required for manual implantation or injection of the IOL. Fold the optic in half on the long axis of the haptics. Insert the leading haptic (haptic and curve always pointing to left) beneath the rhexis margin into the capsular bag. As the folded optic passes through the incision, keep pressed against the posterior lip of the wound to avoid Descemet's membrane tears. Once the leading haptic and part of optic are in the bag, rotate forceps 90° before slowly releasing to allow unfolding. Remove forceps then dial the trailing haptic into the bag with minimal manipulation, or place with McPhersons forceps. Injector systems have the advantage of

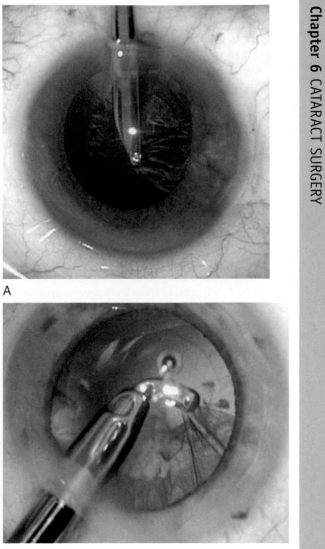

A

B

Fig. 6.15: Cortical clean up. **(A)** Simcoe aspiration of SLM. **(B)** Automated I&A using 90° tip.

avoiding contact between the IOL and ocular surface, and usually permit smaller incisions (Fig. 6.16).

Final steps

Remove all viscoelastic from the AC and behind the IOL to minimize postoperative IOP rise or capsular distension syndrome. Tilt the optic gently with the cannula ('rock and roll') to dislodge viscoelastic from behind the IOL or place the tip behind the optic. Finally, deepen the AC with BSS via a side port and check wound integrity with a sponge. A well-constructed incision is self-sealing and stromal hydration is unnecessary. If wound leaks, suture with 10/0 Nylon or 10/0 Vicryl. Inject subconjunctival antibiotic (cefuroxime 250 mg or gentamicin 25 mg) and steroid (betamethasone 2–4 mg). Protect the eye with a clear shield alone if the blink reflex is present, or else use a pad and shield.

Postoperative care Prescribe oral acetazolomide 250 mg stat and at 6 hours postoperatively, G. dexamethasone 0.1% q.d.s. 4 weeks then taper; G. chloramphenicol 0.5% q.d.s. 2 weeks. Not all surgeons prescribe acetazolamide routinely. Use 6 per day steroids for the first week in Asian, Afro-Caribbean, and diabetic patients who are prone to more vigorous postoperative inflammation. Where the iris has been manipulated (e.g. hooks, iris prolapse) some surgeons add G. ketorolac 0.5% (Acular) q.d.s. 1 month to reduce the risk of cystoid macular oedema.

Patient advice Advise patients to return immediately if they experience visual loss, pain, or redness. Wear the shield at night for 2 weeks. Avoid splashing or rinsing water in the eye for 1 week; avoid swimming until off steroid drops. With self-sealing incisions, limiting heavy lifting and bending is less important, but avoid for 2 weeks.

Follow–up Review on the day of surgery or postoperative day 1 to check IOP, IOL position, and wound integrity. Thereafter, review on day 7–21 primarily to assess visual outcome and inflammation as well as dilated retinal examination. If there are no problems, discharge or list for second eye surgery. Recommend refraction 4–8 weeks postoperatively in routine cases.

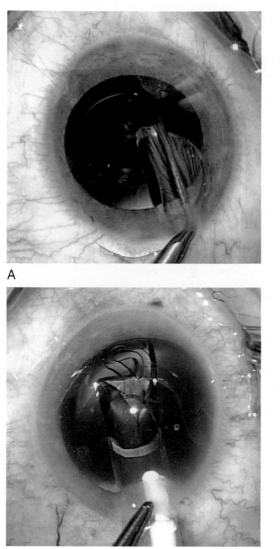

A

B

Fig. 6.16: Insertion intraocular lens. **(A)** Manual insertion of an Acrysof MA60 IOL. **(B)** Injection of Akreos Adaption. (Note leading haptic orientation curving to left being introduced beneath anterior capsule rim).

Difficult Cases

Small pupil Anticipate in diabetes, pseudoexfoliation syndrome (PXF), chronic miotic use, advanced age, and posterior synechniae. Consider the following:

- *Optimise mydriasis*: stop miotics in advance, dilate with cyclopentolate 1%, phenylephrine 2.5% (or 10% but beware BP elevation) plus G. NSAID (e.g. flurbiprofen 0.03%) three times preoperative. If the pupil is still light responsive, give more drops. Intracameral dilute adrenaline is also useful (0.5 mL 1:1000 epinephrine in 500 mL BSS).

- *Highly cohesive viscoelastic*: e.g. Healon GV or 5 helps to splint the pupil open.

- *Posterior synechiolysis*: inject viscoelastic under the pupil margin and sweep the iris free with a cannula or iris repositor. Consider pupil stretch. Remove any pupillary membrane with forceps.

- *Iris hooks* (Fig. 6.17): make limbal stab incisions parallel to the iris (or angled slightly posteriorly) with a 25-gauge orange needle or the tip of an MVR blade; avoid the main wound or side ports. Ensure the proximal two hooks are close to the

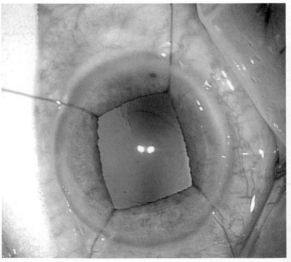

Fig. 6.17: Iris hooks (Courtesy of Mr N Islam).

main incision to avoid 'tenting' and consequent iris trauma by the phako tip. Insert the hooks into the AC, engage the pupil margin and retract. Only adjust to final tension after all hooks are in situ – do not overstretch. If placing hooks is difficult due to a deep AC, indent the globe at the limbus for easier iris capture. To remove hooks, simply disengage the iris and pull. Alternatives include bimanual pupil stretch, multiple small sphincterotomies, and pupil ring expanders.

Zonular weakness/dehiscence Beware in PXF, advanced age, previous trauma or surgery, vitrectomized eyes, high myopia, Marfan's syndrome, homocysteinuria, Weill-Marchesani syndrome, and sulfite-oxidase deficiency. Look for phako- or iridodonesis and identify the location of zonular deficiency preoperatively. Aim to minimize zonular stress. Use viscoelastic generously to tamponade areas of zonular dehiscence. Consider each surgical step in turn:

- *Main incision*: place opposite the zonular weakness if possible.

- *Capsulorrhexis*: initiate the capsulorrhexis toward the weak zonules using the intact zonules for counter-traction. Iris hooks or a second instrument at the capsulorrhexis margin can provide extra stability. Ensure an intact capsulorrhexis is large enough for easy removal of nuclear fragments.

- *Hydrodissection*: ensure good cortical cleavage and hydrodelineation but inject extremely gently.

- *Phako*: use sufficient phako power to avoid 'pushing' the nucleus during sculpting and rotate carefully. Horizontal phako-chop technique produces less zonular stress (p. 248). Beware floppy posterior capsule when removing the last fragments; lower the vacuum and flow rate and consider pulse mode.

- *Cortical removal*: strip the SLM tangentially (c.f. radial) to spread forces. Consider using viscoelastic to keep the capsular bag open or stabilize by preplacing an IOL or capsular tension ring (CTR, see below).

- *IOL implantation*: insert the leading haptic into the bag towards the area of zonular weakness and gently direct the trailing haptic into the bag with MacPherson's forceps (avoid aggressive dialling). Alternatively, inject the IOL so both haptics unfold directly in the bag. Position the IOL with haptics on the axis of zonular weakness to achieve the best centration. If the IOL is significantly decentred, consider a CTR or place in the sulcus. Avoid silicone plate haptic IOLs as they are more likely to decentre.

■ *Capsular tension ring* (CTR): stretches and stabilizes the capsular bag by redistributing forces from weak to intact zonules (Fig. 6.18). Also reduces capsular phimosis, IOL decentration, and possibly PCO. The open ring is made of

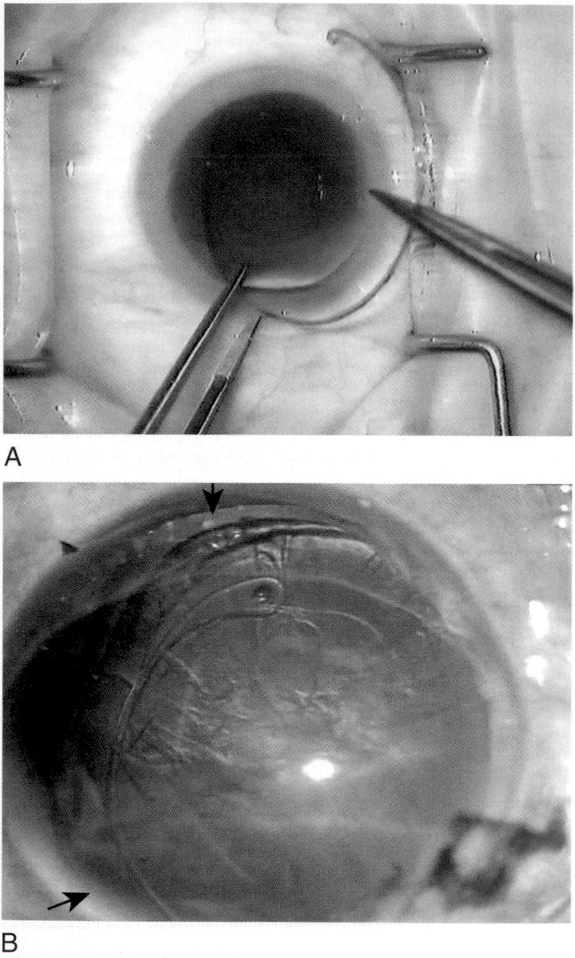

A

B

Fig. 6.18: Inserting capsular tension rings (CTR). **(A)** CTR (Ophthtec) being introduced into the capsular bag via a temporal corneal section. **(B)** CTR (Morcher) insertion before nucleus removal in a patient with anrirdia and 160° zonular dialysis.

PMMA, available in a range of sizes denoted by the diameter of the open ring/compressed ring in millimetres, e.g. 12/10. Insert as large a ring as possible, especially in high myopes. Overlapping of the ends of the CTR is acceptable. Contraindications include incomplete capsulorrhexis or anterior capsule tear, posterior capsule tear if not concentric, and ≥180° zonular dialysis. Insert intact into the bag at any point after capsulorrhexis using forceps or injector. Aspiration of soft lens matter (SLM) trapped under the CTR may be difficult, so delay insertion until after cortical clearance if possible. If zonular loss is marked consider a modified CTR with one or two eyelets positioned anterior to the capsule to allow scleral fixation (e.g. Cionni ring) or, alternatively, consider a sutured PCIOL or ACIOL.

Brunescent lens Dense, large nuclei are at high risk of posterior capsular tear, zonular dehiscence, corneal endothelial damage, and phako wound burns. Use a 'soft shell' viscoelastic technique (see below). Ensure a large capsulorrhexis for safer phako and manipulation. Keep the bottle height low to reduce irrigation volume if surgery is prolonged. Chop techniques reduce phako time and zonular stress. Move the phako tip slowly when sculpting; avoid pushing lens and use sufficient power to emulsify. Beware grooving too deep as the epinucleus is thin or absent. Reduce the total phako time using burst mode or pulse mode (also reduces 'chatter' during fragment removal, i.e. fragments being pushed away from the tip). Dense adhesions may preclude adequate cracking/chopping and residual plate may require separate phako removal.

White cataracts Absent red reflex, release of 'lens milk', and risk of peripheral capsular tears makes capsulorrhexis difficult (Fig. 6.19). Use trypan blue 0.06% (Vision Blue™) to improve capsule visualization. Increased pressure from the intumescent lens may cause the capsulorrhexis to tear peripherally, so aim to make a slightly smaller capsulorrhexis and consider higher-density viscoelastic. See also brunescent lenses above.

High myopia Exclude peripheral retinal breaks pre- and postoperatively. Discuss refractive targeting and the risk of retinal detachment. If the patient desires unaided reading vision, aim for −2.50 DS; for emmetropia aim for −0.50 DS. Beware posterior staphyloma so consider a B-scan cross-check to confirm the axial length (p. 257). Avoid sharp needle LA techniques. The AC is deep, so make a short tunnel incision to avoid distorting the cornea. Capsulorrhexis is more difficult with a deep AC but keep fully formed with viscoelastic to avoid a peripheral tear and do not make it too large. A steep approach with phako makes sculpting

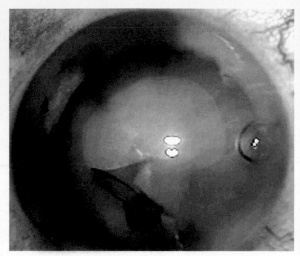

Fig. 6.19: Trypan blue use in white cataract surgery.

and vertical chopping more difficult – a horizontal chop is easier. The depth of the AC can be decreased by permitting some leakage through a side port with the second instrument. Use hydrophilic or hydrophobic acrylic IOLs with square-edged design to reduce posterior capsular opacification (optic diameter ≥6 mm). Avoid silicone IOLs and consider a CTR. Perform second eye surgery in quick succession to minimize the duration of anisometropia/aniseikonia; review refractive outcome from the first eye to check the accuracy of biometry.

Posterior polar cataract This may conceal a defect in the PC. Perform gentle hydrodissection, if any. Consider hydrodelineation alone with viscodissection of cortex after nucleus removal. Ensure a stable AC with low vacuum and bottle height. Avoid divide and conquer; use phako-chop or bowl technique instead (the nucleus is usually soft). Have Sheet's glide/Vectis at hand should a PC defect be present.

Shallow AC/Hypermetropia Make a watertight, long tunnel with three-step incision and small side ports to prevent leaks. Maximize the AC depth and stability with highly cohesive viscoelastic (Healon 5 or GV). Avoid endothelial trauma; use 'soft-shell' viscoelastic method (see below). Reduce the total phako power using chop technique and pulse/burst/cool phako mode. In extremely shallow ACs, a pars plana vitreous tap can create enough working space to perform surgery.

Fuchs' endothelial dystrophy/Guttatae Minimizing endothelial cell loss is paramount. Use a *'soft-shell' technique*: inject dispersive viscoelastic (e.g. Viscoat) adjacent to the endothelium then expand the AC below using cohesive viscoelastic, thus spreading dispersive agent against endothelium. Phako as far from the endothelium as safely possible and reduce total energy with phako-chop and cool/pulse/burst mode. Avoid applying phako power within dispersive viscoelastics as they may coagulate, block aspiration, and cause a phako burn.

Uveitis Explain the increased risks of surgery (relapse of uveitis/cystoid macular oedema, CMO) and the need for careful follow-up. Ideally, uveitis should be controlled for 3 months preoperatively and treatment stable. Pre operative steroids are indicated in patients with posterior uveitis, a history of CMO with anterior uveitis, or CMO following surgery in the first eye. The regimen is usually prednisolone EC 40 mg o.d. for 2 weeks preoperatively and tapered by 5 mg/week postoperatively to the preoperative dose, or, if contraindicated, consider intravitreal triamcinolone at the time of surgery (if not a steroid responder). Use a clear corneal incision, acrylic foldable IOLs, and intensive postoperative topical steroids (G. dexamethasone 0.1% 1–2-hourly). Patients with a history of anterior uveitis not associated with CMO do not usually require prophylactic systemic or topical steroids, but those with chronic anterior uveitis should receive dexamethasone 0.1% b.d.–q.d.s. preoperatively. Patients with Fuchs' heterochromic cyclitis require no topical steroids preoperatively but will require at least q.d.s. dexamethasone 0.1% or equivalent postoperatively.

Glaucoma Be aware that nuclear sclerosis may give the false impression of preserved neuroretinal tissue at the optic disc. Patients with a past history of angle closure glaucoma are likely to have a shallow AC and may get postoperative corneal decompensation. Those with advanced glaucoma may lose VA if postoperative IOP elevation 'snuffs out' the small remaining island of vision; however, avoid oral acetazolamide in those with functioning trabeculectomies as reduced aqueous flow may promote fistula closure. Small pupils are common in those on miotics; where possible discontinue 2 weeks preoperatively. Temporal clear corneal incisions help avoid conjunctival manipulation at the site of existing or future trabeculectomy blebs. Those with functioning trabeculectomy blebs require longer and more intensive postoperative steroids, e.g. dexamethasone 0.1%, 2-hourly for the first week then q.d.s., tapering off over 3 months. Some clinicians advocate subconjunctival 5FU at the time of surgery.

Diabetes See page 469.

Intraoperative Complications

When complications occur during surgery: stop, take a deep breath, and think clearly about what to do next.

Posterior capsule tears

Posterior capsule tears (PCT) during phacoemulsification occur at <1% amongst experienced surgeons, and up to 15% amongst juniors. Identification of predisposing factors, timely recognition, and appropriate management significantly minimizes the associated morbidity. Signs of PCT include sudden deepening of the anterior chamber (AC) and momentary pupil dilatation, direct visualization of the capsule defect or vitreous prolapse, sudden shallowing of the AC during hydrodissection, unstable or immobile lens, and occlusion of the phako handpiece (vitreous occlusion).

Figure 6.20 outlines the management of PCT. If suspected, do *not* immediately remove instruments from eye; instead, lower the bottle height to minimum and assess:

- Extent of the PCT and vitreous loss into the AC.

- Amount of residual lens matter – if the nucleus is remaining, the priority is to safely prevent dropped fragments.

- Remaining capsular support – is sufficient capsule present to secure a PCIOL either in the bag or sulcus?

The key principles are to stabilize the AC, preventing extension of the PCT/further vitreous prolapse, and to perform as few manoeuvres as possible to achieve the desired repositioning of the vitreous. If no vitreous prolapses from a small PCT with intact anterior hyaloid face, it may be possible to convert to a primary posterior capsulorhexis after visco-tamponade and residual nucleus may be removed by careful phako (low vacuum/flow rate), thus avoiding anterior vitrectomy entirely. If there is vitreous loss into the AC, retrieve any free lens fragments manually (Fig. 6.21) but perform anterior vitrectomy (Box 6.3) before attempting to remove any lens material trapped by vitreous. Scissor/swab vitrectomy may be sufficient if the prolapse is minimal (Fig. 6.22).

Posterior dislocation of nucleus or nuclear fragments into the vitreous ('dropped nucleus') Resist the temptation to retrieve dropped lens material as there is a high risk that vitreous traction will cause retinal breaks. Refer to a retinal surgeon for vitrectomy,

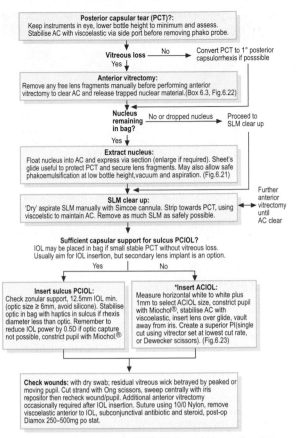

Fig. 6.20: Algorithm for management of posterior capsule rupture.

Posterior capsular tear (PCT)?:
Keep instruments in eye, lower bottle height to minimum and assess. Stabilise AC with viscoelastic via side port before removing phako probe.

Vitreous loss — No → Convert PCT to 1° posterior capsulorrhexis if possible

Yes ↓

Anterior vitrectomy:
Remove any free lens fragments manually before performing anterior vitrectomy to clear AC and release trapped nuclear material.(Box 6.3, Fig.6.22)

Nucleus remaining in bag? No or dropped nucleus → Proceed to SLM clear up

Yes ↓

Extract nucleus:
Float nucleus into AC and express via section (enlarge if required). Sheet's glide useful to protect PCT and secure lens fragments. May also allow safe phakoemulsification at low bottle height,vacuum and aspiration. (Fig.6.21)

SLM clear up: ← Further anterior vitrectomy until AC clear
'Dry' aspirate SLM manually with Simcoe cannula. Strip towards PCT, using viscoelstic to maintain AC. Remove as much SLM as safely possible.

Sufficient capsular support for sulcus PCIOL?
IOL may be placed in bag if small stable PCT without vitreous loss. Usually aim for IOL insertion, but secondary lens implant is an option.

Yes / No

Insert sulcus PCIOL:
Check zonular support, 12.5mm IOL min. (optic size ≥ 6mm, avoid silicone). Stabilise optic in bag with haptics in sulcus if rhexis diameter less than optic. Remember to reduce IOL power by 0.5D if optic capture not possible, constrict pupil with Miochol.®

*Insert ACIOL:
Measure horizontal white to white plus 1mm to select ACIOL size, constrict pupil with Miochol®, stabilise AC with viscoelastic, insert lens over glide, vault away from iris. Create a superior PI(single cut using vitrector set at lowest cut rate, or Dewecker scissors). (Fig.6.23)

Check wounds: with dry swab; residual vitreous wick betrayed by peaked or moving pupil. Cut strand with Ong scissors, sweep centrally with iris repositor then recheck wound/pupil. Additional anterior vitrectomy occasionally required after IOL insertion. Suture using 10/0 Nylon, remove viscoelastic anterior to IOL, subconjunctival antibiotic and steroid, post-op Diamox 250–500mg po stat.

* Alternatively, some prefer secondary sutured PCIOLs (e.g. in corneal decompensation, guttatae, shallow AC, angle pathology, glaucoma) but beware of associated complications (e.g. subluxation, vitreous haemorrhage, RD).

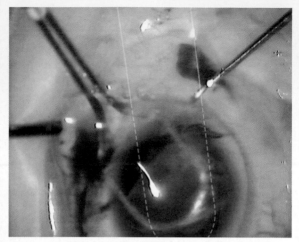

Fig. 6.21: Removal of lens fragment using vectis. Here, a Sheet's glide has been placed over the PC defect to prevent dislocation into the vitreous.

after clearing the AC vitreous and as much SLM as possible. Lens insertion is decided according to local preference but an IOL should usually be placed so that pars plana vitrectomy and fragmatome lens removal can be completed without re-entering the anterior segment (Fig. 6.23).

Postopertively prescribe G. dexamethasone 0.1% preservative free (PF) 1–2 hourly for 1 week then taper slowly over 8 weeks minimum; G. chloramphenicol 0.5% PF q.d.s. 2 weeks; acetazolamide SR 250 mg b.d. p.o. if the IOP is raised or significant viscoelastic is retained. Consider G. ketorolac 0.5% (Acular) q.d.s. 1 month as prophylaxis against cystoid macular oedema (CMO). Review at day 1 for raised IOP, lens and pupil position, wound integrity, and dilated retinal examination. Thereafter, review at day 7, 30, 60 or more frequently as required. Visual rehabilitation is often delayed, but optimal management can minimize the higher risk of CMO, chronic anterior uveitis, IOL decentration, secondary glaucoma, endophthalmitis, and RD.

Suprachoroidal haemorrhage

A rare (0.1%) but devastating complication, due to rupture of bridging vessels crossing the suprachoroidal space. Risk factors

Box 6.3: Anterior vitrectomy (Fig. 6.22)

1. Be familiar with the anterior vitrector before it is required; know how to set up the machine.

2. A bimanual method is preferred by many to limit hydration and further vitreous prolapse. Separate the 20-gauge cutter from the infusion. If there is minimal vitreous prolapse, perform a 'dry' vitrectomy (no infusion), maintaining the AC with viscoelastic. Otherwise, insert the infusion cannula via a side port.

3. Check the vitrector is cutting and aspirating in BSS before using in the eye; if the vitrector blows bubbles, the tubes are incorrectly connected.

4. Insert the vitrector via a corneal section. A pars plana approach 3.5 mm behind limbus is an alternative for experienced surgeons. Set at low vacuum but avoid low cut rates.

5. Place the cutter tip through the PCT and hold steady just behind the capsule, with the cutting port facing anteriorly and visible at all times.

6. Vitreous is difficult to visualize; use pupil asymmetry and iris movement to betray residual vitreous. Intracameral fluorescein (2 drops of 2% unpreserved fluorescein in 2 mL BSS) can be used to stain prolapsed vitreous for easy detection (triamcinolone suspension has also been used for this purpose).

7. Minimize further vitreous loss: avoid shallowing the AC, tamponade with viscoelastic each time before resuming anterior vitrectomy, and lower the bottle height to reduce vitreous hydration. Keep the vitrectomy to the least required to clear the AC to the plane of the PCT and minimize capsular loss.

8. Suture all wounds to ensure positive AC pressure and to decrease the potential for vitreous migration to the wounds.

may include age >65 years, atherosclerosis, anticoagulation (warfarin, aspirin), tachycardia, hypertension, Valsalva manoeuvre, myopia, unstable AC, glaucoma, uveitis, and previous ocular surgery. Early recognition is critical. Look for a sudden shallowing of the AC with positive posterior pressure and iris prolapse. Self-sealing wounds of small incision surgery usually limit the bleed – *never* convert to ECCE as there is a high risk of expulsion of the intraocular contents. Deepen the AC if possible and close the eye *immediately*. Examine the fundus on the table for dark choroidal elevation. Give intravenous 20% mannitol (1 mg/kg over 30 minutes) on the table. If the bleed is limited, surgery may be

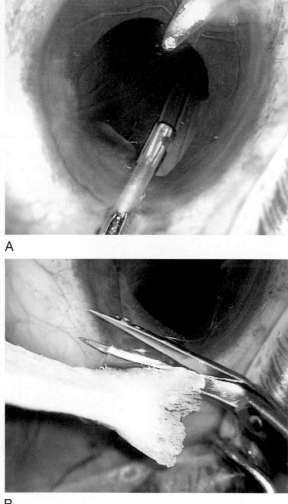

A

B

Fig. 6.22: **(A)** Anterior vitrectomy using bimanual technique with separate cutter and infusion (here a Simcoe is being used as infusion). **(B)** Scissor swab vitrectomy at wound.

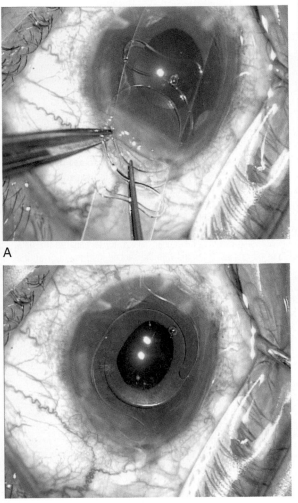

A

B

Fig. 6.23: ACIOL: **(A)** ACIOL is inserted over a Sheet's glide **(B)** ACIOL in situ with haptics in the angle (PI yet to be performed).

completed after waiting at least 30 minutes for the blood to clot. Early drainage via a sclerostomy is controversial and should not be attempted if inexperienced. Postoperatively, arrange a vitreoretinal opinion to exclude RD and consider late drainage of a large suprachoroidal haemorrhage when the clot liquefies. Small haemorrhages may do well but the visual prognosis is usually poor.

Anterior capsule tears/discontinuous capsulorrhexis

Radial capsulorrhexis tears risk extending to the equator and the posterior capsule. To prevent losing a peripherally tearing capsulorrhexis, ensure the AC is fully formed with viscoelastic and attempt to redirect the tearing forces towards the centre by gripping the capsule as close to the tearing point as possible. If the capsulorrhexis is lost under the iris, try to visualize the end-point by retracting the iris with the second instrument or an iris hook. Rescue may also be possible by starting a new tear in the opposite direction to include the deviation. If rescue is not feasible, an experienced surgeon may proceed with 'gentle' phako in the presence of a single tear: use gentle and minimal hydrodissection; avoid overinflation (or collapse) of the AC; use slow bimanual rotation of the nucleus; employ chop techniques and careful cortical aspiration. If the IOL is placed in the bag, position the haptics perpendicular to the tear, or else insert in the sulcus. If phako is too risky, complete the rhexis and convert to extracapsular extraction.

Intraoperative iris prolapse

This is usually due to the wound opening into the AC too posteriorly with a short corneal tunnel. Prolapse is also more likely if the AC is shallow or the iris is 'floppy' – beware patients taking Flomax (tamsulosin). Ensure good wound construction; perform hydrodissection via a paracentesis rather than the main wound if there is a risk of prolapse. In the event of prolapse, tamponade the iris away from the wound with viscoelastic and use an iris repositor via a side port to gently sweep the prolapsed iris back into the AC. If minor prolapse recurs consider proceeding with surgery if iris trauma is minimal. Consider placing iris hooks either side of the wound and subincisionally to secure the iris. Other options include suturing the wound and making a new incision with a longer tunnel, or creating a peripheral iridectomy in the prolapsing iris (beware the risk of postoperative glare from temporal iridectomies). Ensure the corneal wound is well sutured at the end of surgery.

Corneal phako burn

The phako tip heats significantly when emulsification continues without flow of irrigation fluid, resulting in a thermal corneal burn at the main incision, compromising wound integrity and causing significant astigmatism (Fig. 6.24). Wounds frequently require multiple sutures to remain watertight. Phako burns are much less likely using burst mode or hyper-pulse ('cool phaco').

Causes include:

◼ Obstruction to flow by viscoelastic: this results in 'smoke' (emulsified viscoelastic) appearing at the phako tip. Ensure adequate aspiration of viscoelastic before starting phako.

◼ Wound too tight, constricting the infusion sleeve. Enlarge the wound appropriately.

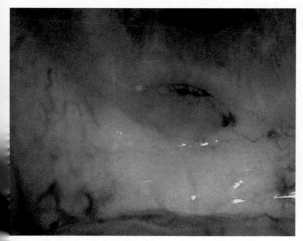

Fig. 6.24: Phako burn. (Courtesy of G. S. Bhermi.)

Postoperative Complications

Although highly successful, modern phako surgery is not without complications (Table 6.4). See page 237 for anaesthetic complications and page 260 for the management of intraoperative complications.

Elevated intraocular pressure Postoperative IOP elevation is common and usually self-limiting. Some surgeons routinely prescribe prophylactic acetazolamide 250 mg p.o. stat postoperatively, repeated at 6 hours. Causes of raised IOP include retained viscoelastic, overpressurized AC on completion of surgery, inflammation, preexisting glaucoma, posterior capsule (PC) rupture, and vitreous loss. Less common causes include pupil block (p. 325) and malignant glaucoma (p. 317). Short-term topical IOP lowering agents and/or systemic acetazolamide is usually successful in treating elevated IOP. Late (>2 weeks, typically 4–6 weeks) postoperative IOP rise after uncomplicated surgery is usually secondary to steroid response (p. 310) – stop steroids and use a topical NSAID (or G. rimexolone 1%) if required. Exclude chronic inflammation and retained lens matter.

Wound leak Prevention is better than cure! Causes include poor wound construction, phako burn, inadequate suture closure, and postoperative trauma. If the AC remains deep, observe or insert a bandage contact lens. If there is persistent or brisk leak, iris prolapse, flat AC or excess against-the-wound astigmatism, return to theatre to re-suture wound.

Table 6.4: Complications of phako surgery			
Intraoperative	**Incidence %**	**Postoperative**	**Incidence %**
Zonular/PC rupture	2.68	Uveitis	2.4
Vitreous loss	1.35	Endophthalmitis	0.06
Iris trauma	0.68	Wound gape/iris prolapse	0.06
Choroidal haemorrhage	0.1	Raised IOP	0.28 (open angle)
AC haemorrhage	0.09	Clinical cystoid macular oedema	0.6
		Retinal detachment	0.02

Johnston et al. UK 8 Centre Electronic Patient Record Audit. In Royal College of Ophthalmologists Cataract Surgery Guidelines 2004.

Postoperative iris prolapse This may be avoided with well-constructed, self-sealing wounds or adequate suture closure in those at risk (shallow AC, 'floppy iris' in those on tamsulosin (Flomax), intraoperative prolapse, risk of rubbing eye postoperatively). G. pilocarpine 4% in the early postoperative period may reduce minor incarceration but surgery is usually required if the iris is prolapsed through the wound. Reposition viable iris if not epithelialized (<48 hours), excise any nonviable tissue, and suture the wound. Intensive topical steroids and antibiotic are required to reduce the risk of severe inflammation or infection.

Decentred, subluxed, or unstable intraocular lens This may be asymptomatic, or result in reduced best-corrected vision, dysphotopsia, diplopia, glare, uveitis-glaucoma hyphaema syndrome. Causes include loss of capsular support (anterior rhexis tear, PC tear, zonular dehiscence), asymmetric haptic placement, and pupil capture (if rhexis larger than optic or sulcus PCIOL). According to symptoms and signs, management is by early or late IOL repositioning, PCIOL exchange with or without fixation (iris or scleral), or replacement with an ACIOL. Minimize intervention if the endothelial count is low and beware the eccentric pupil (c.f. IOL subluxation). An IOL dislocated into the vitreous does not necessarily require retrieval but may be removed via a vitrectomy if the mobile lens gives troublesome symptoms. Refer routinely for vitreoretinal review.

Corneal decompensation Risk factors include preexisting endothelial compromise (symptomatic diurnal variation in vision, guttatae, pachymetry >630 μm) and intraoperative endothelial trauma. Exclude postoperative IOP rise. To minimize endothelial cell loss, use highly retentive viscoelastic protection, reduce phako energy with pulse, burst, or cool phako mode, and use chop techniques. Allow at least 3 months for resolution of oedema and assess vision and pachymetry before considering corneal graft surgery. Consider interim treatment with topical hypertonic saline (G. sodium chloride 5% q.d.s. or Oc. sodium chloride l0% nocte).

Rhegmatogenous retinal detachment The reported incidence after uncomplicated phako surgery ranges from 0.2–3.6% (average 0.7%). The excess risk in the first 10 years is probably 5.5, with most occurring in the first year. The risk is increased with PC rupture or vitreous loss (4.5–13-fold), high myopia (10-fold), peripheral lattice degeneration, ocular trauma, or previous retinal detachment. Some studies show increased risk in myopic males compared to females.

Refractive surprise See page 230.

Cystoid macular oedema See page 492.

Endophthalmitis See page 382.

Posterior capsular opacification (PCO) The most common complication (<10% at 2 years) occurring months to years after cataract surgery due to proliferation and migration of residual lens epithelial cells across the PC. Symptoms include gradual blurring, glare, or reduced contrast sensitivity. PCO may be asymptomatic. Exclude coexisting disease accounting for visual loss. Patient-, surgical-, and IOL-related factors influence the risk of developing PCO.

- *Patient factors*: young age (virtually 100% occurrence in children) and uveitis.

- *Surgical factors*: in the bag IOL fixation and 360° overlap of the capsulorrhexis margin onto the anterior optic surface provide biomechanical barriers to posterior lens epithelial cell migration. Good cortical clean-up reduces the risk but routine anterior or posterior capsule polishing may not.

- *IOL factors*: barriers to cell migration include square-edged optic and contact between the optic and posterior capsule (facilitated by angled haptics; large optic diameter; convex posterior optic surface; bioadhesive IOL material, e.g. hydrophobic acrylic c.f. silicone or PMMA).

Treatment involves Nd:YAG laser posterior capsulotomy (Box 6.4 and Fig. 6.25) or rarely surgical removal.

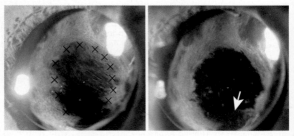

Fig. 6.25: Inverted-'U' (horseshoe) Nd:YAG laser posterior capsulotomy. Avoids visual axis and minimizes floaters post laser. Yellow stars represent position of laser shots. Note capsule flap remains attached inferiorly and folds backward (white arrow).

Box 6.4: Nd:YAG posterior capsulotomy

1. Consent.

   Benefit: Improve VA and contrast sensitivity, reduce glare, improve view of the fundus for management of posterior segment disease.

   Risk: IOP rise, inflammation, IOL pitting (not usually visually significant unless in the visual axis); subluxation or posterior dislocation of the IOL (especially silicone plate haptic IOLs). Rarely bleeding, iris damage, endophthalmitis (release of loculated bacteria), corneal decompensation, macular oedema (less likely if capsulotomy is delayed ≥3 months postoperatively); retinal detachment (up to 4.1% within 4 years, excess risk 3.9), especially if axial length >24 mm.

2. Check the pupil position and visual axis on the slit lamp before dilating the pupil.

3. Instil topical anaesthetic before applying a capsulotomy contact lens (e.g. Abraham lens).

4. Set the laser to a single pulse. Defocus by +1.50 D. Minimize laser energy: start with ≤1 mJ, increase the power until sufficient to open the capsule (rarely need >2.5 mJ). Focus on or just behind capsule with the helium–neon aiming beam.

5. Start peripherally to avoid pitting the IOL in the visual axis. Aim to clear the visual axis to the largest physiological mydriatic pupil size or more if a clear peripheral fundal view is important, e.g. diabetic retinopathy. An inverted-'U' (horseshoe) opening avoids the potential of pitting in the visual axis (unlike a cruciate opening) and minimizes 'floaters' (unlike full-'circular' capsulotomy). Treating areas under tension allows the capsule to spring apart, minimizing the number of shots (and total energy) required. Usually requires 30–40 shots.

6. For prophylaxis against post-YAG IOP spike, instil 1 drop apraclonidine 1% before and after treatment. Alternatively, a single dose of oral acetazolamide SR 250 mg may be given. Check IOP 1 hour post laser.

7. To minimize inflammation, prescribe a short course of topical steroid, e.g. G. dexamethasone 0.1% q.d.s. 5–7 days.

8. Warn about new floaters, and distinguish from retinal detachment symptoms.

Follow-up is not routinely required, but patients with raised IOP at 1 hour despite prophylactic treatment should be monitored for glaucoma.

Optometry and General Practice Guidelines

General comments

Age-related cataracts produce a gradual reduction in acuity. The diagnosis is seldom difficult using slit lamp examination. The red reflex is often altered when viewed with a direct ophthalmoscope, although nuclear sclerotic cataracts may be less evident than cortical lens opacities or posterior subcapsular cataracts. If the vision deteriorates below the patient's requirements and they would like to discuss surgery, then arrange routine referral. Direct referral by optometrists using local guidelines is increasingly favoured in the UK.

Optometrists

■ If symptoms are disproportionate to VA using standard high-contrast charts, check contrast sensitivity, low-contrast VA, and glare sensitivity. These may give a better indication of 'real world' visual function.

■ Where possible, include the following when referring:

1. Visual symptoms attributable to cataract, including the effect on the patient's desired lifestyle, occupation, and driving.

2. Any known ocular comorbidity.

3. Up-to-date spectacle refraction and best corrected VA in each eye.

4. Any relevant medical or social history and any special circumstances.

General practitioners

■ Remember the cataractogenic effect of long-term corticosteroid use (including eye drops, face cream, oral or inhaled steroids).

■ Consider reduced VA as a cause of falls in the elderly. Gradually progressing cataracts may mean patients are unaware of very poor VA.

- Exclude diabetes mellitus, especially in younger patients with cataract.

- Remember to record Snellen VA. Where possible, refer to an optometrist to confirm the diagnosis of cataract, and for best corrected VA with updated refraction before considering surgery.

- Identify systemic disease which may compromise surgery or the anaesthetic, e.g. orthopnoea, respiratory or cardiovascular disease.

- Provide a list of current medications. Flomax (tamsulosin), anticoagulants and antiplatelet drugs are particularly relevant.

- Poorly controlled hypertension or diabetes increases the risk of complications and may result in cancellation of surgery. Initiate measures to improve control prior to referral, and monitor in the run-up to surgery.

- Explain that smoking increases the risk of cataract. Stopping may slow progression.

Chapter 7

GLAUCOMA

Pharmacology of Intraocular Pressure-Lowering Drugs

Background Glaucoma describes a group of disorders with characteristic structural optic neuropathy (disc cupping) and associated visual field loss. Intraocular pressure (IOP) is often, but not always elevated.

Recognized types of glaucoma include:

- Primary open-angle glaucoma.

- Angle-closure glaucoma.

- Secondary glaucoma (due to uveitis, trauma, etc.).

- Congenital glaucoma.

Reducing IOP is often the most effective means of preserving the visual field.

IOP-lowering medications Prostaglandin agonists have superceded beta blockers as the first-choice therapy due to greater efficacy at lowering IOP and fewer side effects. If the first-choice monotherapy alone is not effective or not tolerated, it is preferable to switch to another drug that can be initiated as monotherapy, such as a beta blocker.

Pilocarpine has been less prescribed in recent years because of the ocular side effects and the frequent daily dosage, but is still useful in primary angle closure with plateau iris configuration, in acute angle closure with pupillary block mechanism, and in aphakic glaucoma.

If monotherapy is well tolerated but insufficient to reach the target IOP, consider adding a second drug or using a combined drug preparation. The commonly prescribed combination drugs are:

- Timolol 0.5% and dorzolamide 2% (Cosopt) – this has additive effect with pilocarpine.

- Latanoprost 0.005% and timolol 0.5% (Xalacom).

Side effects and precautions Occlusion of the nasolacrimal duct may help to reduce the incidence of the side effects shown in the Table 7.1. For drug use in pregnancy, see page 702.

Pharmacology of intraocular pressure-lowering drugs

Table 7.1: Common side effects

Category	Generics	Main mechanism of action	Most common or severe side effects	Contraindications (CI), precautions (P), and theoretical risks (T)
Prostaglandin F2α analogues	Latanoprost Travaprost Bimatoprost	Increased uveoscleral outflow (IUSO)	Increased skin and iris pigmentation, excessive lash growth, aphakic cystoid macular oedema. Rarely: reactivate herpes keratitis, uveitis. Latanoprost less likely to cause red eye than Bimatoprost or Travaprost.	T: risk of abortion (See p. 702).
Nonselective β antagonists	Timolol Levobunolol Carteolol Metipranolol	Reduced aqueous production (RAP)	Bradycardia, arrhythmia, heart failure, bronchospasm, syncope, nocturnal hypotension, headache, depression. Mild corneal hypoaesthesia with prolonged use.	CI: asthma, chronic obstructive airways disease (COAD), bradycardia, heart block, heart failure. Avoid in normal pressure glaucoma. T: patients on oral hypotensives.
Selective β1 antagonist	Betaxolol	RAP	Similar to other β antagonists but theoretically fewer respiratory side effects.	P: asthma, COAD, bradycardia, heart block, heart failure.
Alpha2 agonists	Brimonidine Apraclonidine	RAP & IUSO RAP	Allergy and red eye, taste disturbance. Respiratory failure and fatigue in children. Fatigue may also occur in adults.	CI: Oral monoamine oxidase (MAO) inhibitor users and children.

Table 7.1: Common side effects—cont'd

Category	Generics	Main mechanism of action	Most common or severe side effects	Contraindications (CI), precautions (P), and theoretical risks (T)
Parasympathomimetics	Pilocarpine	Increased aqueous outflow	Miosis, pseudomyopia, brow ache, ciliary spasm. Rarely pupil block. Theoretical increased risk of retinal detachment.	P: Urinary outflow obstruction, asthma. T: Parkinsonism, peptic ulcers.
Carbonic anhydrase inhibitors (CAI)	Brinzolamide Dorzolamide	RAP	Blurred vision, aesthenia, paraesthesia, induced myopia.	CI: sulphonamide allergy, severe renal impairment. P: corneal endothelial dysfunction.
Oral CAI	Acetazolamide	RAP	Paraesthesia, nausea, vomiting, diarrhoea, depression, electrolyte imbalance. Rarely, blood dyscrasias, metabolic acidosis, renal stones.	CI: suprarenal gland failure, electrolyte imbalance, severe liver disease. P: reduce dose if renal failure (liaise with renal physicians).
Hyperosmotics	Glycerol (1.0–1.5 g/kg p.o.) Mannitol (1.0–1.5 g/kg i.v.)	RAP	Hyperglycaemia (glycerol), pulmonary congestion, electrolyte imbalance, dehydration, headache, chest pain (mannitol), disorientation, coma.	CI: diabetes. P: renal failure, elderly patients with renal or cardiovascular disease.

History

Ask about:

- Active problems, mode of presentation, and the patient's worries.

- Presenting IOPs, if recorded at source of referral.

- Past ophthalmic history (e.g. uveitis, trauma). Surgery and complications, especially glaucoma, cataract, retinal procedures, and refractive surgery (alters corneal thickness and IOP measurements). Refractive error. Contact lens usage (may be affected by surgery and influence choice of medication).

- Medical history for conditions linked with glaucoma (hypotensive crises, migraine, Raynaud's phenomenon) and those affecting the choice of medication (bradyarrhythmias, asthma, renal stones, sickle cell disease).

- Medication used previously and currently, especially: systemic beta blockers; other antihypertensive medication; systemic, inhaled, or topical steroids; and bronchodilators. Any side effects of ocular medications.

- Ethnic/racial group and preferred language.

- Family history of glaucoma or blindness.

- Occupation. Are driving authorities aware of the diagnosis?

- Social support and care arrangements.

Optic Disc Examination

Background Identification of characteristic optic disc changes enables a diagnosis of glaucoma to be made, and the detection of disease progression.

Examination Measure the vertical disc size by reducing the height of the focused light beam to the same size as the disc. Note the beam height (mm) and lens used (magnification factor). Measure the cup-to-disc ratio (CDR). Normal CDR varies with disc size (Fig. 7.1). Assess the rim for focal thinning or notches. Check the 'ISNT rule': normal rim thickness inferior > superior > nasal > temporal.

Other features: tilting, parapapillary atrophy, disc haemorrhages, and 'bayoneting' (double angulation) or 'baring' (exposing) of blood vessels. Nerve fibre layer defects are best seen using either white or red-free light, carefully focused, particularly in superotemporal or inferotemporal nerve fibre bundles. Record all observations. Asymmetric CDR is suspicious of glaucoma if the discs are the same size.

Imaging A baseline record of disc appearance (photograph or scanning laser ophthalmoscope image) aids detection of change.

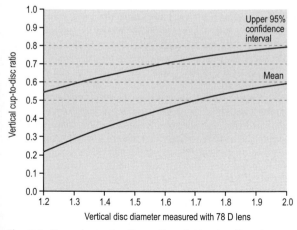

Fig. 7.1: Normal cup-to-disc ratio relative to disc size (Courtesy of DF Garway-Heath).

Gonioscopy

Background Examine the drainage angle of all patients with suspected glaucoma or ocular hypertension, both at diagnosis and periodically thereafter.

Equipment Goldmann one- or two-mirror lenses are steeper than corneal curvature (K) and require a coupling medium. Four-mirror lenses (Zeiss, Posner, Sussman) are flatter than K. Steeper-than-K lenses provide a stable, clear view and are easier to use. They can be used to perform dynamic (compression) examination. Four-mirror lenses are superior for difficult dynamic examinations.

Examination Dim ambient illumination and ensure adequate topical anaesthesia. Apply a low-viscosity coupling fluid (e.g. Viscotears or hypromellose 0.5%) to the Goldmann lens. Use a narrow slit beam, 1 mm long to avoid pupil constriction and widening of the angle. Identify Schwalbe's line at the apex of the corneal wedge reflex (Fig. 7.2). The trabecular meshwork lies immediately posterior to this. Estimate the geometric width of the angle (in degrees) between the surface of the trabecular meshwork and a line tangential to the peripheral one-third of the iris. Note the profile of the iris (plateau, concave, regular, steep), its first point of contact with corneoscleral coat and its point of true insertion (modified Spaeth classification). The angle width is often recorded as 1 = 10 degrees, 2 = 20 degrees. Care is necessary with shorthand notation, as this may lead to confusion with the inferior grading system that describes the angle structures visible (I, II, III and IV; IV being the widest, most open angle). The angle structures visible are heavily influenced by orientation of the eye and gonioscope. It is preferable to include a short explanatory note.

After assessing the angle width, widen the beam and examine the four quadrants again for the presence of pigment (intratrabecular, diffuse or geographic, blotchy deposits on trabecular surface), Sampaolesi's line (granular pigment on Schwalbe's line), and abnormalities such as neovascularization, membranes, angle recession or iridodialysis. Peripheral anterior synechiae are identified by using a Goldmann lens; ask the patient to look towards the mirror and gently indent the cornea with the edge of the lens. If the angle does not open, perform indentation gonioscopy with a four-mirror lens to differentiate between appositional and synechial angle closure. A normal angle is shown on page 297.

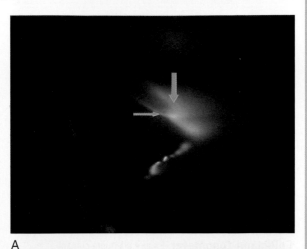

A

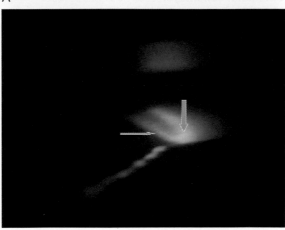

B

Fig. 7.2: Gonioscopy showing a wide-open angle **(A)** and a closed angle **(B)**. The corneal wedge is formed by the junction of the reflex from the corneoscleral junction (broad arrow) and the corneal endothelium (thin arrow). The apex of the wedge indicates the location of Schwalbe's line. The trabecular meshwork is visible posterior to this in the top image. See also Fig. 7.13.

Intraocular Pressure (IOP)

Background IOP is the cardinal modifiable risk factor for glaucoma. The prevalence of glaucoma rises with IOP but 30–50% of cases have normal IOP. Mean IOP rises with age in Caucasians, and tends to be highest in the morning. Glaucoma is associated with greater IOP fluctuations. IOP is measured by flattening or indenting the cornea, hence corneal abnormalities (scars, extremes of thickness) may significantly influence results. Inaccuracies of ±6 mmHg may occur at the extremes of corneal thickness. The use of correction tables and formulae to adjust for the effect of corneal thickness is controversial.

Equipment Goldmann (routine use), Perkins applanation tonometer (for immobile patients), and Tonopen (may offer advantages in scarred/abnormal corneas).

Goldmann tonometer Ensure adequate corneal anaesthesia and that the prism is clean and free from contaminants. Avoid excess fluorescein. If corneal astigmatism is >3.0 D, rotate the prism so the minus cylinder axis on the prism graduation corresponds to the red mark on the prism holder. If necessary, hold the lids against the orbital rim but avoid pressure on the globe. Be aware, breath-holding increases IOP. If the mires pulsate, measure at the midpulse amplitude. Note the time of measurement.

Calibration: mount the tonometer on the slit lamp with the prism inserted. Fit the calibration bar into the socket on the side of the tonometer. Graduations on the bar correspond to different IOPs: centre (0 = 0 mmHg), second (2 = 20 mmHg), third (6 = 60 mmHg). The longer part of the calibration bar is on the side opposite the prism (Fig. 7.3). Dialing the appropriate reading should cause the bar to pivot with adjustments ±2 mmHg either side of the correct reading.

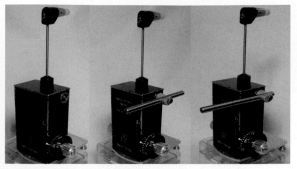

Fig. 7.3: Goldmann tonometer with calibration bar attached showing calibration to 0, 20, and 60 mm Hg (left to right).

Interpreting Humphrey Visual Field Tests

Background Static, white-on-white, semi-automated perimetry is the standard method for identifying and assessing progression of functional visual loss from glaucoma.

Single field test Ask, is the field: 1. Reliable and 2. Glaucomatous?

- The best measure of reliability given by the machine is the false-positive level: high levels of fixation losses and false negatives may not indicate unreliability.

- Causes of artefact include inattention (producing a 'clover-leaf' field), small pupil size, uncorrected refractive error, lens rim, lid/brow, media opacities, and macular disease.

- Characteristic sites of early glaucomatous damage are paracentral, nasal, and arcuate.

- 'Raw' thresholds give the height of the 'hill of vision' (in dB of attenuation: high dB values mean a dim stimulus was seen) at test locations.

- Total deviation compares the patient's 'hill of vision' to age-matched normals.

- Pattern deviation highlights focal rather than diffuse loss (total deviation shows both).

- Global indices attempt to summarize plots in a single number: MD (mean deviation) for total deviation, PSD (pattern standard deviation) for the pattern of deviation.

- The Glaucoma Hemifield Test compares corresponding clusters in superior and inferior hemifields. Repeatable abnormality suggests glaucoma.

- *Always evaluate fields in the light of other clinical findings, especially the optic disc appearance. If in doubt, repeat.*

Field series Ask if a field defect is: 1. Progressing and 2. If so, how fast?

- Ideally, all fields in the series should be same type, e.g. all Standard Full Threshold (FT) or all SITA. If the series is mixed FT/SITA use Pattern Deviation for progression.

- Some clinicians feel that clinical judgement alone is insufficient to decide about progression. Consider using glaucoma change software (Figs. 7.4, 7.5):

  1. Statpac2 (recently upgraded to Glaucoma Progression Analysis) compares fields with baseline for significant change.

  2. PROGRESSOR models the behaviour of each test location over time to detect significant progression.

- At least five fields are needed for a reliable decision.

- Sources of error include fluctuation (short- and long-term), learning effects, inappropriate change criteria, inappropriate frequency of testing, artefact (see Single field test, above), poor reliability (see Single field test, above), and field loss beyond the dynamic range of the perimeter.

Monocular field determines management. Binocular field determines quality of life.

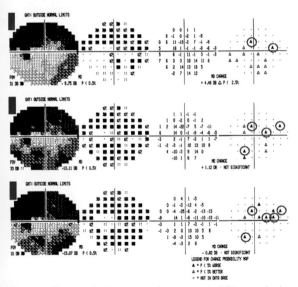

Fig. 7.4: Statpac 2 glaucoma change probability analysis. The test locations circled in blue show significant deterioration in two out of the three fields shown. Those circled in red showing significant deterioration in each of the three consecutive fields.

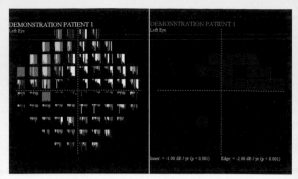

Fig. 7.5: PROGRESSOR output for the same visual field series shown in Fig. 7.4. The left pane shows the cumulative graphical output with each test location represented by a bar graph in which the length of the bar relates to the depth of the defect, and the colour representing the probability value of the regression slope. The right pane shows the test locations that satisfy progression criteria. Note that the pattern of progressing points is similar to the circled points in Fig. 7.4.

Primary Open Angle Glaucoma

Background A progressive optic neuropathy associated with distinctive, excavated disc appearance and a pattern of visual field loss localizing damage to the optic nerve head. Usually bilateral, but often asymmetric. Affects 2% of people over 40 years of age. Risk factors include Black African or Caribbean origin, positive family history, myopia, and increasing age. Elevated IOP is the most important modifiable risk factor for development of primary open angle glaucoma (POAG).

Symptoms Typically asymptomatic until advanced visual field loss occurs.

History Ask specifically for a family history of glaucoma and glaucoma blindness. Exclude causes of secondary glaucoma (history of trauma, uveitis, or steroid usage).

Examination

■ *Slit lamp*: the anterior segment is normal in POAG. Exclude signs of secondary glaucoma, e.g. pigment dispersion, pseudoexfoliation, neovascularization, anterior segment dysgenesis, angle closure and aphakia. The risk of POAG increases with the level of IOP.

■ *Gonioscopy*: by definition the angle is open, not occludable, and with no peripheral anterior synechiae. Gonioscopy is essential to differentiate POAG from other forms of glaucoma.

■ *Optic disc*: progressive, pathological loss of neuroretinal rim and associated nerve fibre layer defects, manifesting as enlargement of the cup-to-disc ratio.

Investigations

■ *Visual field*: look for progressive field loss anatomically consistent with the area of neuroretinal rim loss. Monitor with regular automated perimetry every 3–4 months if progression is suspected.

■ *Optic disc imaging*: a baseline photograph or scanning laser ophthalmoscope image is very useful for future comparison and detection of change.

■ *Central corneal thickness*: affects measured IOP, with thick corneas registering higher IOP (thin cornea vice versa). Mean thickness is $\approx 550\,\mu m$ (SD, $35\,\mu m$).

Diagnosis Moderate/advanced POAG is easily diagnosed with typical disc and field change. Early glaucoma is more difficult and may need monitoring for months or years before progression confirms the diagnosis.

Differential diagnosis

- *Ocular hypertension*: IOP >21 mmHg but no glaucomatous optic neuropathy.

- *Normal pressure glaucoma* (NPG): IOP <21 mmHg with characteristic progressive glaucomatous optic neuropathy. Identifying NPG as a subset of POAG is controversial as the risk gradually increases through the range of IOP.

Treatment All current treatments principally aim to lower IOP and reduce or eliminate glaucomatous progression. Options are medical, laser, or surgery.

- *Casualty*: Only start treatment if the diagnosis is certain and IOP is >28 mmHg, or if there is advanced disc damage. Start with single therapy regardless of IOP. Topical prostaglandin analogues are used as first-line treatment. Arrange routine clinic referral.

- *Clinic*: Treatment is tailored to the patient's circumstances (consider age, stage of glaucoma, etc.). Aim initially for a 30% IOP reduction medically. Stop treatment if not effective and use alternatives. Avoid polypharmacy. Monitor regularly for disc and field progression. If IOP reduction is not adequate to stop progression on maximal medical therapy (two or three drops) consider laser trabeculoplasty (p. 296) or trabeculectomy surgery (p. 289). The 'target pressure' for an individual patient is the estimated IOP needed to prevent progression: it may be different in each eye and may vary with time and changing circumstances (Fig. 7.6).

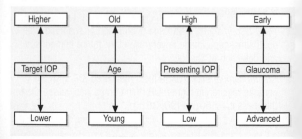

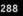

Fig. 7.6: Factors influencing the target IOP.

Trabeculectomy I: Surgical Technique

Indications Progressive glaucomatous field and/or disc changes. Failure to achieve target IOP. Failure or inability to use regular medication.

Anaesthesia

- *General anaesthetic*: children, anxious adults, complex/long procedures, high preoperative IOP (>30 mmHg).

- *Local anaesthetic*: use low volumes of anaesthetics combined with hyaluronidase to prevent pressure elevations. Subconjunctival anaesthesia is feasible combined with intracameral anaesthetic.

Consent

- *Benefit*: Stabilize but not improve vision. Reduced dependence on medication.

- *Risk*: Blindness ('wipe-out' in advanced glaucoma, endophthalmitis, suprachoroidal haemorrhage), loss of one line of Snellen acuity is likely, 12–66% chance of cataract progression at 3 years (most in first year), long-term possibility of blebitis ± endophthalmitis and need for surgical bleb revision, problems wearing contact lenses. Failure to control IOP and continued dependence on medication occurs in 10–30%.

Preoperative eyedrops

- *Steroids and NSAIDs*: topical application 24–72 hours before surgery in patients with conjunctival hyperaemia, who require iris manipulation or if fibrinous uveitis is possible.

- *IOP-lowering agents*: consider stopping aqueous suppressants in advance with outpatient IOP monitoring.

Technique See Box 7.1.

Box 7.1: Trabeculectomy

1. Superior limbus, under the lid, is the only acceptable site (document lid position preoperatively).

2. Place a 7/0 corneal traction suture (semicircular needle).

3. Use spring scissors to make a limbal conjunctival incision ('fornix-based flap'), at least 10 mm long.

4. Posteriorly, dissect a 15×15 mm subconjunctival pocket.

5. Lift conjunctiva and separate its attachments to muscle tendon.

6. Create a 4×3 mm scleral pocket by lamellar dissection (50% thickness) (Fig. 7.7).

7. Cut side incisions to within 1 mm of the limbus (Fig. 7.8).

8. Soak 4–6 sponges with mitomicin C (0.2 or 0.5 mg/mL) or 5FU (50 mg/mL) if required.

9. Fold and insert sponges into the subconjunctival and scleral pockets. Treat as large an area as possible but avoid the conjunctival wound edges (Fig. 7.9). After 3 minutes remove sponges and irrigate with 20 mL of balanced saline solution (BSS).

10. Preplace 10/0 Nylon sutures on the posterior corners of the scleral flap.

11. Make an oblique paracentesis. Consider continuous anterior chamber infusion in 'high-risk' patients.

12. Create a small (1 mm) limbal keratectomy with punch, or blade and scissors under the scleral flap (Fig. 7.10).

13. Create a peripheral iridectomy.

14. Suture the flap watertight with a combination of permanent, releasable or adjustable sutures (especially important with MMC use) (Fig. 7.11).

15. Test outflow by injecting BSS into the paracentesis, before conjunctival closure. Rotate any 'permanent' scleral flap sutures.

16. Close conjunctiva with 10/0 Vicryl purse-string sutures at the corners, and mattress sutures through conjunctiva and limbus.

17. Inject subconjunctival steroid and antibiotic, 180° away from the trabeculectomy site.

18. Ensure careful postoperative management. (see p. 294)

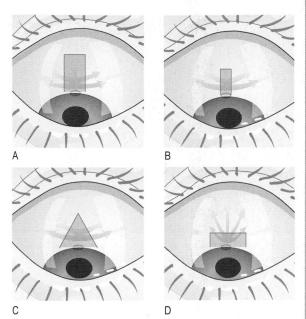

Fig. 7.7: Scleral flap design. Long, narrow, and triangular flaps **(A, B, C)** encourage aqueous flow laterally towards the limbus, increasing the risk of conjunctival thinning. A short, broad flap **(D)** is preferred, as it directs aqueous flow posteriorly, away from the limbal conjunctiva.

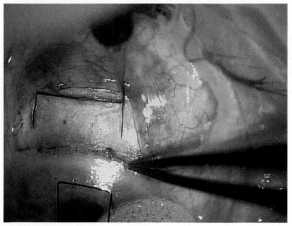

Fig. 7.8: Scleral flap. Limited side cuts help prevent 'aqueous jets' at the limbus which can produce conjunctival thinning.

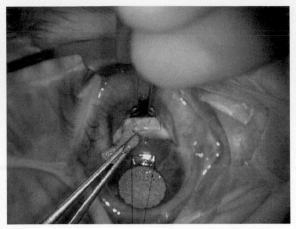

Fig. 7.9: Mitomycin-soaked sponge being inserted under the conjunctiva while protecting the conjunctival edge with a clamp.

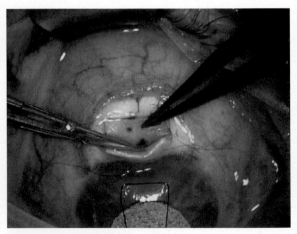

Fig. 7.10: Small sclerostomy with iris presenting prior to iridectomy. Note preplaced Nylon sutures.

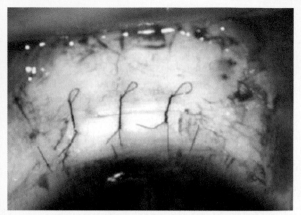

Fig. 7.11: Releasable sutures tied with four throws. The apex of the loop extending into the cornea is buried in a shallow corneal groove.

Trabeculectomy II: Postoperative Care

Background Careful postoperative care is essential to the success of glaucoma surgery. Typically, topical therapy includes: prednisolone acetate 1% 2-hourly for 2 weeks, tapering off over 12 weeks, topical antibiotics for 4 weeks and subconjunctival 5FU ± betnesol if the bleb is failing.

Signs of impending bleb failure Increased bleb vascularity, reduction of conjunctival microcysts, progressive IOP elevation or focal bleb encapsulation (Fig. 7.12).

Subconjunctival 5FU Used to modify postoperative wound healing, following a needling or re-exploration procedure, or to prevent failure after cataract surgery. Use topical amethocaine, povidone-iodine 5% and a lid speculum. Inject one-tenth of 1 mL of 50 mg/mL 5FU in an insulin syringe (integral 29-gauge needle) posterior to the bleb. This may be combined with 1–2 mg Betnesol. Stop before the injection meets the drainage area. Leave the needle in place for a few seconds (this helps to hydrate and seal the injection site). Irrigate any leakage.

Post-trabeculectomy complications

- *Shallow/flat anterior chamber*: differentiate high and low IOP. High IOP indicates aqueous misdirection (See below, and p. 317). Low IOP suggests over-drainage. Prevent by suturing the flap tight initially and avoiding early release of scleral flap sutures. Exclude conjunctival wound leaks. Dilate with atropine 1%. Most cases settle without intervention. Hypotony maculopathy requires revision of flap. If there is lens–corneal touch, consider reforming the anterior chamber with gas or viscoelastic.

- *Choroidal effusion*: treat with atropine and frequent topical steroids. Drain effusions if there is lens–corneal touch with corneal oedema, bleb failure with increasing IOP, marked anterior segment inflammation, or apposition of the effusions ('kissing choroidals'). Consider other causes of effusions such as scleritis and nanophthalmos.

- *Raised intraocular pressure*: usually due to inadequate aqueous outflow. Treatment depends on the site of obstruction. Obstruction may occur in several sites at once:

  1. *Aqueous misdirection* (malignant glaucoma): indicated by very shallow anterior chamber. Ensure the peripheral iridectomy is patent. Use atropine 1%, phenylephrine 10%

(if no contraindication), and aqueous suppressants ±
hyperosmotics. Surgical vitrectomy may be necessary.

2. *Blockage of fistula*: causes include a tight scleral flap,
   fibrin and blood, and iris/ciliary body/vitreous incarceration
   in the sclerostomy. Manage with gentle massage at the
   posterior lip of the scleral flap. Remove releasable sutures,
   loosen adjustable sutures or perform argon laser suture
   lysis. Pilocarpine may help. Argon or YAG laser
   obstructions in the sclerostomy.

3. *Cyst or capsule formation*: use intensive topical steroids
   and topical aqueous suppressants. Needling of an
   encapsulated bleb may only be of temporary benefit.

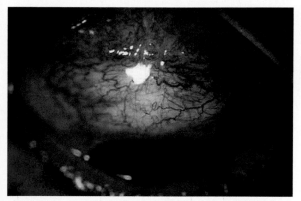

Fig. 7.12: Inflamed bleb with increased vascular diameter
and tortuosity (cork-screw vessels). This appearance
suggests a high risk of failure.

Argon Laser Trabeculoplasty

Indications Inadequate IOP control. Specifically, to lower IOP where surgery is contraindicated or to decrease dependency on topical medication (poor compliance, adverse effects).

Contraindications Uveitic glaucoma; angle-closure glaucoma; poor angle visualization; patient unable to sit at laser or maintain a steady gaze.

Consent

- *Benefit*: reports suggest 65–90% get a 7–10 mmHg drop, with 10% attrition/year.

- *Risk*: elevated IOP, pain, vasovagal attacks, peripheral anterior synechiae (PAS), visual field loss, iritis, haemorrhage, and corneal burns.

Technique See Box 7.2.

Box 7.2: Argon laser trabeculoplasty

1. Continue all glaucoma medications before and after treatment.

2. Instil G. proxymethacaine 0.5%, G. pilocarpine 2–4%, G. apraclonidine 0.5%.

3. Select a Goldmann model gonioscope.

4. Target the circular aiming beam at the junction of pigmented and nonpigmented meshwork (Fig. 7.13).

5. Use continuous wave laser at 50 microns, 0.1 sec.

6. Increase power in 100 mW increments (maximum 1200 mW), until the meshwork blanches with a tiny bubble. Pigmented meshwork requires less energy.

7. Equally space 50 burns over the superior 180° (inferior 180° for re-treatment).

8. Document the area treated.

9. Prescribe G. prednisolone 0.5% q.d.s. 1 week.

10. Check IOP at 1.5 hours, treat acute pressure spikes.

11. Review at 1 and 4–6 weeks.

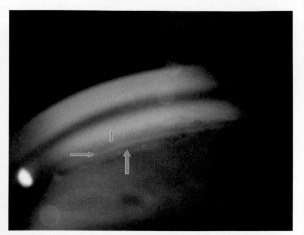

Fig. 7.13: Gonioscopy showing ciliary body band (upward arrow), scleral spur (horizontal arrow), junction of pigmented and non-pigmented trabecular meshwork (downward arrow).

Trans-scleral Cyclodiode Laser Treatment

Background Cyclodiode aims to reduce IOP by cyclodestructive trans-scleral diode laser.

Indications Advanced glaucoma with uncontrolled IOP, often with a poor visual prognosis.

Contraindications Exercise caution if there is low aqueous flow (e.g. uveitic glaucoma, previous cyclodestructive procedures): the risk is hypotony.

Technique See Box 7.3.

Follow-up The full effect takes 4 weeks. Continue glaucoma therapy until reviewed.

Box 7.3: Trans-scleral cyclodiode laser treatment

1. Give a sub-Tenon's or peribulbar block.

2. Avoid areas of subconjunctival haemorrhage (risk of conjunctival burns).

3. Transilluminate the globe to locate the ciliary body, as its position may be highly variable, especially in eyes with congenital glaucoma or multiple previous operations.

4. Use a diode laser and the appropriate probe. Position the heel of the probe at the anterior border of the ciliary body.

5. Apply two rows of five burns (one slightly posterior to the other) per quadrant. Avoid the long ciliary nerves (3 and 9 o'clock positions).

6. Standard settings are 1.5 Watts for 1.5 seconds. Reduce power if popping occurs.

7. Prescribe G. prednisolone 1% 6–8 times daily and strong analgesia, e.g. coproxamol or ibuprofen, as postoperative pain is common.

Glaucoma Drainage Implants

Indications Uncontrolled IOP, especially after failed trabeculectomy, extensive conjunctival scarring, and as a primary procedure for certain secondary glaucomas.

Surgery A reservoir explant is sutured to the sclera, usually superotemporally. This connects to the anterior chamber by a tube inserted through a tight stab incision (25-gauge) behind the limbus. This should lie just anterior to, and parallel with, the plane of the iris, touching neither the iris nor cornea. The tube is occluded with an external Vicryl ligature to prevent drainage until a fibrous capsule has formed around the explant. An additional intraluminal 'Supramid' stent suture (3/0) is often used. The extracameral course of the tube is covered with donor sclera, cornea, or sometimes an autologous scleral flap. Sulcus or pars plana tubes are sometimes used.

Follow-up

■ *Early complications*:

1. Raised IOP: manage medically and avoid early ligature or stent removal

2. Hypotony due to inadequate ligation or oversized entry site – both require surgery. Tube occlusion with iris indicates a precipitous IOP drop.

■ *Late complications*:

1. Hypotony when the ligature absorbs

2. Tube erosion (Fig. 7.14)

3. Iris or corneal contact.

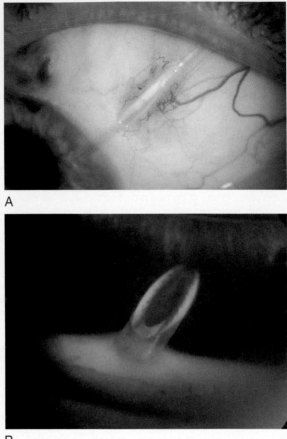

A

B

Fig. 7.14: Glaucoma drainage implants with the tube eroded through the conjunctiva **(A)** and in contact with the iris **(B)**.

Normal Pressure Glaucoma

Background Normal pressure glaucoma (NPG) describes the presence of glaucoma damage with IOP in the statistically 'normal' range. An IOP of 21 mmHg is controversially used to define NPG, probably representing the lower end of a spectrum of IOP associated with glaucoma. NPG is usually bilateral, but often asymmetric. Patients are older on average than those with high IOP, with a female preponderance.

Symptoms Typically asymptomatic until advanced visual field loss occurs. May have associated vasospasm.

History Ask specifically for a history of migraine or peripheral vasospasm, e.g. Raynaud's phenomenon.

Examination

- *Slit lamp*: normal anterior segment. IOP remains <21 mmHg on phasing (repeated IOP measurement throughout the day).

- *Gonioscopy*: normal open angle.

- *Optic disc*: glaucomatous cupping, but focal ischaemic notches and disc haemorrhages are more likely.

Investigations

- *Visual field*: look for progressive optic nerve head pattern of defects on automated perimetry.

- *Optic disc imaging*: a baseline photograph or scanning laser ophthalmoscope image is needed to detect change.

- *Central corneal thickness*: a thin cornea is associated with lower measured IOP.

- Consider ambulatory blood pressure monitoring for nocturnal 'dips'.

Differential diagnosis Confirm the presence of IOP in the normal range and glaucomatous optic neuropathy. Exclude other causes of optic neuropathy and specifically consider:

- Primary open angle glaucoma (POAG) with high IOP.

- Previous elevated IOP causing stable, nonprogressive signs of optic neuropathy.

- Nonglaucomatous optic neuropathy.

- Other lesions of the visual pathway.

Treatment Many patients are elderly with slow disease progression and may not benefit from treatment. The indication for treatment is progressive disease likely to cause significant loss of vision in the patient's lifetime.

■ Objectives:

1. *Lower IOP*: with medication, laser trabeculoplasty or trabeculectomy. The 'target pressure' or estimated IOP needed to prevent progression will be lower than in POAG.

2. *Improve optic nerve head blood flow*: prevent nocturnal hypotension (from systemic medication or nocturnal topical beta blockers), treat significant carotid insufficiency, and treat vasospasm (with calcium channel blockers in collaboration with a physician). Carbonic anhydrase inhibitors theoretically improve blood flow.

3. *Neuroprotection*: currently unproven.

4. *Monitor* regularly for disc and field progression.

Pseudoexfoliation Syndrome

Background Pseudoexfoliation syndrome (PXS) is characterized by the deposition of grey flecks of amyloid-like fibrillar material on the lens capsule and many extraocular tissues. It is more common with increasing age, with geographical and racial clustering. Associated trabecular dysfunction may cause elevated IOP and pseudoexfolative glaucoma (PXG).

Symptoms May be an incidental finding or present late with glaucomatous field loss. Two-thirds are unilateral on presentation.

Signs Radial lens–iris contact may rub off pseudoexfolation (PXF) material leaving a 'bull's-eye' pattern (a clear intermediate zone). Central iris transillumination occurs due to abrasion of iris pigment epithelium, and PXF material may be seen on the iris and pupil margin (Fig. 7.15). Gonioscopy shows 'salt and pepper' pigmentation on the trabecular meshwork and pigment deposition anterior to Schwalbe's line (*Sampaolesi line*). The pupil often dilates poorly.

History and examination Record family history, VA, IOP, iris transillumination, gonioscopy, RAPD, and disc examination (with pupils dilated). Note cataract density and postdilation pupil size. Look for phacodonesis – lens subluxation may occur due to weak zonules.

Investigations Arrange baseline disc imaging and visual fields. Further investigations are not routinely required.

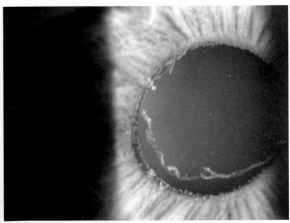

Fig. 7.15: Pseudoexfoliation.

Treatment Manage ocular hypertension and glaucomatous optic neuropathy as for primary open angle glaucoma (p. 287). Argon laser trabeculoplasty may be effective but may also fail abruptly. Routine trabeculectomy is usually effective. Cataract surgery may be complicated ($\approx$fivefold increase in vitrectomy rate) due to weak zonules and small pupils, so manage accordingly (p. 254). Postoperative capsule phimosis may be significant.

Follow–up With PXF only (no glaucomatous optic neuropathy or ocular hypertension), review 12 monthly. For PXG, review 3–12 monthly as indicated by the stability of IOP, disc, and field.

Pigment Dispersion Syndrome

Background Pigment dispersion syndrome (PDS) is characterized by pigment shedding from iris pigment epithelium and deposition on other intraocular structures. It is more common in Caucasians, myopes, and the 35–50 age group, and can occur with an autosomal dominant inheritance pattern with variable penetrance. Posterior bowing of the midperipheral iris results in abrasion of the iris by lens zonules. Pigment deposits in the trabecular meshwork are associated with raised IOP and glaucoma.

Symptoms Transient visual blurring or halos often following physical exertion. May present late with glaucomatous field loss.

Signs Pigment loss results in iris transillumination, typically seen as radial spokes in the midperiphery (Fig. 7.16). Pigment deposition on the corneal endothelium is usually concentrated in the vertical midline by aqueous convection (Krukenburg spindle). The anterior chamber is deep. Gonioscopy shows diffuse pigment deposition around 360° of the trabecular meshwork. The angle is

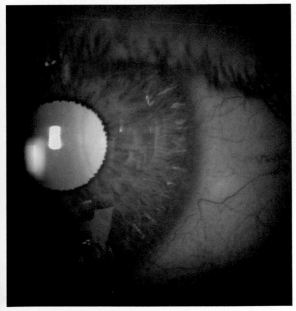

Fig. 7.16: Pigment dispersion syndrome with peripheral iris transillumination (Courtesy of K Barton).

open and the peripheral iris may be appreciably bowed posteriorly. Pigment granules may be seen on the iris surface and among zonular insertions at the lens equator (Scheie stripe).

Differential diagnosis Angle pigmentation can occur in angle closure, and following trauma, iritis, and in pseudoexfoliation. Iritis may cause iris transillumination.

History and examination Ask about visual disturbance, particularly following exercise. Record family history, VA, IOP, corneal pigment deposits, anterior chamber depth and cellular activity, iris transillumination, gonioscopy, RAPD, and disc examination (with pupils dilated). Exclude peripheral retinal holes, especially if prescribing pilocarpine.

Investigations Request a baseline disc image and visual field.

Treatment Consider IOP measurement following exercise. Pigment dispersion may 'burn out' prior to causing elevated IOP. Iris–zonule contact may be reduced by low-dose pilocarpine, but this is often not tolerated. Treatment with laser peripheral iridotomy is controversial. Manage pigmentary glaucoma as for primary open angle glaucoma (p. 287). Argon laser trabeculoplasty may be effective but has a high failure rate; use low-power settings. Trabeculectomy is often effective.

Follow–up With PDS only (no glaucomatous optic neuropathy or ocular hypertension), review 6–12 monthly; for pigmentary glaucoma, 3–12 monthly as indicated by stability of the IOP, disc and fields.

Neovascular Glaucoma

Background A secondary glaucoma with open angle and angle-closure mechanisms resulting from iris neovascularization.

Symptoms Redness, pain, photophobia and decreased VA.

Signs Poor VA, high IOP, conjunctival congestion, corneal oedema, iris new vessels (NVI or rubeosis iridis), ectropion uveae, vessels crossing trabecular meshwork on gonioscopy, and peripheral anterior synechiae (PAS). Rubeosis iridis is shown on page 440.

Differential diagnosis For the causes of rubeosis iridis, see page 440.

Investigations Fluorescein angiography is not usually necessary. Arrange Carotid Doppler if relevant.

Treatment

- *Control IOP*: as shown in the treatment algorithm (Fig. 7.17). Arrange physician review as required.

- *Urgent panretinal photocoagulation* (PRP): using slit lamp, indirect, or endolaser. For technique see page 434. Consider cryotherapy or trans-scleral diode laser retinal ablation if an inadequate fundal view prevents laser treatment under direct vision.

- *Medical treatment*: topical glaucoma medication is required in eyes with navigational vision or better. If the eye is painful with no useful navigational vision, manage with G. dexamethasone 0.1% q.d.s., G. atropine 1% b.d.

- *Surgical treatment*: for eyes with good potential visual function, consider glaucoma drainage devices (GDD), or mitomycin C (MMC) augmented trabeculectomy only if the eye is uninflamed.

- *Ciliary ablation by diode laser*: see page 298.

- *Retrobulbar alcohol or enucleation*: reserved for painful blind eyes not controlled medically or with cyclodestruction.

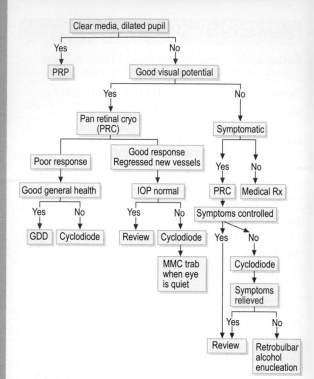

Fig. 7.17: Neovascular glaucoma treatment algorithm.

Uveitic Glaucoma

Background Ten percent of uveitic eyes develop secondary glaucoma.

Signs Look for keratic precipitates, flare, iris atrophy/nodules, and posterior synechiae. Gonioscopy may show peripheral anterior synechiae, pigment, or debris in the angle.

Management Problems include frequent recurrence, variable IOP, pupillary membranes and secondary cataracts precluding disc assessment and reliable field testing, and the need for long-term steroid treatment. Collaborate with uveitis specialists and physicians, especially for immunosuppression. Treatment depends on the mechanism(s):

■ *Secondary open angle glaucoma*: treat medically and control the uveitis.

■ *Closed angle glaucoma with pupil block*: examine the other eye to rule out primary angle closure. Treat as acute angle closure but without miotics. Surgical iridectomy is preferable to laser.

■ *Steroid pressure response*: see next page.

■ *Closed angle without pupil block*: medical management of IOP.

■ *All mechanisms*: if medical therapy fails, consider mitomycin C-augmented trabeculectomy. Do not combine cataract and filtering surgery. Use postoperative steroids and 5FU judiciously, using the minimum steroid potency and dosage. If enhanced filtration surgery fails then consider drainage tubes.

Steroid Pressure Response and Associated Glaucoma

Background Usually caused by topical steroids, especially prednisolone and dexamethasone, but may be caused by intraocular, periocular, inhaled, intranasal, or systemic steroids. G. dexamaethasone 0.1% q.d.s. for 6 weeks is associated with an IOP rise of >6 mmHg in 35% of normal adults versus 95% of patients with primary open angle glaucoma (POAG). Higher IOP rises occur in POAG patients and their first-degree relatives.

Classification Low response (<6 mmHg IOP rise); intermediate response (6–15 mmHg); and high response (>15 mmHg). Diagnosis is confirmed by IOP fall on steroid reduction.

Symptoms Often asymptomatic unless there is advanced field loss or very high IOP.

Signs Raised IOP, usually after 4–6 weeks of steroids (rarely before 2 weeks, except in children). Optic disc cupping with visual field loss may suggest steroid-induced glaucoma.

History and examination Record the steroids used, their concentration, frequency and duration, IOP, and optic disc assessment. Perform gonioscopy. Exclude posterior subcapsular cataract.

Differential diagnosis Undiagnosed or coexisting ocular hypertension / POAG.

Investigations Disc imaging and visual field assessment.

Treatment See Box 7.4

Follow–up The rate of IOP fall is variable (days to months). Occasionally, IOP rise is permanent.

Box 7.4: Treatment of steroid pressure response and associated glaucoma

- Reduce the potency and frequency of steroid treatment.
- Consider fluorometholone or rimexolone (less steroid response in adults).
- Treatment as for POAG if IOP remains above target (p. 287).
- Consider topical NSAIDs for the management of inflammation.

Phacolytic and Phacomorphic Glaucoma

Background Disease of the lens may cause raised IOP. Identifying the underlying mechanism is important before deciding on the appropriate therapeutic options.

Classification

- *Phacolytic*: leakage of protein from mature or hypermature cataract through an intact capsule obstructing trabecular meshwork.

- *Phacomorphic*: secondary angle closure from lens intumescence. Increases relative pupil block.

Symptoms Unilateral pain, reduced VA, lacrimation, and photophobia.

Signs Intumescent mature or hypermature (Morganian) cataract, conjunctival hyperaemia, corneal oedema, and IOP >21 mmHg. Note VA.

History Record duration and severity of symptoms, previous history of cataracts, ocular surgery or uveitis.

Examination

- *Phacolytic*: angles open on gonioscopy, intense anterior chamber flare with small white particles of lens matter.

- *Phacomorphic*: closed angles on gonioscopy, shallow anterior chamber, typically with contralateral eye showing deeper anterior chamber and open angles.

Differential diagnosis

- *Symptomatic primary angle closure*: characteristically has symmetrically narrow angles. A mature/hypermature cataract is not present.

- *Inflammatory/uveitic glaucoma*: exclude other uveitides by thorough examination.

- *Phacoanaphylactic glaucoma*: granulomatous uveitis with keratic precipitates and hypopyon is usual, with a history of cataract surgery.

Investigations B-scan ultrasonography (±ultrasound biomicroscopy [UBM]) is useful in defining the anatomical relationships and excluding retrolental disease. Record axial length, AC depth, lens thickness, or PC configuration in both eyes.

Box 7.5: Phacolytic and phacomorphic glaucoma treatment

- Topical beta blockers (e.g. timolol 0.25% b.d.,), and/or topical alpha agonist (e.g. apraclonidine 0.5% t.d.s.).

- Oral carbonic anhydrase inhibitors (e.g. acetazolamide 500 mg stat dose, then 250 mg q.d.s).

- Topical steroid (e.g. prednisolone 1% 2-hourly).

- Cycloplegics (e.g. cyclopentolate 1% t.d.s.).

Treatment The immediate aim is to control IOP and inflammation (Box 7.5).

Hyperosmotic agents (e.g oral glycerol 50% 1 ml/kg) may be necessary. Miotics *must* be avoided, since they may shift the iris–lens diaphragm forward, exacerbating angle closure, and possibly increase inflammation. The definitive treatment is cataract extraction as soon as IOP and inflammation are controlled.

Traumatic Glaucoma

Background Trauma may lead to early or late IOP elevation, progressing to glaucomatous optic neuropathy. Hyphaemas may cause very high IOP. The trabecular meshwork may be directly damaged (alkalis, siderosis, angle recession) but this may not reduce outflow for many years. Angle-recession results in glaucoma in 5% (10% of those with 360° recession). Traumatic cataract, significant iris injury, and lens subluxation/dislocation are also important risk factors for glaucoma.

Symptoms Acutely: pain, reduced vision, or halos. May present late with glaucomatous field loss.

Signs Iris sphincter ruptures, deep anterior chamber, anterior chamber cells (hyphaema, ghost cells), flare, or phacodonesis. Gonioscopy may show peripheral anterior synechiae, angle recession (Fig. 7.18), cyclodialysis clefts, or blood. Look for 360° angle recession by comparing both eyes. Exclude vitreous haemorrhage and posterior segment sequelae of trauma.

Differential diagnosis Primary open angle glaucoma.

History and examination Record the details of the injury and subsequent treatment; VA; IOP; iris defects; AC depth and cellular activity; pupil size; gonioscopy; RAPD; and dilated disc examination. If the injury resulted from a workplace accident or alleged assault, make careful and complete notes. Carefully examine the orbit, anterior segment, posterior segment and peripheral retina for other injury.

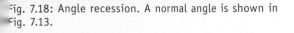

Fig. 7.18: Angle recession. A normal angle is shown in Fig. 7.13.

Investigations Baseline visual field and optic disc photography/imaging.

Treatment

■ *Casualty*: If the IOP is elevated, commence medical treatment. Request early clinic review.

■ *Clinic*: Anterior chamber wash out (hyphaema), vitrectomy (ghost cells), or cataract extraction (lens trauma) may be necessary if the IOP is not responsive. Treatment is determined by the likely mechanism of pressure rise. Argon laser trabeculoplasty is unlikely to be effective. Routine trabeculectomy has a high failure rate due to prior inflammation and conjunctival scarring. Mitomycin C trabeculectomy or a glaucoma drainage device (e.g. Molteno Tube) are often considered as a primary procedure.

Follow-up As indicated by IOP, disc and field. Annual IOP measurement is required for eyes with angle recession. Always check IOP when reviewed, even years later.

Glaucoma Following Vitreoretinal Surgery

Background Temporarily raised IOP after vitreoretinal surgery is common. Progression to glaucoma occurs in <5% of cases. Risk factors include preexisting glaucoma, trauma, angle recession, steroid response, high myopia, pigment dispersion syndrome, chronic inflammatory disease, proliferative retinopathies, use of silicone oil, and vitreous haemorrhage.

Mechanism

- *Scleral buckling procedures*: ciliary body rotation with angle closure; anteriorly placed buckle causing angle closure; high buckle with vortex vein compression; shed photoreceptor outer segments occluding outflow (Schwartz-Matsuo syndrome).

- *Vitrectomy*: ghost cell glaucoma; retained lens material; pigment dispersion after cryotherapy; chronic inflammation; neovascular glaucoma.

- *Vitrectomy with intravitreal tamponade*: pupil block with overfill of tamponade and direct angle closure or intratrabecular obstruction and damage from emulsified silicone oil.

Signs Look for raised IOP, corneal oedema, cells or emulsified silicone oil in the anterior chamber, and iris bombé. Gonioscopy may show an open or closed angle, peripheral anterior synechiae, or new vessels. Check the patency of any inferior iridectomy in aphakic silicone-filled eyes.

Natural history IOP often settles when postoperative inflammation resolves. Steroid response within 2 weeks of surgery is unlikely. Removal of emulsified silicone oil does not affect IOP.

Medical management

- *Open angle*: first-line treatment is topical beta blocker and alpha-adrenergic agonists b.d. Consider prostaglandin agonists o.d. if postoperative inflammation is not severe. Oral acetazolamide may be required.

- *Closed angle*: difficult to control medically. Aqueous suppressants are first line, such as oral acetacolamide 250 mg q.d.s. orally, topical beta blocker b.d. and an alpha-adrenergic agonist.

- *Pupil block*: mydriatics, e.g. atropine 1% b.d.

Surgical management Overfill of tamponade with pupil block requires partial removal of gas or silicone. Glaucoma surgery is often needed in eyes with closed angles and aphakic eyes. Trans-scleral diode laser ciliary ablation is used in most cases, but more than one treatment is often needed. Consider drainage tube implants if there is potential for good navigational vision (VA >6/60 and/or visual field >10 degrees).

Prognosis No perception of light in 50% of eyes with IOPs persistently >30 mmHg or hypotony after treatment. Optic disc cupping may progress despite IOP control. Cases with closed angles have the poorest prognosis.

Aqueous Misdirection ('Malignant Glaucoma')

Background Characterized by axial shallowing of the anterior chamber and raised IOP. Occurs in 2% of patients undergoing trabeculectomy for angle closure. May occur after any type of intraocular surgery. Crowding of the ciliolenticular space (possibly from anterior rotation of ciliary body) is believed to block aqueous flow. Posterior aqueous diversion into the vitreous increases retrolenticular pressure and shallowing of the anterior chamber. Risks are high in nanophthalmic eyes.

Symptoms Unilateral pain, reduced vision, lacrimation, and photophobia.

Signs Shallow or flat anterior chamber, IOP >21 mmHg. Choroidal detachment, haemorrhage, or signs of pupil block are absent.

History Ask about the duration/severity of symptoms, previous history of angle closure, and recent ocular surgery.

Examination Record VA and IOP. Shallowing of the anterior chamber is axial, unlike iris bombé in pupil block. Exclude hypotony/overdrainage or choroidal effusions. Confirm patency of any iridotomy.

Differential diagnosis

■ Symptomatic angle closure.

■ *Choroidal detachment*: IOP is typically low with choroidal elevation visible on fundoscopy.

■ *Choroidal/vitreous haemorrhage*: sudden onset of elevated IOP associated with severe pain. Blood may be visible.

Investigations Arrange preoperative biometry ± ultrasound to identify nanophthalmic eyes prior to glaucoma surgery (axial length <21 mm, scleral thickness ≥2 mm). B-mode ultrasound is useful in excluding choroidal detachment or haemorrhage.

Treatment Identify high-risk eyes preoperatively: suture the scleral flap watertight using releasable sutures, and give postoperative cycloplegia.

Established cases:

■ Cycloplegia: G. atropine 1% t.d.s. and phenylephrine 10% b.d.

■ Reduction of aqueous production:

1. Topical beta blockers (e.g. timolol 0.25% b.d.) and topical alpha agonist (e.g. apraclonidine 0.5% t.d.s).

2. Oral carbonic anhydrase inhibitors (e.g. acetazolamide 250 mg q.d.s.).

■ *Reduction of vitreous volume*: if unresponsive consider hyperosmotic agents (e.g. oral glycerol 50% 1 mL/kg, or intravenous mannitol 2 g/kg).

In 50% of cases, IOP is lowered and the anterior chamber deepens with atropine and ocular hypotensive drugs. If unsuccessful, or when lens–cornea touch is present, laser and/or surgical intervention is required.

Laser/surgical management YAG laser disruption of the posterior capsule/anterior hyaloid is performed in pseudophakic eyes. It is important to extend the capsulotomy to the periphery. If this fails, pars plana vitrectomy is effective in two-thirds of cases. In phakic eyes, direct argon laser through an existing peripheral iridectomy may shrink the ciliary processes: trans-scleral diode can also be used. Vitrectomy alone has a poor success rate. Combined cataract extraction with primary posterior capsulotomy and anterior vitrectomy is recommended in any patient with even mild lens opacity. With no opacity, clear lens extraction is an option. The treatment algorithm in Figure 7.19 outlines the management of malignant glaucoma.

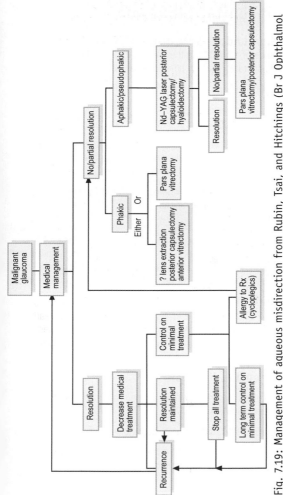

Fig. 7.19: Management of aqueous misdirection from Rubin, Tsai, and Hitchings (Br J Ophthalmol 1997) with permission.

Congenital Glaucoma

Background Congenital glaucoma is a rare disease with an incidence of 1:20000 in the Caucasian population. Cases are usually sporadic, but can be autosomal recessive.

Classification

- *Primary congenital glaucoma* (isolated trabeculodysgenesis): the most common form of neonatal glaucoma.

- *Secondary to ocular disease*: anterior segment dysgenesis (Axenfeld-Rieger's syndrome, Peters anomaly), aniridia, aphakic glaucoma, and uveitic glaucoma.

- *Secondary to systemic disease*: metabolic, chromosomal, and connective tissue disorders.

Clinical features Classic triad of epiphora, photophobia, and blepharospasm. May also present with enlarged cornea (buphthalmos), corneal clouding, or after screening in families with early-onset glaucoma. Late presentation may lead to reduced vision and nystagmus, strabismus and rapidly progressing myopia.

History and examination Record any complications during pregnancy and labour, age at onset of symptoms (earlier onset indicates worse prognosis), developmental milestones, family history, and consanguinity. Full examination usually requires anaesthesia.

Differential diagnosis

- *Enlarged cornea*: axial myopia, megalocornea, and connective tissue disorders.

- *Haab's striae*: birth trauma, posterior polymorphous dystrophy.

- *Corneal oedema/opacity*: congenital hereditary endothelial dystrophy, sclerocornea, infections, metabolic, e.g. mucopolysaccharidoses.

- *Watering/red eye*: conjunctivitis, nasolacrimal obstruction and ocular inflammation. All have normal IOP and an absence of disc cupping.

Examination under anaesthesia (EUA) EUA is performed using ketamine anaesthesia. The gold standard for IOP measurement is Perkins' tonometry (without fluorescein, in case goniotomy required). Important findings include:

- *Cornea*: note oedema/opacity, posterior embryotoxon, and horizontal corneal diameter (>11 mm in newborn or >12 mm in

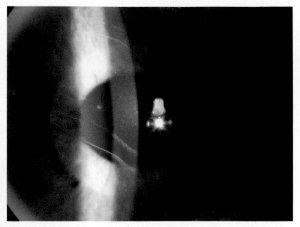

Fig. 7.20: Haab's striae.

children under 1 year is suspicious of glaucoma; >13 mm is abnormal at any age, as is disc asymmetry). Haab's striae (Fig. 7.20) are linear ruptures in Descemet's membrane that are a characteristic of raised IOP in children, usually occurring in the first 18 months of life.

■ *Gonioscopy*: look for any secondary causes and anterior segment dysgenesis.

■ *Cup-to-disc ratio* (CDR): >0.3 in a newborn or >0.5 at any age is suspicious, as is asymmetry. Do not dilate pupils in case goniotomy is required.

■ *Refraction* (progressive myopia) and B-scan are essential to assess axial length and coexistent disease.

■ *Systemic evaluation* and blood can be taken for genetic studies if indicated during EUA.

Treatment Surgical therapy is the mainstay of treatment although initially IOP can be controlled medically. Beta blockers or pilocarpine are usually first line; avoid brimonidine. Goniotomy is the operation of choice in primary congenital glaucoma and often requires corneal epithelial debridement with alcohol. The success rate is up to 90%, although surgery may need repeating. Trabeculectomy is preferred if goniotomy fails or is not possible. All patients require anti-scarring agents due to a high rate of failure. Broad iridectomy is useful if there is central opacity. Tube drainage devices are used if trabeculectomy fails or as a primary therapy in aphakia and uveitic glaucoma. Cyclodestruction is used if surgery fails, there is poor visual prognosis, or surgery is not technically possible. There is a significant risk of intraocular inflammation and phthisis, particularly if used on multiple occasions. Occlusion therapy and correction of refractive error are essential.

Follow-up Intensive surveillance is required, particularly postoperatively. This is usually carried out in specialists units. Education, social support, and counselling are important in managing the family as a whole.

Bleb-Related Infection

Background Bleb related infection is a potentially blinding, late complication of glaucoma filtering surgery. It refers to a spectrum of disease ranging from blebitis (isolated bleb infection) to bleb-related endophthalmitis (BRE). The organisms usually responsible for BRE (*Streptococcus* and *Haemophilus* spp.) are different to, and more virulent than, those of early postoperative endophthalmitis. Thin-walled, cystic, leaking blebs are at risk.

Early and aggressive antimicrobial therapy often permits retention of functional VA and a filtering bleb.

Symptoms Redness, photophobia, pain, reduced VA, and discharge.

Signs Bleb opalescence or mucopurulent infiltrate with surrounding conjunctival injection ('white on red'), ±bleb leak, and intraocular inflammation and purulent discharge (Fig. 7.21).

History and examination Ask about the duration and severity of symptoms (prodrome of a few days suggests blebitis; sudden onset with rapid progression suggests BRE), ocular trauma (accidental or iatrogenic, e.g. bleb needling), contact lens use, and risk factors such as blepharitis, trichiasis, and dry eyes. Record VA and test for the presence of a bleb leak using 2% fluorescein (Seidel's test).

Differential diagnosis Bleb leak alone may produce mild ocular discomfort and AC activity. Recent corticosteroid withdrawal or rapid tapering may result in rebound inflammation. In both these cases the bleb is clear, the AC reaction mild, and VA unchanged.

Investigations Blebitis associated with ≥1+ AC cells is considered as BRE, even in the absence of vitritis. BRE requires anterior chamber tap plus vitreous biopsy. A conjunctival swab is not indicated as cultures often correlate poorly with intraocular cultures. A B-scan is indicated if vitritis cannot be excluded or the fundal view is inadequate.

Treatment See Box 7.6.

Follow–up Following an episode of bleb-related infection, surgery is advisable but its risks and benefits must be evaluated for each patient. Surgical revision of the bleb usually involves bleb excision with conjunctival advancement. If present, scleral thinning or a defect must also be repaired with a scleral or Tenon's graft to avoid the recurrence of cystic blebs. Treat chronic blepharitis, ocular surface, and lid disorders. Prophylactic topical antibiotics are not advised.

Box 7.6: Treatment of bleb-related infection

- Instil povidon-iodine 5% into the conjunctival sac.

- G. ofloxacin hourly and G. cefuroxime hourly (day and night) for at least 24 hours, reducing frequency as clinically indicated.

- Ciprofloxacin 750 mg b.d. p.o. and co-amoxiclav 625 mg t.d.s. p.o. (azithromycin 500 mgs b.d. p.o. if penicillin allergy) for 7 days.

- Review patients with blebitis or bleb-related infection within 6 hours to exclude progression to bleb-related endophthalmitis (BRE).

- Intravitreal vancomycin 2 mg and either amikacin 0.4 mg or ceftazidime 2 mg in cases of BRE.

- G. prednisolone 1% q.d.s. (once the course of infection is clear in blebitis).

- Prednisolone 1 mg/kg p.o. commenced 12 hours after admission.

- Consider intravitreal dexamethasone 0.4 mg to minimize inflammation-related retinal toxicity in cases of BRE.

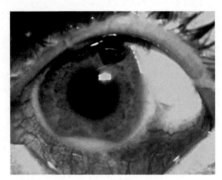

Fig. 7.21: Bleb-related endophthalmitis.

Primary Angle Closure

Background Angle closure is contact between the iris and trabecular meshwork accompanied by a significant impairment of aqueous outflow. It may be primary (PAC) or secondary, with 75% of primary cases due to pupil block. Frequently associated with glaucomatous optic neuropathy. The symptomatic form ('acute' angle closure) is a common ophthalmic emergency.

Classification The traditional classification of acute, intermittent, chronic, and latent phases fails to identify the disease stage and mechanism of closure. Classify as follows:

- ◼ Stage.

  1. Narrow angles (angle closure suspect).

  2. Primary angle closure: a narrow angle with either high IOP or peripheral anterior synechiae (PAS).

  3. Angle closure with glaucomatous optic neuropathy (PACG).

- ◼ Mechanism of angle closure.

  1. Pupil block.

  2. Anterior, non-pupil-block (includes plateau iris).

  3. Lens induced.

  4. Causes behind the lens.

  Nuclear sclerosis is almost invariably present. This is part of the primary disease and distinct from phakolytic/phakomorphic glaucoma (p. 311).

Symptoms Blurring of vision sometimes accompanied by halos around lights, redness and periocular or hemicranial pain. There may be nausea and vomiting. However, angle closure is often asymptomatic, especially in Asian people.

Signs Signs mirror symptoms in acute disease; VA is reduced, there is circum-limbal injection with corneal oedema, raised IOP, and an immobile pupil. Refraction is often (but not always) hypermetropic.

History and examination A positive family history is common. Dynamic gonioscopy is essential to make the diagnosis. Record the estimated geometric angle width, angle structures visible, iris profile (steep, regular, or plateau), iris pigment on the trabecular meshwork, and extent of PAS. Asymmetry between the two eyes suggests a secondary cause.

Differential diagnosis Consider: primary open angle glaucoma; phakolytic and phakomorphic glaucoma; irido-ciliary cysts; retinopathy of prematurity; uveitis; nanophthalmos; Weill-Marchesani syndrome; Marfan's syndrome; persistent hyperplastic primary vitreous and lens subluxation; posterior segment pathology; iatrogenic causes. PAC is extremely uncommon below the age of 30. In older people, rule out neovascularization and hypertensive uveitides. Consider posterior segment disease and iatrogenic causes (including vitreoretinal surgery). Numerous drugs can precipitate angle closure (topical mydriatics; anticholinergic agents including bronchodilators; antispasmodics; antidepressants; proprietary cold and flu medication; anticonvulsants).

Investigations B-mode ultrasound is invaluable in identifying posterior segment disease (e.g. ciliary effusions) when the fundal view is inadequate.

Emergency management of symptomatic PAC In acute, symptomatic cases, pressure control by medical and/or laser treatment is the immediate priority. If topical medication and acetazolamide are unsuccessful in lowering the IOP in symptomatic cases, laser iridoplasty should be considered (see below).

- Admit the patient if symptomatic and IOP >40 mmHg in an eye with useful vision.

- Stat: G. levobunolol 0.5%, G. apraclonidine 0.5%, G. prednisolone 1%, acetazolamide 500 mg i.v., lie the patient supine. Analgesics/antiemetics as required.

- Check IOP at 30 minutes.

    1. *If responding*: Diamox 250 mg q.d.s. p.o.; G. prednisolone 1% 2 hourly; G. pilocarpine 2% q.d.s. (4% if dark irides). Avoid intensive pilocarpine.

    2. *If not responding*: consider laser iridoplasty (see below) or glycerol 50% 1 g/kg bodyweight p.o., or mannitol 20% 1 g/kg i.v..

- Unless there is a clear reason not to, perform laser iridotomy in both eyes as soon as corneal clarity allows (Box 7.7).

Subsequent management is targeted at the specific mechanism of closure. If there is a visually significant cataract, removing this will open the angle. If the angle remains partially closed after laser iridotomy, either laser iridoplasty (Box 7.8) or topical pilocarpine may be used. However, this area of management is currently controversial, and some glaucoma specialists opt for careful observation.

The presence of >6 clock hours of PAS extending across the trabecular meshwork and glaucomatous optic neuropathy both suggest that laser and medical treatment are unlikely to control IOP satisfactorily. A trabeculectomy will frequently be needed. Because of the poor success rate, trabeculectomy should be avoided soon after an acute attack, unless absolutely necessary.

Follow–up Once IOP is controlled, review patients at one week, 1 month, then annually.

Box 7.7: YAG laser iridotomy

This is the cornerstone of management

1. Premedicate with G. apraclonidine 0.5% and pilocarpine 2% (4% for dark brown irises) 30 minutes and 5 minutes before.

2. Use a Wise or Abraham's lens. Try to treat in the base of an iris crypt (Fig. 7.22).

3. Create an iridotomy that will be covered by the upper lid. Avoid treating in an area under the marginal tear strip; this may cause glare.

4. If bleeding occurs, a little pressure with the contact lens helps to stop this.

5. Argon pretreatment is useful in patients with thick brown irises: 10–40 shots, 0.05–0.1 s, 50 microns, 200 to 1000 mW power. Avoid charring.

6. YAG laser energy varies with the machine and patient, typically 1–3 mJ, 10–20 shots.

7. Iridotomies should be ≈200 microns in diameter.

8. Check IOP 2 hours post laser. Prescribe G. prednisolone 1% hourly for 24 hours, then q.d.s. 7 days.

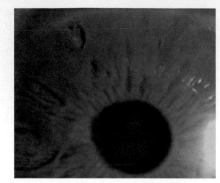

Fig. 7.22: Laser iridotomy in the 11 o'clock position.

Box 7.8: Laser peripheral iridoplasty

Applying large, slow-contraction burns to peripheral iris is useful in both symptomatic and asymptomatic cases. Premedication and lenses are as for iridotomy.

1. Select a 500 micron spot size, 0.5 sec for all iris colours. Power: 100 mW increasing as required.

2. End point: brisk contraction of the stroma without charring or a pop.

3. Target the peripheral iris but ensure there is a gap between the endothelium and iris. This may mean starting in the midperipheral iris and spiralling out to the far periphery as a gap opens with treatment.

4. Apply 5 evenly spaced shots per quadrant.

If used for medically unresponsive cases of acute angle closure, *a peripheral iridotomy must be completed at the earliest opportunity* within hours of pressure normalization. Monitor pressure and give topical steroids as for iridotomy.

Optometry and General Practice Guidelines

General comments

Cases of suspected open angle glaucoma require routine referral for assessment by an ophthalmologist, or preferably a glaucoma specialist. Acute angle closure and bleb-related infections are emergencies that require prompt action and immediate ophthalmology review.

Optometrists

Glaucoma is a progressive optic neuropathy in which the optic nerve head has characteristic changes and there is typically a corresponding visual field loss. Intraocular pressure (IOP) and age are the major risk factors but IOP on its own is not a good predictor of glaucoma (5% of the normal population have IOPs >21 mmHg and about one-third of those with open angle glaucoma have IOPs <22 mmHg). Other risk factors are ethnicity (Afro-Caribbean) and family history (a first-degree relative with glaucoma).

Consider the cup-to-disc ratio (CDR) in relation to the disc size (a large CDR may be normal if the disc is also large; see p. 279) and look for notches and variations from the normal distribution of rim thickness (see Jonas' ISNT rule, p. 279). An IOP consistently >24 mmHg caries a 9% risk of progressing to glaucomatous optic neuropathy. A modest (20%) reduction of the IOP reduces this risk to 4%. Refer on a routine basis, or manage in line with local protocols.

General practice

The optometry guidelines also apply. Headaches and eye pain are not generally associated with glaucoma, unless the IOP is very high. If unable to assess disc and fields effectively, recommend review by an optometrist. Topical beta blockers are contraindicated in people with asthma and chronic airways disease. Note that steroids, both systemic and topical (eye, nose, skin), have the potential to generate a steroid-induced increase in IOP. People using these agents regularly for more than 6 weeks should have their IOP monitored. In general, steroid eyedrops are for short- to medium-term use, but with some exceptions, including blind painful eyes, some chronic corneal diseases, and chronic uveitis.

The following guide to referral urgency is not prescriptive, as clinical situations vary.

Immediate

- Suspected blebitis   p. 323
- Acute angle closure   p. 325
- IOP >40 mmHg   p. 325

Soon (within 1 month)

- Advanced glaucomatous disc damage (CDR >0.8 and advanced field loss)   p. 279
- IOP >35 mmHg on any occasion   p. 287

Routine

- IOP consistently in mid 20s with normal disc and fields   p. 287
- Suspected glaucomatous optic disc changes (any IOP)   p. 279
- Repeatable, suspected glaucomatous field loss (any IOP)   p. 284
- Pigment dispersion syndrome   p. 305
- Pseudoexfoliation   p. 303
- Suspected narrow angles (asymptomatic)   p. 325

Chapter 8

UVEITIS

History and Examination

Uveitis is an umbrella term for intraocular inflammation which has a varied clinical phenotype. The diagnosis is predominately clinical, reliant upon meticulous history taking and examination. The aetiology may be primarily inflammatory, infective, or malignant, or, in about 40% of patients, it remains undetermined (organ-specific autoimmune disease), even after appropriate clinical assessment and investigation. Anatomically, uveitis can be classified into anterior, intermediate, posterior, or panuveitis.

History A comprehensive ocular and systemic history is paramount. Note age, sex, country of origin, and ethnicity. Ask about the duration and pattern of symptoms, which may be unilateral or bilateral, acute, recurrent, or chronic, and previous eye surgery or trauma. Document a full past and current medical problem list, BCG vaccination history, any prior, recent and/or concurrent infections, and all drugs and dosages. Personal details including foreign travel, occupation, pets, social and family circumstances, are all relevant. Additional questions such as pregnancy, pregnancy intention, breastfeeding, sexual history, and intravenous drug usage may also be appropriate. Enquire about skin, joint, respiratory, gastrointestinal, genitourinary, and neurological symptoms of associated systemic disease.

Examination

- *Slit lamp examination*: note the following: pattern of conjunctival/episcleral/scleral injection; corneal epithelial or stromal disease; size, appearance, and distribution of keratic precipitates (KPs); cells, flare, fibrin, hypopyon; iris atrophy/ nodules; cataract; posterior and peripheral anterior synechiae; rubeosis. Measure IOP.

- *Dilated fundoscopy*: both slit lamp and indirect ophthalmoscope examination are mandatory in all patients to assess for: vitreous cells; 'snowballs'; 'snowbanking' (which is in the retinal periphery and may be missed on slit lamp examination alone); disc oedema or hyperaemia; vasculitis (arterial, venous, or both); perivascular exudates; cystoid macular oedema; retinitis; choroiditis or choroidal infiltrates;

chorioretinal scars; retinal detachment (rhegmatogenous, serous, and tractional).

■ If VA is worse than 6/9 a cause must be sought.

Acute Anterior Uveitis

Background Acute anterior uveitis (AAU) is the commonest form of acute uveitis accounting for ≈75% of all cases of intraocular inflammation. It is often recurrent, has numerous causes, and is associated with HLA-B27 in 60% of cases.

Symptoms Onset over hours or days of redness, pain, and photophobia. Usually unilateral but may be simultaneously or sequentially bilateral.

Signs

Ocular: Conjunctival (predominately perilimbal) injection and anterior chamber flare and cells are the hallmarks of AAU. Cells are graded by the number observed in an oblique 1 × 1 mm slit beam:

0	(−)	10–20 cells	(2+)
1–5 cells	(±)	20–50	(3+)
5–10 cells	(1+)	>50	(4+)

Flare is graded as 0–4, with grade 4 representing fibrin deposition. The cornea may show epithelial or stromal changes consistent with herpes zoster virus or less commonly herpes simplex virus infection. Keratic precipitates (KPs) may be large and greasy looking ('mutton fat') or fine and small (Fig. 8.1).

Fibrin, hypopyon, iris abnormalities (posterior synechiae [PS], peripheral anterior synechiae [PAS], atrophy, nodules), and raised or low IOP, are variable findings. Posterior segment signs are restricted to a few anterior vitreous cells (spillover) and cystoid macular oedema (CMO). CMO is uncommon, but the most important cause of visual loss.

Systemic: variable, dependent upon any associated disease.

History and examination Ask about the pattern of anterior uveitis (unilateral, bilateral, recurrent) and associated systemic disease, particularly back and joint pain, skin lesions, and gastrointestinal and urinary tract symptoms linked with HLA-B27 disorders. Occupational and travel history may suggest brucellosis (abattoir workers, vets), leptospirosis (farmers and sewage workers), or Lyme disease (USA, Scandinavia, Eastern and Middle Europe). Record VA and grade cells and flare. The pattern of signs provides clues to the aetiology:

- *Hypopyon*: HLA-B27, Behçet's disease, rarely candida infection, and malignancy.

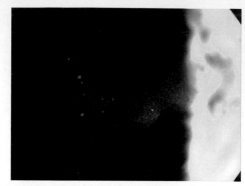

Fig. 8.1: Acute anterior uveitis. Anterior chamber cells with flare and keratic precipitates.

- *Keratic precipitates*: large 'mutton fat' KPs suggest sarcoidosis or TB.

- *Iris atrophy*: sectorial in herpetic infections.

- *Iris nodules*: sarcoidosis, syphilis or TB.

  Look for complications of uveitis: raised IOP (common in herpetic uveitis, Posner-Schlossman syndrome, and toxoplasma chorioretinitis), PS, and CMO. Full, dilated examination is mandatory in casualty to exclude acute retinal necrosis and other posterior segment disease.

Differential diagnosis

- *HLA-B27-positive AAU*: systemic associations include ankylosing spondylitis, Reiter's syndrome, psoriatic arthritis, and inflammatory bowel disease.

- *Systemic disease*: sarcoidosis, Behçet's syndrome.

- *Infection*: herpetic (zoster and simplex), tuberculosis, syphilis, and other systemic infections.

- *Ocular syndromes*: Posner-Schlossman syndrome (intermittent low-grade inflammation, elevated IOP often >40 mmHg, open angle and no PS. Responds quickly to topical steroids and IOP-lowering medications.)

- *Drug induced*: rifabutin, cidofovir.

- *Trauma*: contusion, intraocular foreign body.

- *Lens induced*.

- *Postoperative*.

■ *Masquerade syndromes* (p. 371).

■ *Idiopathic*

If VA is worse than 6/9 seek posterior segment disease, and if the fundal view is inadequate to exclude intraocular infection refer directly to a uveitis clinic.

Investigations Investigate in clinic, not casualty. Unilateral disease with unremarkable history and examination requires no investigation at first presentation. For recurrent, bilateral, or poorly responsive disease and no suggestive aetiology, restrict initial investigations to CXR, serum ACE, and syphilis serology. Confirmation of HLA-B27 status in a fit person may spare further investigation. Consider additional investigations, e.g. Lyme, *Brucella*, and *Leptospira* serology, but only if specifically suggested by the history and signs. If VA is worse than 6/9 and no cause is found, arrange fluorescein angiography or OCT to exclude CMO. If there are symptoms of associated systemic disease, refer for appropriate medical evaluation.

Treatment Attacks of AAU typically last from several days to 6 weeks, but less than 3 months by definition.

■ *Casualty*: The majority of patients can be managed with cycloplegia (G. cyclopentolate 1% t.d.s.), and intensive topical steroid therapy, initially G. prednisolone 1% or G. dexamethasone 0.1% hourly for week 1, 2-hourly for week 2, 6 times daily week 3, q.d.s. for week 4, then reduced every week by one drop/day until clinic review at 6 weeks. Add steroid ointment nocte if inflammation is more marked. Subconjunctival Mydricaine II (0.3 mL) may break new PS. Reserve subconjunctival betamethasone (4 mg in 1 mL) for severe AAU, usually 4+ cells or fibrin/hypopyon. Tissue plasminogen activator (TPA) is rarely required but has a rapid effect in breaking down fibrin in cases with severe fibrinous response refractory to topical and subconjunctival steroids. Instil povidone-iodine 5% and topical anaesthetic into the conjunctival sac then inject 12.5 mcg in 0.1 mL directly into the anterior chamber using an insulin syringe and needle This can be performed either on the slit lamp or with the patient lying down. No paracentesis is required and the injection can be repeated if necessary. Instruct patients to return quickly if there is a deterioration of vision and persistent pain. For the treatment of uveitic glaucoma see page 309. If an exact aetiology is determined, alternative or additional treatment may be required. Anterior uveitis following trauma is typically relatively mild and usually settles rapidly with less-intensive treatment, e.g. G. dexamethasone 0.1% q.d.s. tapered off over 2–3 weeks.

■ *Clinic*: If the inflammation is settling, continue to slowly taper off topical steroids. Reintroduce hourly steroids and above regimen for exacerbations during the tapering period. Rarely, oral steroids are required for very severe cases resistant to subconjunctival and maximal topical treatment, or CMO unresponsive to local steroid injection (p. 343).

Follow–up All children, patients with severe inflammation (fibrin, hypopyon), raised IOP, known steroid responders, and definite or suspected CMO with reduced VA, should be seen within 1 week. Otherwise, arrange clinic review within 6 weeks and then discharge those with uncomplicated and resolved AAU. Advise patients that recurrences are common and to attend casualty if they are symptomatic.

Chronic Anterior Uveitis

Background Arbitrarily defined as anterior uveitis persisting for >3 months. Unlike acute anterior uveitis, it is not associated with HLA-B27.

Symptoms May be asymptomatic or present with only blurred vision.

Signs As for acute anterior uveitis, but the eye may be white and there is a higher incidence of complications (posterior synechiae; peripheral anterior synechiae; raised IOP; cataract; cystoid macular oedema, CMO).

Differential diagnosis

- *Systemic disease*: juvenile idiopathic arthritis; sarcoidosis.

- *Ocular syndromes*: Fuchs' heterochromic cyclitis.

- *Infective*: herpes zoster ophthalmicus (HZO), herpes simplex virus (HSV), syphilis.

- *Chronic idiopathic anterior uveitis*: accounts for ≈50% of cases.

- *Postoperative inflammation*: especially cataract surgery.

Clinical features Patients may have anterior vitreous cells and CMO but no other posterior segment signs. Two well-recognized types of chronic anterior uveitis are Fuchs' heterochromic cyclitis (FHC) and herpetic uveitis.

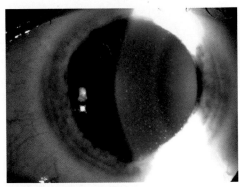

Fig. 8.2: Fuchs' heterochromic cyclitis with stellate keratic precipitates.

■ *Fuchs' heterochromic cyclitis* (FHC): features include white eye; characteristic translucent round or stellate keratic precipitates (KPs) scattered over the whole endothelium (Fig. 8.2); heterochromia (variable); iris stromal atrophy is typically diffuse; PS are absent; cataract is common; raised IOP (25%); vitreous cells and floaters may be considerable; CMO is rare.

■ *Herpetic uveitis*: seek a history of vesicles of HSV or HZO rash, corneal changes (p. 178, p. 182), Sectorial iris atrophy is common. Assess for complications at each visit.

Investigations Arrange CXR, sACE, and syphilis serology if no suggestive aetiology.

Treatment

■ *Casualty*: Treat acute exacerbations and refer to clinic as for AAU (p. 333). Use a weaker steroid (G. prednisolone 0.5% q.d.s.) covered with Oc. aciclovir five times daily for HSV uveitis, even if there is no active epithelial disease.

■ *Clinic*: Taper steroids slowly over months and attempt to stop. In steroid responders, G. rimexolone 1% (Vexol) may control inflammation without raising IOP. Add topical apraclonidine 0.5% t.d.s. and dexamethasone 0.1% if inflammation recurs. FHC does not require topical steroids.

Follow–up Assess and manage complications as they arise. Review after several weeks if topical steroids are stopped to exclude recurrence as this may be asymptomatic. For patients with FHC and normal IOP, arrange baseline disc imaging (photo or HRT) then annual glaucoma screening with an optometrist. Monitor those with elevated IOP in clinic.

Intermediate Uveitis

Background Intermediate uveitis is inflammation centred on the pars plana and peripheral retina. Pars planitis is defined as intermediate uveitis with 'snowbanking' and no systemic association. There is no racial or sex bias, with onset typically in childhood or young adult life. Pars planitis rarely presents over the age of 40 years.

Symptoms Bilateral in >80%, although asymmetry is not uncommon and about one-third present with unilateral disease. The history is frequently vague, but floaters from vitreous opacification or blurred vision from cystoid macular oedema (CMO) are common.

Signs The eye is white and the anterior segment usually quiet, or it may demonstrate slight flare, a few cells, and several small keratic precipitates (KPs). Vitreous signs predominate. Cells and opacities are invariable and may aggregate to form 'snowballs' concentrated over the inferior peripheral retina (Fig. 8.3). 'Snowbanking' is the appearance of a white plaque, typically overlying the inferior pars plana and retina but it can encompass the entire peripheral fundus (Fig. 8.4).

   CMO occurs in 25% and is the most important threat to vision. Other findings include mild vasculitis and sheathing of peripheral retinal venules, diffuse retinal oedema, optic disc or peripapillary swelling, and neovascularization of the disc or 'snowbank'.

History and examination The diagnosis is made by recognizing vitreous signs, an absence of focal choroidal and retinal lesions, or the presence of systemic diseases associated with pars planitis (see differential diagnosis below). Sarcoidosis

Fig. 8.3: Intermediate uveitis with 'snowballs'.

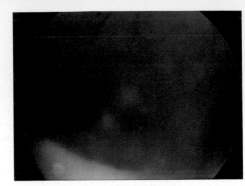

Fig. 8.4: Pars planitis with 'snowbank'.

and syphilis can be indistinguishable from idiopathic intermediate uveitis. A history of optic neuritis or other neurological features points to multiple sclerosis. Record VA at each visit. Assess for complications: CMO, posterior synechiae, raised IOP, cataract, vitreous haemorrhage from posterior vitreous detachment (most common) or neovascularization (less common), and epiretinal membrane formation.

Differential diagnosis

- *Idiopathic*: overwhelming majority.

- *Systemic disease*: sarcoidosis, multiple sclerosis, syphilis, inflammatory bowel disease, amyloidosis.

- *Ocular disease*: senile vitritis (affects the middle-aged or elderly, usually women).

- *Masquerade syndromes*: particularly large cell lymphoma (consider particularly in patients aged over 60 years although it may occur in younger patients).

Investigations If the history and examination are unremarkable, restrict investigations to CXR, sACE, and syphilis serology, with other tests only as indicated.

Treatment It is important not to overtreat. The main indication is VA of ≤6/12 due to CMO or vitritis. Refer suspected systemic disease to a physician.

- *Casualty*: Treat anterior uveitis with tapering topical steroids and cycloplegics. If VA is reduced from CMO, arrange urgent clinic referral; otherwise, review within 8 weeks.

- *Clinic*: Topical, periocular, intravitreal, and systemic steroids all have a role according to the pattern of disease and driven by the acuity and presence of CMO (p. 343). In pars planitis, neovascularization is secondary to inflammation, whereas in intermediate uveitis it may be secondary to inflammation, ischaemic retinal vasculitis, or a combination of both. Fluorescein angiography helps with the distinction. Steroids (oral or consider periocular injection in unilateral disease) are used to treat neovascularization secondary to inflammation, and argon laser is used if there is an ischaemic drive to new vessel formation. It may be appropriate to use oral prednisolone for 2 weeks prior to panretinal photocoagulation to dampen the inflammatory response.

Follow–up The majority have a chronic course lasting years with subacute exacerbations and low-grade remissions requiring long-term, periodic follow-up.

Posterior Uveitis

Background Posterior uveitis may reduce vision in several ways:

- *Reversible*: cystoid macular oedema (CMO); retinal or disc neovascularization, choroid neovascular membrane, disc swelling, cataract, epiretinal membranes, vitreous changes and retinal detachment.

- *Irreversible*: macular ischaemia, optic atrophy, glaucoma, and retinal scars.

History and examination Exclude anterior uveitis and its sequelae (p. 333) with slit lamp examination. Dilate and assess vitreous involvement. Use an indirect ophthalmoscope to look for peripheral vitreous condensations ('snowballs'), 'snowbanking', and any associated neovascularization. Define the primary site of inflammation: choroiditis, chorioretinitis, retinitis, or retinochoroiditis. Establish the pattern of vascular involvement. Venous vasculitis is a common and non-specific sign, it may be ischaemic, and sheathing may persist after inflammation subsides. Arterial involvement is less common but associated with serious systemic diseases such as collagen/vascular disease (systemic lupus erythematosus, Wegener's granulomatosis, polyarteritis nodosa) and Behçet's syndrome. A combination of arterial and venous vasculitis occurs in Behçet's syndrome, toxoplasmosis, syphilis, and acute retinal necrosis. Scars are associated with toxoplasmosis, sarcoidosis, presumed ocular histoplasmosis syndrome, punctuate inner choroidopathy, multifocal choroiditis, or may represent Dalen-Fuch's nodules (sympathetic ophthalmia, Vogt-Koyanagi-Harada syndrome, sarcoidosis). Determine the cause(s) of any visual loss.

Treatment

- *Casualty*: Exclude infection (e.g. varicella-zoster virus, metastatic endophthalmitis), treat anterior uveitis, and refer urgently to a uveitis clinic, the same day if vision is threatened.

- *Clinic*: Treat anterior uveitis accompanying posterior uveitis with topical steroids and mydriatics (p. 333). Regardless of the aetiology, the treatment of posterior uveitis is similar, once infection and neoplasia (such as lymphoma) are excluded. Not all patients require treatment; treat only if the eye is being damaged or the vision threatened. The most common indications are vitritis and CMO, but also retinitis, serous retinal detachment, papillitis, optic neuritis, and retinal neovascularization. Control inflammation with the minimum effective dose and duration of treatment. Consider: location and immediacy of the threat to vision; whether the disease is potentially reversible; if unilateral or bilateral; systemic factors including age, general health, and pregnancy; patient compliance and preference. In general, use periocular steroids if the patient is not a steroid responder, particularly in unilateral disease. Otherwise, use oral steroids in the first instance with the addition of ciclosporin or mycophenolate if unable to induce remission or reduce the relapse rate. If the disease is still not controlled, consider intravitreal triamcinolone if not a steroid responder (sometimes necessary despite known steroid response). Alternatively, use a combination of steroids/ciclosporin/mycophenolate.

Corticosteroids are the mainstay of management.

▨ *Local administration*: topical steroids treat anterior uveitis and anterior vitreous cells but not posterior segment inflammation. In contrast, local steroid injections (periocular or intravitreal) are effective in posterior uveitis and should be used whenever possible. The commonest indications are unilateral or bilateral asymmetric disease, especially where high-dose systemic steroids are contraindicated, e.g. pregnancy, or while obtaining diabetic or hypertensive control. Periocular steroids can take several weeks to work and are unsuitable when there is an immediate threat to vision. They are also contraindicated in steroid responders. Local injections are most useful in controlling vitritis and chronic CMO.

Posterior sub-Tenon triamcinolone (40 mg in 1 mL) or orbital floor methylprednisolone (Depomedrone 40 mg in 1 mL) appear equally effective. These can be repeated after 6 weeks but the mean time to best VA is 9 weeks. Discontinue if there is no response after 3 injections. Intravitreal triamcinolone (Kenalog 4 mg in 0.1 mL) is more potent and is given using the same technique as intravitreal antibiotics (p. 385). Measure IOP 15 minutes after injection. The risk of steroid-induced glaucoma is ≈30%, but may be up to 80% in patients under 30 years, so check IOP after 3 weeks when steroid response is usually first seen. Injections can be repeated after 3–4 months if the IOP is normal.

▨ *Systemic steroids*: use if the disease is bilateral, vision threatening, or local steroids have failed, but discuss the risks versus benefits. If the vision is threatened that day or VA ≤6/60, a typical starting dosage is prednisolone 80 mg o.d. (or 1–2 mg/kg) for 1 week, then, if responding, 60 mg o.d. 1 week, 40 mg o.d. 2 weeks, and thereafter guided by clinical effect. If VA is 6/12–6/18 and the visual threat is less severe, consider 40 mg o.d. (0.5–1 mg/kg) for 2 weeks then 30 mg o.d. 2 weeks. The required duration of treatment is difficult to predict. Aim to taper slowly, usually over months, to avoid reactivation. If unilateral reactivation occurs, consider local steroid injection to avoid increasing oral steroids. Some patients require indefinite treatment.

■ *Side effects*: hypertension, hypokalaemia, diabetes, osteoporosis, cushingoid appearance, and peptic ulceration. Cover with omeprazole 20 mg o.d. or ranitidine 150 mg b.d. Review drug interactions in the British National Formulary or equivalent.

■ *Baseline tests*: weight, BP, blood glucose, FBC, U&E, and CXR if indicated (history of TB/TB risk). Steroid-induced bone loss is worse at very high doses and aggravated by ciclosporin. Significant loss occurs in the first 6 months, so if this duration of treatment is likely then prescribe alendronate (Fosamax) 70 mg once weekly from the outset. Alternatively, reserve alendronate for high-risk patients and use calcium supplements (Calcichew D3 Forte b.d.) for lower-risk cases (avoid in sarcoid). A baseline bone scan will help define the risk.

■ *Monitoring*: measure weight, BP, and blood glucose at each visit. Check FBC (microcytic anaemia from GI blood loss, neutrophilia and lymphopaenia) and U&E (hypokalaemia) every 1–3 months. Advise patients to carry a steroid card and seek medical attention if they develop fever or lose their tablets.

Second-line agents Steroid-sparing agents are used to augment or help reduce steroid treatment, e.g. when steroid dose ≤10 mg produces frequent relapses. At all ages, balance the risk of lymphoma from treatment and try to avoid second-line agents in unilateral disease.

■ *Young healthy patients*: ciclosporin 3–7.5 mg/kg/day p.o. in two divided doses is the most widely used second-line agent although some clinicians prefer to avoid it for long-term use, selecting azathioprine or mycophenolate instead. Ciclosporin takes 2–6 weeks to work, depending on the dose. Renal impairment, liver disease, hypertension, and abnormal FBC are relative contraindications. Review drug interactions in the British National Formulary or equivalent. Arrange baseline BP, U&E and creatinine, LFTs, FBC, and urine dipstick for protein and blood. If diastolic pressure rises to >95 mmHg, or creatinine by 30% above baseline, reduce the dose by 25% immediately. Once stable, monitor BP and U&E every 3 months. Tacrolimus has a similar mode of action to ciclosporin; it is more potent but has a high incidence of renal toxicity. Methotrexate and azathioprine are often selected as third-line drugs. Cyclophosphamide and chlorambucil both have significant toxic side effects, so avoid unless absolutely necessary for severe destructive scleral inflammatory disease refractory to other agents, e.g. Wegener's granulomatosis.

- *Older patients* (>55–60 years) are generally less tolerant of ciclosporin in the long term (nephrotoxicity and hypertension). Mycophenolate (Cellcept) 0.5–1 g p.o. b.d. is increasingly used, or azathioprine 2–3 mg/kg/day in divided doses (recommended maximum of 100 mg b.d.). For azathioprine check TPMT (thyopurine methyltransferase) before starting and in carriers reduce to 0.5–1 mg/kg, or if low, avoid. Allow 3–6 weeks for effect and monitor FBC/LFTs.

Follow–up Varies but generally see patients starting systemic treatment at 1–4 weeks to monitor disease, side effects, and compliance. As inflammation settles, increase progressively to 3-monthly review. Advise patients to attend if symptoms recur. Monitor closely if there is a relapse, if re-introducing high-dose steroids, or starting second-line agents.

Sarcoidosis

Background A systemic granulomatous disease commonest in Asian and Afro-Caribbean patients. Multiple sites may be affected but particularly the lungs, lymph nodes, skin, liver, and eyes.

Symptoms Those of anterior, intermediate, or posterior uveitis. Systemic disease may be asymptomatic.

Signs These include: unilateral or bilateral acute or chronic anterior uveitis; intermediate uveitis; inferior preretinal nodules; patchy periphlebitis and sheathing; venous occlusion and neovascularization; small, round, usually inferior, chorioretinal lesions (Fig. 8.5); optic nerve involvement (granulomas, papilloedema with CNS involvement); secondary cataract/glaucoma. Look for iris infiltration with a velvety appearance and large, pink, peripheral nodules which tend to produce peripheral anterior synechiae.

History and examination Include extraocular assessment for lung, skin, bone, joint and muscle, salivary gland, and CNS involvement. Ask about cardiac pain.

Differential diagnosis Depends on the pattern of ocular/systemic signs. Exclude TB (risk of reactivation with systemic steroids) and syphilis. Consider other causes of multifocal choroiditis (p. 342). Arteriolar involvement is rare and suggests Behçet's disease, toxoplasma chorioretinitis, syphilis, or acute retinal necrosis.

Investigations Arrange CXR, sACE, syphilis serology, Mantoux/Heaf test if there is a risk of TB (best done by a physician). Biopsy skin/conjunctival lesions if obvious clinically. Refer those with systemic symptoms to a physician.

Treatment and follow-up Use topical, periocular, or systemic steroids as appropriate. Neovascularization may be secondary to ischaemia or inflammation, requiring laser or steroids, respectively, or sometimes both. Long-term follow-up is usually needed. Patients may go into remission but relapses are common.

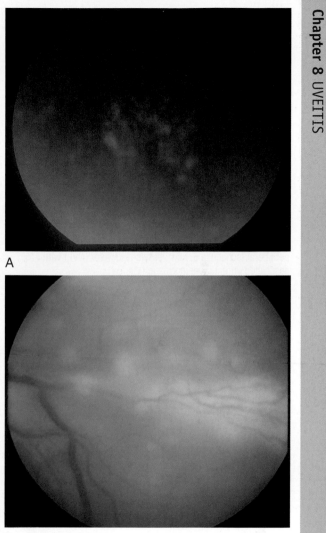

A

B

Fig. 8.5: Sarcoidosis with chorioretinal lesions **(A)** and severe retinal periphlebitis ('candlewax drippings') **(B)**.

Tuberculosis

Background At-risk groups include patients from Asia or those who are immunosuppressed, including HIV. Ocular manifestations may be due to direct infection or a hypersensitivity response to TB elsewhere.

History Many patients are systemically well. Pain, redness, blurred vision, and floaters are variable. Ask about BCG vaccination, previous TB/TB risk assessment, and evidence of a TB focus.

Examination Look for: conjunctival phlycten; nondescript anterior uveitis or associated with iris nodules; variably sized keratic precipitates; solitary choroidal granulomata (Fig. 8.6); multifocal choroiditis (lesions characteristically variable in size); subretinal abscess; retinitis; retinal vasculitis from infection (nonocclusive) or a hypersensitivity response with widespread peripheral ischaemia ± new vessels elsewhere (NVE) with associated vitreous haemorrhage (VH).

Differential diagnosis The diagnosis is often presumptive but exclude other granulomatous disease, especially sarcoidosis and Eales' disease (widespread peripheral venous occlusion, NVE/ vitreous haemorrhage, but no anterior chamber/vitreous cells).

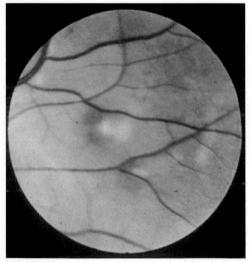

Fig. 8.6: TB choroidal granuloma.

Investigations CXR, Heaf/Mantoux test (by a physician), and sACE (overlap with sarcoidosis).

Treatment and follow-up Manage with a specialist physician. Treatment may include TB chemotherapy, oral steroids for active inflammation, retinal laser for new vessels, and topical steroids for conjunctival phlycten and anterior uveitis. Adjust (double) steroid treatment for patients on rifampicin.

Behçet's Disease

Background A chronic systemic inflammatory disease most frequent in young men of Japanese, Arabic, or Mediterranean origin (particularly those from Turkey and Greece). Major diagnostic criteria are:

- Recurrent oral ulcers (have to be present)
- Genital ulcers
- Skin lesions (erythema nodosum and pustules)
- Positive pathergy test
- Uveitis

Symptoms Pain and photophobia, or rapid-onset floaters and blurred vision.

Signs Transient hypopyon is common and may accompany anterior uveitis. Chronic panuveitis with severe acute recurrences is characteristic, as is an ischaemic vasculitis involving both arteries and veins. White necrotic retinitis may be accompanied by retinal infiltrates, oedema, and haemorrhage (Fig. 8.7). Second eye involvement may be delayed for years.

Differential diagnosis Reiter's syndrome, Crohn's disease, other causes of arterial vasculitis (collagen/vascular disorders).

Investigations None. Clinical diagnosis.

Treatment and follow–up See page 342 for the treatment of uveitis. Second-line agents are often required from the outset and the long-term prognosis is guarded. Recurrent posterior uveitis may result in retinal vascular attenuation and secondary optic atrophy. Lifelong follow-up is typical for posterior segment disease.

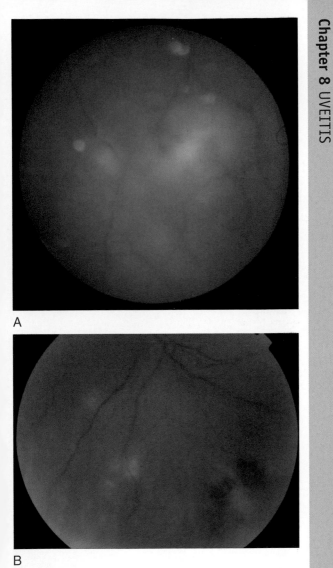

A

B

Fig. 8.7: Behçet's disease with active retinitis (**A**) and vascular occlusion (**B**).

Vogt-Koyanagi-Harada Syndrome

Background A systemic disease with ocular and skin involvement more common in Asian, Hispanic, and Japanese patients.

Symptoms Bilateral, synchronous or sequential blurred vision, with variable redness, pain, and photophobia. Patients may have a prodromal illness of pyrexia, headache, malaise, auditory or meningeal symptoms.

Signs Serous retinal detachments overlying diffuse or multifocal choroiditis, with vitritis, disc oedema or hyperaemia (characteristic pink disc) (Fig. 8.8). Anterior uveitis is common. Cutaneous signs (alopecia, poliosis, vitiligo) may develop later. Check colour vision and exclude an RAPD.

Differential diagnosis Consider sympathetic ophthalmia, posterior scleritis, sarcoidosis, and masquerade syndromes. Acute multifocal posterior placoid pigment epitheliopathy (AMPPE) rarely causes serous detachment.

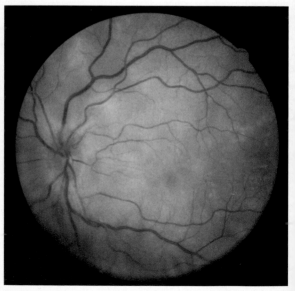

Fig. 8.8: Vogt-Koyanagi-Harada syndrome with swollen pink disc and choroidal lesions.

Investigations A clinical diagnosis. Fluorescein angiography shows pinpoint areas of enlarging hyperfluorescence with late staining of the disc and subretinal fluid. If a meningo-encephalitic picture occurs, request a neurological opinion, or if the eye lesions are atypical. B-scan ultrasound may help exclude posterior scleritis.

Treatment and follow–up For the treatment of posterior uveitis see page 342. Second-line agents may be required to allow steroid dose reduction if inflammation is severe or prolonged. The length of treatment depends on the optic neuritis. Retinal detachments usually settle rapidly, leaving considerable RPE mottling or a 'sunset glow' fundus. Choroidal granulomas leave Dalen-Fuchs' nodules (Fig. 8.9). It is often possible to stop systemic treatment after 1 year. Recurrences are typically as an anterior uveitis only and respond to topical treatment.

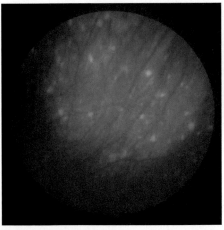

Fig. 8.9: Dalen-Fuchs' nodules.

Sympathetic Ophthalmia

Background Bilateral panuveitis following penetrating ocular injury, surgery, or nonpenetrating cyclodestructive procedures.

Symptoms Bilateral subacute discomfort or visual loss usually 1–12 months after the inciting event (range 5 days to 60+ years).

Signs Typically bilateral granulomatous panuveitis with diffuse choroidal involvement or multiple yellow-white Dalen-Fuchs' nodules, often with papillitis or peripapillary oedema (See Fig. 8.9). There is a broad spectrum of disease activity that may appear confined to the anterior segment.

Differential diagnosis Vogt-Koyanagi-Harada syndrome, multifocal choroiditis, phakoanaphylactic uveitis, and sarcoidosis.

Investigations A clinical diagnosis, although in apparently isolated anterior disease consider ICG angiography to exclude choroidal involvement.

Treatment The treatment of posterior uveitis is detailed on page 342. There is no role for enucleation of the traumatized eye if there is visual potential. Use topical steroids alone for inflammation limited to the anterior chamber. Systemic steroids are usually required and second-line agents may also be needed. Recurrences are likely, often with fresh Dalen-Fuchs' nodules or peripapillary oedema.

Follow-up It is unlikely that treatment can be stopped for at least 1 year. There is a reasonable long-term visual prognosis, but a high risk of cataract and glaucoma.

Presumed Ocular Histoplasmosis Syndrome

- Presumed ocular histoplasmosis syndrome (POHS) affects all ages with no sex bias.

- The characteristic triad is of peripapillary atrophy, multiple atrophic 'histo-spots' (Fig. 8.10), predominately around the posterior pole and often with internal pigment clumping, and serous or haemorrhagic disciform detachment due to choroidal neovascularization (CNV), usually associated with a macular 'histo-spot'.

- Linear streaks of chorioretinal atrophy are sometimes seen.

- Vitreous cells are absent.

- Usually asymptomatic until CNV develops.

- The diagnosis is clinical but request a fluorescence angiogram if CNV is suspected.

- Focal argon laser is appropriate for juxta- and extrafoveal CNVs. Oral steroids are of no benefit. Photodynamic therapy is unproven. As the CNV is type II, it may benefit from surgical removal. The role of anti-VEGF agents has yet to be fully determined.

- Offer an Amsler chart to monitor the other eye.

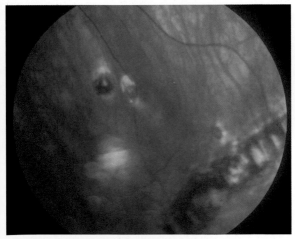

Fig. 8.10: Presumed ocular histoplasmosis.

Multifocal Choroiditis and Panuveitis

■ Affects all ages.

■ Acute, usually bilateral onset of anterior chamber and vitreous inflammation with lesions of varying size and age in the periphery, posterior pole, or both. Acute lesions are pale yellow or grey (Fig. 8.11).

■ Exclude sarcoidosis.

■ Usually follows a relapsing–remitting course.

■ VA is good unless cystoid macular oedema or choroidal neovascularization occur.

■ Cystoid macular oedema may respond to systemic steroids.

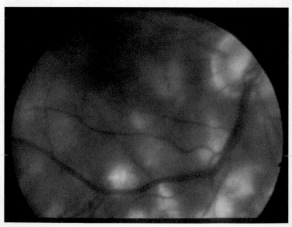

Fig. 8.11: Multifocal choroiditis.

Punctate Inner Choroidopathy

- Punctate inner choroidopathy (PIC) usually affects young myopic females.

- Presents with bilateral acute blurring of vision or photopsia with small yellow or grey spots around the posterior pole at the level of the choroid or RPE.

- Few if any vitreous cells are present.

- Fluorescein angiography of acute lesions shows early hyperfluorescence and late staining.

- Recurrences are uncommon but can occur.

- There is a high risk of choroidal neovascularization which may respond to systemic or intravitreal steroids, or photodynamic therapy. The role of anti-VEGF agents has yet to be fully determined.

- Provide an Amsler grid and instructions.

Acute Multifocal Posterior Placoid Pigment Epitheliopathy (AMPPE)

- Primarily affects young adults of either sex.

- Causes acute, usually bilateral, blurred vision.

- One-third of cases are preceded by a viral prodrome.

- Cream-coloured, ill-defined lesions occur at the level of the choriocapillaris or RPE, most commonly at the posterior pole (see p. 424).

- A mild vitritis occurs in 50% and anterior chamber cells in a minority.

- Severe hypertension may produce choroidal infarcts that mimic AMPPE so check BP.

- Fluorescein angiography shows early blockage of choroidal fluorescence with late staining. ICG angiography shows areas of choriocapillary hypoperfusion (p. 424).

- The disease is usually self-limiting but may recur.

- The benefit of systemic steroids is unproven but they are often given if VA is reduced at presentation.

- Ask about severe headaches as these suggest cerebral vasculitis, which may be fatal. If present, refer promptly to a neurologist.

Birdshot Chorioretinopathy

■ Usually occurs in HLA-A29-positive Caucasians aged 40–70 years.

■ Gradual bilateral onset.

■ Oval, cream-coloured, ill-defined lesions occur around the posterior pole and midperiphery (Fig. 8.12); these may take years to appear. Choroidal neovascularization may occur.

■ Often associated with moderate vitritis, vasculitis, cystoid macular oedema, and disc oedema.

■ A chronic progressive course usually requires systemic steroids and second-line agents for visual loss from cystoid macular oedema.

■ Loss of retinal function (ERG) precedes VA change and dictates therapy.

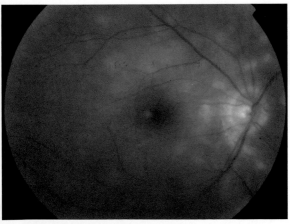

Fig. 8.12: Birdshot chorioretinopathy.

Multiple Evanescent White Dot Syndrome (MEWDS)

■ Typically causes acute unilateral visual loss or paracentral scotoma in young adult females, often following a flu-like illness.

■ Small white spots occur at the level of the RPE or retina, mostly within and around the vascular arcades and disc, showing early hypofluorescence and late staining on fluorescein angiography. The macula has a granular appearance due to tiny punctate yellowish or orange spots (Fig. 8.13). ICG angiography typically shows multiple hypofluorescent areas in late films which are more extensive than the lesions seen clinically.

■ Vitreous cells may be present, as may an RAPD, disc swelling, and blind spot enlargement.

■ MEWDS resolves spontaneously over weeks to normal or near normal acuity.

■ The fundus changes also resolve, and may be absent unless examined acutely. ICG angiography may, however, be abnormal for several weeks before reverting to normal.

■ Recurrences are rare.

■ There is no proven treatment.

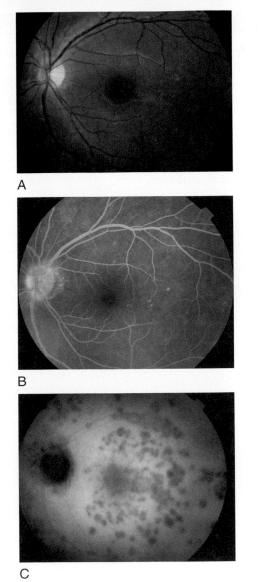

A

B

C

Fig. 8.13: MEWDS (A) with fluorescein angiogram (B), and ICG (C).

Serpiginous Choroidopathy

- Rare, usually bilateral disease mostly affecting Caucasians of either sex. Also called geographic choroidopathy.

- Presents typically as a middle-aged adult with active choroidal inflammation adjacent to previous scars (Fig. 8.14). May present at a younger age (>10 years) .

- Has a slow stepwise progression with spread from the peripapillary area towards the periphery.

- Active lesions show early blockage with late staining on fluorescein angiography.

- Often treated with systemic steroids for vision-threatening lesions, although not of proven benefit.

- Extrafoveal choroidal neovascularization is sometimes treated with argon laser with steroid cover.

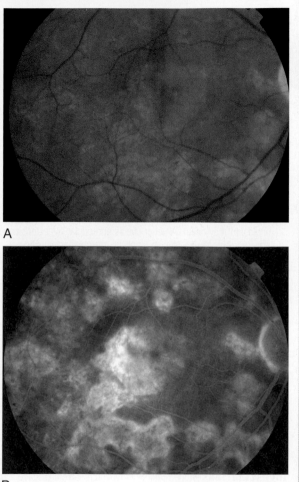

A

B

Fig. 8.14: **(A,B)** Serpiginous choroidopathy.

Toxoplasmosis

Background Usually represents a reactivation of healed early acquired/congenital toxoplasmosis and is less frequently a manifestation of acute recently acquired infection.

Symptoms Blurred vision, or floaters due to vitritis.

Signs

■ *Inactive disease*: characteristically an atrophic chorioretinal scar of variable size with pigment clumping.

■ *Active disease*: focal yellow-white area of active necrotizing retinitis, with poorly demarcated edges, adjacent to the edge of an old inactive scar (Fig. 8.15), with associated vitritis. Localized arterial and venous vasculitis are common, and occlusion may occur. Anterior uveitis and ocular hypertension are frequent. Neuro-retinitis, papillitis, retrobulbar neuritis, punctate outer retinal toxoplasmosis, massive granuloma, and diffuse unilateral toxoplasmosis are less frequent. VA is directly affected if there is involvement of the fovea, papillomacular bundle, or optic nerve, or indirectly as a consequence of cystoid macular oedema, epiretinal membrane, or as a result of vascular occlusion and ischaemia/ neovascularisation. Choroidal neovascularization, and tractional and rhegmatogenous retinal detachments are rare. Recently acquired toxoplasma retinitis is not associated with chorioretinal scarring and is typically solitary, discrete, and unilateral.

History and examination Acute acquired infection is usually asymptomatic. Record VA, the degree of vitritis, and the location of the active retinitis. Look for inactive scars in the fellow eye.

Investigations None required in typical recurrent disease. If recently acquired disease is suspected, the diagnosis is confirmed by high IgM antibody titre which reverts to IgG after 3–9 months. When treatment is indicated, request baseline BP, BM, FBC, U&E, and LFT to monitor the side effects of antibiotics and steroids (p. 343). Request a head CT in immunocompromised patients.

Treatment The disease is self-limiting and not all lesions require intervention. Treat the following lesions:

■ Active lesions inside or straddling the temporal vascular arcades;

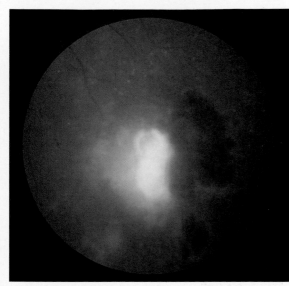

Fig. 8.15: Toxoplasma retinitis.

■ Threat to a major retinal vessel

■ Within one disc diameter of the optic disc or causing disc swelling

■ Multifocal lesions

■ Sufficient vitritis to obscure the macular view

The most-used combination is pyrimethamine (50 mg p.o. loading dose, then 25 mg o.d.) in conjunction with folinic acid (15 mg twice weekly) to alleviate marrow toxicity, sulphadiazine (2 g p.o. loading dose then 1 g q.d.s.), and systemic steroids, typically prednisolone 60 mg o.d. and tapered as inflammation subsides. Some clinicians feel that loading doses are unnecessary. The treatment length is guided by the clinical response but is usually 4–6 weeks. Systemic steroids should not be given without antibiotics, and local steroids injections are contraindicated. Female patients with primary disease need to be advised that there is a risk of passing the infection to the fetus for 6 months and the need for contraception as appropriate.

Follow-up If no treatment is required, review in 1 week initially and reassess. Review weekly on treatment with FBC at each visit.

As inflammation subsides, the edges of active lesion harden off and are replaced by a chorioretinal scar with clearing of vitritis. Overall, 30% retain 6/12 vision or better. Discharge when the retinitis is quiescent. Advise patients that treatment cannot prevent recurrences (mean, 2.7 yr) and that they should return to casualty if symptoms recur.

Acute Retinal Necrosis

Background Acute retinal necrosis (ARN) is most frequently caused by varicella zoster virus (VZV) but is also reported with herpes simplex virus (HSV) I and II and rarely cytomegalovirus (CMV). Patients may be healthy or immunocompromised.

Symptoms Often there is no systemic disease although some may have evidence of recent or concurrent VZV or HSV infection. Onset is typically unilateral with visual loss, often with ocular or periocular discomfort. Sequential bilateral involvement occurs in up to one-third of cases, usually within 3 months, but may be delayed for several years. Patients may get recurrent anterior uveitis.

Signs Characterized by focal, well-demarcated, whitened areas of peripheral retinal necrosis outside the major vascular arcades (Fig. 8.16), which rapidly progress circumferentially to become confluent. Vascular occlusion, both arterial and venous, is an important clinical feature. Optic nerve head swelling is common. Vitritis is always present and may obscure the fundal view. There is a high incidence of retinal breaks just anterior to normal retina. Anterior uveitis is present in all patients, keratic precipitates may be large, and IOP is often elevated. Immuncompromised patients, particularly those with HIV infection, may have a more aggressive

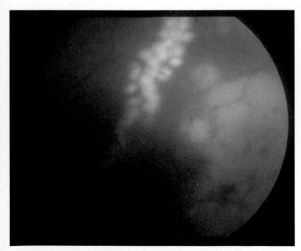

Fig. 8.16: Acute retinal necrosis peripheral to an argon laser demarcation line.

form (previously called progressive outer retinal necrosis) but with less inflammation (p. 374).

Investigations Consider vitreous biopsy and VSV, HSV I & II, Epstein Barr, and CMV PCR in all patients to confirm the diagnosis. Request baseline FBC, U&E, and LFTs. If bilateral at presentation, inquire about sexual history/HIV risk and arrange testing as appropriate with infectious disease clinicians. Spontaneous VZV preceding ARN indicates immunocompromise until proved otherwise.

Differential diagnosis

- *Behçet's disease*: features retinal necrosis and arterial and venous vasculitis, but also extraocular features.

- *Pars planitis*: may produce significant peripheral retinal whitening and vitritis but onset is not acute and ischaemia is absent.

- *Syphilis*: may cause retinal whitening, arteritis, and vitritis.

- *Toxoplasmosis*: can cause large peripheral white lesions and significant vitritis but typically there is a chorioretinal scar.

Treatment Early initiation of antiviral therapy is important. Admit for i.v. aciclovir 10 mg/kg infused over 1 hour t.d.s. for 1 week. Renal toxicity is the most important side effect; monitor U&Es and fluid balance, ensuring adequate intake (i.v. fluids if necessary) and output. As retinitis subsides, whitened necrotic retina is replaced by RPE scarring and atrophy. Systemic steroids (1 mg/kg and rapidly tapered) are usually introduced after 24 hours of i.v. aciclovir if significant vitritis limits the fundal view or there is optic nerve involvement. To prevent rhegmatogenous retinal detachment, some clinicians recommend prophylactic argon laser behind the posterior edge of involved retina (3 rows of 500 µm light/moderate burns) as soon as visualization is adequate. Others now feel that this is not helpful and have discontinued laser prophylaxis. If immunosuppressed, arrange physician review. I.V. aciclovir is followed by oral therapy (800 mg five times daily) for 6 weeks, aiming to stop any systemic steroids during this time. Some clinicians prescribe 12 weeks aciclovir since second eye involvement tends to occur in this interval. In immunosuppressed patients, the course of both i.v. and oral aciclovir may need to be prolonged. Avoid systemic steroids. Consider systemic or intravitreal foscarnet (2.4 mg in 0.1 mL) in severe cases, or those that relapse on aciclovir.

Follow–up Usually for 3–5 years to assess for second eye involvement and rhegmatogenous retinal detachment. Proliferative vitreoretinopathy is common.

Cytomegalovirus Retinitis

Background Usually occurs in association with severe immunocompromise, either iatrogenic, from malignancy, or most commonly, AIDS (CD4+ count almost always <50 cells/µL). In the majority, the cause of the underlying immunosuppression is already established, but CMV retinitis is the presenting feature in 2% of patients with AIDS.

Symptoms Visual loss or scotomas from posterior pole involvement. May be asymptomatic.

Signs Full-thickness necrotizing retinitis with haemorrhage, often with accompanying retinal vasculitis (Fig. 8.17). Slowly progressive (250–300 µm/week) and usually more rapid towards the retinal periphery than the posterior pole, so areas are characteristically sectorial. The edge of lesions are the most active, with expansion resembling a 'brush-fire'. Visual loss occurs when retinitis involves the optic nerve or macula, or from rhegmatogenous retinal detachment, serous macular detachment, or cystoid macular oedema.

Differential diagnosis Small focal areas of involvement may be mistaken for cotton-wool spots of HIV retinopathy (these wax and wane, whereas CMV retinitis is progressive without

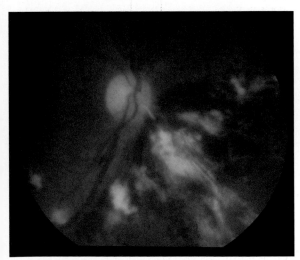

Fig. 8.17: Cytomegalovirus retinitis with severe haemorrhage and vasculitis.

treatment) or other herpes virus retinitis. HIV retinopathy is rare in black patients.

Investigations Inquire about sexual history/HIV risk and arrange testing as appropriate with an infectious disease clinician. Check VDRL (often positive). If the diagnosis is in doubt, arrange a vitreous biopsy PCR at the time of the first intravitreal injection.

Treatment Start treatment immediately and manage jointly with physicians. Drugs used for the treatment of CMV retinitis are virostatic and cannot prevent recurrence. Aim to induce remission with induction, then maintenance therapy while monitoring for relapse. Antivirals may be given locally either by intravitreal injection (ganciclovir, foscarnet) or implant (ganciclovir), or systemically either i.v. (ganciclovir, foscarnet, cidofovir) or orally (ganciclovir, valganciclovir).

Follow–up Watch for recurrence and second eye involvement. Within 1–2 week of induction expect a loss of retinal whitening and resolution of oedema, exudate, and haemorrhage, leaving retinal atrophy and RPE scarring. Reactivation may be more difficult to detect and may manifest as a smouldering border with a small area of retinal whitening, merely changes in the whiteness of the border, or a recurrence of perivascular sheathing. Serial photographs are invaluable.

Masquerade Syndromes

Background Masquerade syndromes are disorders which mimic intraocular inflammation but have an underlying cause which may be malignant, infective, or a miscellany of other causes. These include drug-induced, retained intraocular foreign body, Schwartz syndrome (rhegmatogenous retinal detachment and anterior chamber 'cells'), ghost-cell glaucoma following vitreous haemorrhage, ocular ischaemic syndrome, and retinitis pigmentosa. Many are apparent from the history and examination, or due to their atypical clinical features, or failure to respond to steroids.

Lymphoma Always consider in patients over 60 years who present for the first with intraocular inflammation. Suspect if there is marked vitritis but good VA. Usually bilateral with both an anterior chamber reaction and vitritis (classically 'veils'), sometimes with subretinal or intraretinal infiltration. The majority of patients have CNS non-Hodgkin's lymphoma but there can be systemic spread, although this tends initially to produce choroidal disease. The eye may be the only organ involved. If suspected, arrange a vitreous biopsy for cytology, CNS imaging, and CSF cytology. Treatment comprises ocular and CNS irradiation and chemotherapy. Cystoid macular oedema is uncommon.

Leukaemia All forms of leukaemia may involve the eye. Manifestations include direct retinal and optic nerve infiltration, and serous retinal detachment overlying choroidal infiltrates. Subhyaloid haemorrhage, Roth spots, vascular dilatation or tortuosity, and cotton wool spots are secondary to thrombocytopenia and anaemia. Anterior segment involvement is less common but includes acute anterior uveitis with hypopyon ('white eye'), diffuse iris infiltration, or iris nodules. If suspected, refer to a haematologist.

Retinoblastoma See page 407.

Melanoma Choroidal melanomas may cause signs of both anterior and posterior segment inflammation. Amelanotic choroidal tumours may simulate an inflammatory mass. Ultrasound and fluorescein angiography are useful in establishing the diagnosis. Iris tumours may be mistaken for inflammatory nodules. Diffuse iris melanomas may cause heterochromia.

Metastases Most commonly from lung and breast. Usually present as an isolated choroidal lesion which when flat may resemble an inflammatory focus but patients can present with endophthalmitis. Anterior segment metastases are rare but may cause an anterior uveitis, pseudohypopyon, or iris nodules.

Uveitis in Children

Background Most types of uveitis can be seen in children and are managed in a similar way to adults depending on the anatomic location, severity, threat to vision, and complications present. For example, children may get recurrent acute anterior uveitis associated with HLA-B27 and diseases such as ankylosing spondylitis. Although uncommon, Fuchs' heterochromic cyclitis has been reported even in young children. Children may get sympathetic ophthalmia following trauma and disorders such as Vogt-Koyanagi-Harada syndrome. Infective disorders such as chickenpox can cause a uveitis, and metastatic endophthalmitis can occur from any septic site. Reactivation of toxoplasmic retinochoroiditis is uncommon in children, and the commonest cause of posterior uveitis in the under 16 age group is pars planitis.

Juvenile idiopathic arthritis is associated with uveitis that may be asymptomatic, so review all children at diagnosis. The risk of uveitis depends on the type of arthritis (systemic versus polyarticular versus pauciarticular). Uveitis in systemic disease is rare. ANA+ve pauciarticular females aged <7 years are at highest risk. Review high-risk children (those aged <7 years who are ANA+ve, with pauci- or polyarticular arthritis) 3 monthly, medium-risk 6 monthly, and low-risk (systemic disease) yearly. The high-risk group become medium-risk after 4 years follow-up. The medium-risk group becomes low-risk after 4 years. All go to low-risk after 7 years. The characteristic chronic anterior uveitis has a high ocular morbidity if not well controlled; band keratopathy, posterior synechiae, cataract, cyclitic membranes, and macular oedema can all occur. Posterior synechiae at presentation indicate severe disease. Topical steroids and mydriatics are the mainstay of treatment in children with anterior uveitis. Steroid response may occur in addition to open angle glaucoma and raised IOP secondary to pupillary occlusion. Usually, cataract removal is by lensectomy because of cyclitic membrane formation; systemic steroid cover for this is helpful.

Uveitis in Pregnancy

Patients with uveitis who wish to get pregnant need to consider the risks and benefits of any systemic medication. Acetazolamide is commonly avoided. Prednisolone ≤15 mg daily is probably safe in the first trimester and throughout pregnancy. There are fewer data on other immunosuppressive agents so avoid if possible, but as with transplant patients azathioprine, ciclosporin, and mycophenolate can be used in pregnancy at the lowest effective dose. Many of the drugs can be found in breast milk, and this information must be given to mothers wishing to breast feed. For drug use in pregnancy see page 702.

Immune-mediated uveitis may get better during pregnancy, stay the same, or get worse. The same applies to postpartum uveitis. Periocular steroids may be used during pregnancy and breastfeeding, and can be given bilaterally if necessary. Although some drug is absorbed systemically by this route, the amount is extremely small and is not thought to harm the fetus.

Patients with reactivation of toxoplasma retinochoroiditis present no infective risk to their babies, but consider which drugs can be used safely. Patients developing primary toxoplasma infection, even if apparently in the eye alone, must be made aware that this is a systemic infection which carries a serious risk of fetal involvement, the extent of which depends on the stage of the pregnancy.

HIV

Background The ocular manifestations of HIV vary with the level of immunocompromise, reflected in the presence of HIV virus in the blood (viral load) and CD4$^+$ count. A CD4$^+$ count >1000 cells/mL is normal; <50 cells/μL is extremely low with a high risk of serious ocular infection, particularly cytomegalovirus (CMV) retinitis. Highly active antiretroviral therapy (HAART) markedly improves CD4$^+$ counts and reduces opportunistic infections, but lymphoma has become more common.

History and examination Ask about systemic illnesses, infections, interventions, medications, and duration of HIV infection. A minimum routine examination includes VA, eyelids, conjunctival fornices, anterior segment, and dilated fundoscopy including peripheral retina. Examination specifically to exclude uveitis and CMV retinitis.

Clinical features The following are associated with HIV infection:

- *Blepharitis*: often severe.

- *Molluscum contagiosum*: usually extensive.

- *Premature presbyopia*.

- *Conjunctival Kaposi's sarcoma*: signifies AIDS.

- *Conjunctival squamous cell carcinoma*: more common in Africa.

- *Herpes zoster ophthalmicus*: a common presenting feature of AIDS in developing nations.

- *HIV retinopathy*: cotton-wool spots and dot haemorrhages are common and inconsequential (Fig. 8.18).

- *Uveitis*: can be of infective, inflammatory, or malignant aetiology. Improved immunity following antiretroviral therapy may cause an immune recovery uveitis that is a leading cause of new visual loss. As the CD4$^+$ count drops, infections become increasingly important, particularly syphilis, toxoplasmosis, herpes simplex, and herpes zoster. HIV itself can cause a panuveitis. Lymphoma may cause a masquerade-type of uveitis that may have CNS or systemic involvement. Syphilitic uveitis can occur at any CD4$^+$ count and in the presence of HIV may indicate tertiary syphillis.

- *CMV and varicella-zoster retinitis* (previously called PORN or progressive outer retinal necrosis): both CMV retinitis and

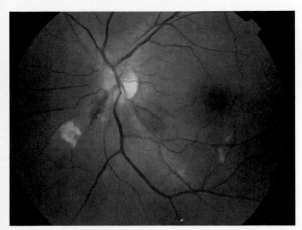

Fig. 8.18: HIV retinopathy.

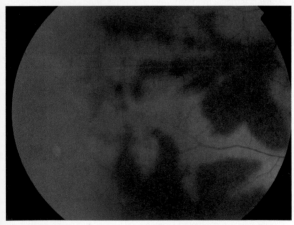

Fig. 8.19: Varicella-zoster retinitis (progressive outer retinal necrosis).

PORN can occur with little or no intraocular inflammation (a useful diagnostic clue). PORN (Fig. 8.19) tends to be more aggressive than acute retinal necrosis (ARN) that occurs in immunocompetent patients.

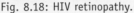 *Toxoplasmosis*: retinal lesions may be bilateral and multifocal; 56% have CNS involvement.

- *Metastatic bacterial or fungal endophthalmitis*: particularly following sepsis, surgery, or intravenous drugs use.

- *Tuberculosis*: increasing incidence in the HIV population. Ocular manifestations include uveitis and optic nerve involvement. Choroidal granulomas are an indication of miliary TB.

- *Pneumocystis choroiditis*: implies systemic infection and requires systemic treatment. No additional ocular treatment is required. *Pneumocystis* very rarely causes conjunctivitis, orbital masses, and optic neuropathy.

- *Retrobulbar neuritis*: due to *Cryptococcus*, syphilis, histoplasmosis, or herpes zoster.

- *Toxic optic neuropathy*: from drug therapy, especially dideoxyinosine and ethambutol.

- *Papillitis*: secondary to CMV, syphilis, or toxoplasmosis.

- *Cortical visual loss*: causes include non-Hodgkin's lymphoma, toxoplasmosis, and progressive multifocal leucoencephalopathy.

- *Cryptococcal meningitis*: may cause visual loss through raised intracranial pressure. Optic nerve sheath fenestration may help.

- *Reiter's disease*: comprises a triad of urethritis, arthritis, and conjunctivitis. Treat conjunctivitis with topical steroids. Add antibiotics if it looks infective.

Follow up In patients with CD4$^+$ counts <50 cells/µL, perform dilated fundoscopy every 6 weeks or earlier if they develop floaters, field loss, or blurred vision. The need for regular screening decreases with CD4$^+$ counts >200 cells/µL.

Episcleritis

Background A self-limiting condition of unknown aetiology.

Clinical features Episcleritis is often mistaken for scleritis. In episcleritis, congestion is limited to the radially orientated superficial episcleral vessels within Tenon's capsule (Fig. 8.20). In anterior scleritis, the irregular-crossing deep episcleral vessels on the scleral surface are also involved and there is accompanying scleral thickening. G. phenylephrine 10% only produces blanching of the superficial episcleral venous plexus. The onset of episcleritis is typically more acute, the sensation is not of pain but grittiness, there is no corneal or intraocular involvement, and vision is unaffected.

Management Offer reassurance. Treatment is not routinely required as symptoms usually resolve. If frequently recurrent, oral NSAIDs such as Froben 50 mg p.o. t.d.s. may help but have side effects (gastric/duodenal ulceration, exacerbation of asthma). Topical steroids are sometimes useful, e.g. fluorometholone 0.1% q.d.s. 2 weeks.

Follow up Not required, but explain that recurrences are common.

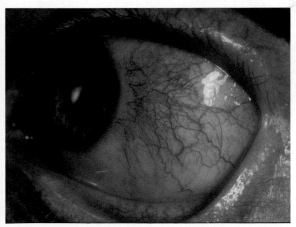

Fig. 8.20: Mild episcleritis.

Scleritis

Background Less common than episcleritis. Scleritis has frequent (≈50%) systemic associations and is vision threatening. Systemic therapy is essential. Broadly classified into anterior and posterior scleritis.

Anterior scleritis Has a subacute onset of severe ocular and periocular pain, often worse at night, with redness, photophobia, and globe tenderness (Fig. 8.21). Deep episcleral vessels on the surface of the sclera are dilated with vascular closure in necrotizing disease. The sclera may have a bluish tint that is best appreciated with the naked eye and bright room light. Avascular areas are best seen with red-free (green) slit lamp light. May be diffuse, nodular, or necrotizing.

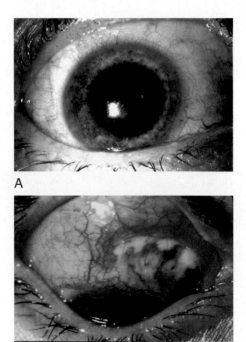

A

B

Fig. 8.21: Scleritis. Mild anterior diffuse scleritis **(A)** and necrotising anterior scleritis **(B)** with uveal tissue visible beneath thinned sclera.

■ Diffuse

  a. May involve small or large areas of sclera.

  b. The most common type of scleritis.

  c. Pain may be severe.

  d. Not usually sight threatening and usually resolves.

■ Nodular

  a. Part of the inflamed sclera is raised in one or more nodules.

  b. May progress.

  c. Commonly recurs.

■ Necrotising

  a. Least frequent but most severe type of anterior scleritis.

  b. Female preponderance.

  c. Associated with vascular closure and pale regions of scleral necrosis within areas of active scleritis.

  d. Scleromalacia perforans is a very rare form of necrotizing anterior scleritis which occurs without inflammation, is asymptomatic, bilateral, and seen only in advanced rheumatoid arthritis (RA), usually in females. Perforation of the thinned and translucent sclera is unusual without trauma. There is no ocular treatment.

■ Associations

  a. *Local*: ocular surgery, infection (toxoplasmosis, acanthamoeba, herpes simplex virus, varicella-zoster virus, bacterial), and masquerade syndrome (ocular surface carcinoma, intraocular tumour).

  b. *Systemic* (50%): most commonly RA but also other collagen/vascular disorders including Wegener's granulomatosis, polyarteritis nodosa (PAN), systemic lupus erythematosus (SLE).

Posterior scleritis May be nodular or diffuse. Presentation is with pain and reduced vision. Rarely, there is conjunctival chemosis with some limitation of movement and proptosis. Posterior segment signs are variable and may include serous retinal detachment, swollen optic disc, subretinal mass lesion, choroidal folds, and choroidal detachment. Approximately one-third of patients have associated anterior scleritis. Local associations are as for anterior scleritis. Systemic associations (30%) include

RA, Wegener's granulomatosis, PAN, SLE, relapsing polychondritis, and neoplasia.

Differential diagnosis Episcleritis may overlay scleritis, so it is important not to miss the scleritis. For distinguishing features, see page 377.

Investigations There is a high incidence of systemic associations. If there is a suggestive history and general examination arrange urine dipstick for blood and protein, FBC, ESR, CRP, RhF, ANA, U&E, LFTs, and ANCA (if Wegener's granulomatosis suspected). Discuss with physicians. In many cases the diagnosis is already established. In patients with suspected posterior scleritis, B-scan ultrasonography is very useful in demonstrating either diffuse or nodular scleral thickening (>2 mm) with an adjacent echolucent area from oedema in Tenon's space. Fluorescein angiography in patients with serous retinal detachment typically shows multiple small foci of leakage at the level of the RPE which may look similar to Vogt-Koyanagi-Harada syndrome.

Management

Casualty: Treat anterior non-necrotizing scleritis, and mild posterior scleritis with no visible posterior segment abnormalities with Froben 100 mg p.o. t.d.s. (combined with omeprazole 20 mg p.o. o.d. if there is a history/risk of gastric/duodenal ulceration). Review in 1–2 weeks. Reduced pain indicates a good response, and treatment can then be tailed off, but warn of the risk of recurrence. If pain and inflammation persist, refer to clinic and consider oral prednisolone 0.5–1 mg/kg o.d., then tapered off. Necrotizing scleritis, and posterior scleritis associated with retinal or choroidal detachment, disc swelling, or subretinal mass lesion, require same-day specialist review. If there is hypertension, protein or blood on urine dipstick, or associated systemic disease, then consult urgently with physicians; systemic disease is potentially life threatening.

Clinic: High-dose oral steroids (prednisolone 1 mg/kg) are recommended for necrotizing anterior scleritis and posterior scleritis with visual loss or threat. Consider admission and pulsed i.v. methylprednisolone 0.5–1.0 g for 1–3 days followed by oral steroids in severe cases. Adjunct immunosuppressive therapy is often required for those with systemic disease or when scleritis is resistant to steroids alone. Cyclophosphamide may be necessary in very severe necrotizing disease, as may occur in Wegener's granulomatosis. Surgical treatment may be required either for diagnostic (infection, masquerade syndrome) or therapeutic (cataract, corneal/scleral grafts) indications.

Ideally, surgery is undertaken when scleritis has been controlled medically and under corticosteroid cover (prednisolone 40 mg p.o. o.d. 2 weeks preoperatively). Clear corneal incisions are less likely to require high-dose steroid cover than scleral tunnels.

Endophthalmitis

Background Endophthalmitis is vitreous and/or anterior chamber inflammation of presumed infective origin. Classified as exogenous (after surgery, keratitis, or trauma) or endogenous (also called metastatic).

Exogenous Postoperative Endophthalmitis

Clinical features

- *Acute onset* (0–17 days): ocular pain, reduced vision and headache with lid oedema, conjunctival hyperaemia, chemosis, purulent discharge, corneal oedema, anterior chamber reaction, hypopyon, and poor red reflex.

- *Delayed acute* (18–60 days): due to less virulent organisms or from a suture track, wound dehiscence, or vitreous wick.

- *Chronic* (>60 days): usually a capsular bag infection with a low-virulence organism (often *Propionibacterium acnes* or *Staphylococcus epidermidis*). Presents with reduced vision and minimal pain. May have signs of steroid-responsive iritis, capsular plaque, granulomatous uveitis, or localized vitritis. Hypopyon uveitis following YAG capsulotomy is a classic presentation. Endophthalmitis may occur years after trabeculectomy (p. 323).

History and examination Assess severity, which relates to the speed of onset, VA at presentation, RAPD, and fundal view. Measure the hypopyon height.

Differential diagnosis Assume all severe postoperative inflammation is infective endophthalmitis unless there is another obvious cause, especially in patients with no history of uveitis. If in doubt and VA is 6/12 or worse, admit for 6–12 hours of half-hourly, topical, preservative-free dexamethasone 0.1% and reassess 2 hourly.

Investigations Lid and conjunctival swabs are of no value. Take a corneal scrape if keratitis is present. Arrange aqueous and vitreous samples in all patients (including those with perception of light vision at presentation) (Box 8.1). If there is no fundal view, arrange ultrasound prior to sampling. If not immediately available, proceed with biopsy but arrange ultrasound at the first opportunity. Request baseline FBC, U&E, weight, blood sugar, and blood pressure measurements before starting on systemic steroids.

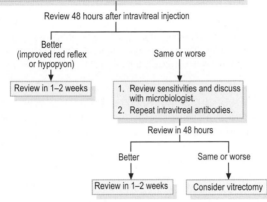

1. Intravitreal biopsy and antibodies as soon as possible, preferably at first hospital contact. For technique, see Box 8.1.
2. Moxifloxacin 400mg od PO for 10 days.
3. Gutte dexamethasone 0.1% preservative free hourly, steroid ointment nocte, chloramphenicol 0.5% qds, cyclopentolate 1% tds.
4. Analgesia
5. Anterior chamber tissue plasminogen activator (12.5mcg in 0.1ml) if there is severe fibrinous response.
6. Subconjunctival 0.3 ml Mydricaine II if poor pupil dilation.
7. Review Gram/Giemsa stain the same day.
8. After 24 hours start enteric coated prednisolone 1 mg/kg/day with ranitidine 150 mg bd. Steroids are contrindicated in fungal endophthalmitis so check Gram and Giemsa stain. *Candida* spp are Gram positive but other fungi are only detected with Giesma stain.

Review 48 hours after intravitreal injection

Better
(improved red reflex
or hypopyon)

Review in 1–2 weeks

Same or worse

1. Review sensitivities and discuss with microbiologist.
2. Repeat intravitreal antibodies.

Review in 48 hours

Better

Review in 1–2 weeks

Same or worse

Consider vitrectomy

Fig. 8.22: Treatment of acute postoperative endophthalmitis.

Treatment

■ For children, discuss the drug dose and selection with a pharmacist. For adults, see Fig. 8.22.

■ Moxifloxacin may have an antibiofilm effect on coagulase-negative staphylococci and a better spectrum of activity than ciprofloxacin, but use ciprofloxacin 750 mg b.d. 10 days if not available.

■ Consider periocular steroids if systemic steroids are contraindicated.

■ Chronic endophthalmitis usually responds to treatment, but some cases recur when treatment is stopped, as organisms may be sequestered behind the lens. Re-treat with intravitreal and systemic antibiotics but if inflammation recurs again then arrange IOL and total capsule removal. Send samples at each stage for microbiology and histopathology. Avoid systemic steroids that may mask ongoing inflammation.

▪ *The Endophthalmitis Vitrectomy Study (EVS)*[1] was a large randomized, controlled trial that suggested early vitrectomy with intravitreal antibiotics may improve the final VA for patients with PL vision. Recent local experience suggests that early vitrectomy results in a worse prognosis for those with PL vision but many other centres follow the EVS recommendations.

Some reports advocate intravitreal ceftazidime 2 mg in 0.1 mL instead of amikacin for Gram-negative cover, because of the risk of aminoglycoside retinal toxicity. Avoid combining vancomycin and ceftazidime in the same syringe.

Some reports advocate intravitreal dexamethasone 0.4 mg but the evidence is not clear.

Follow-up Manage patients as day-cases if they can cope; otherwise admit. If admitted, consider discharge when there is clinical improvement, typically after 48 hours, and then review within 2 weeks. Follow up all patients for 3–6 months, as they may require additional procedures, e.g. vitrectomy for vitreous debris. Final VA is <6/60 in 22–77%. Patients with an acute presentation, good presenting VA, and negative cultures tend to have a better prognosis.

Endogenous Endophthalmitis

Endogenous endophthalmitis is haematogenous spread of infection to the eye. Commonest in the elderly, debilitated, diabetics, those with indwelling foreign bodies (urinary or i.v. catheters, prosthetic heart valves), immunosuppressed (iatrogenic or disease) and i.v. drug users. Patients may or may not be acutely ill and can present with either a fulminating or low-grade endophthalmitis. Manage in combination with a physician to identify the source, predisposing disease, and treatment options. Request blood cultures.

▪ *Endogenous bacterial endophthalmitis*: If the organism is not known obtain aqueous and vitreous taps (Box 8.1) and give oral and intravitreal antibiotics as described for exogenous infection.

▪ *Endogenous fungal endophthalmitis*: The majority are diagnosed on clinical grounds, most typically in i.v. drug users or following a septic or other hospital episode involving intravenous cannulation, or broad-spectrum antibiotics. Collections of cells may be seen in the choroid, retina, or vitreous. These may form 'puff-balls' (*Candida* spp.) or hyphae (*Aspergillus* spp.). Fungal endophthalmitis is uncommon after intraocular surgery or secondary to penetrating injury. *Candida* species are by far the most common (Fig. 8.23). Aspergillus

Box 8.1: Aqueous and vitreous tap and intravitreal antibiotic injection

1. Contact the microbiology department to ensure Gram staining is done the same day.

2. Instil G. proxymetacaine then tetracaine (amethocaine), then povidone-iodine 5% into the conjunctival sac and on the lid margins. Allow dwell time for bacterial/fungal killing.

3. Administer subconjunctival or more usually peribulbar anaesthesia (lidocaine 2%).

4. Prepare then draw up the required concentration of antibiotics, combined into a 1 mL syringe (change the needle, as this gets blunt going through the rubber bungs):

   a. *Vancomycin*: 2.0 mg in 0.1 mL.

   b. *Amikacin*: 0.4 mg in 0.1 mL (beware dilution errors).

   c. *Amphotericin B*: 5–10 mcg in 0.1 mL *only if fungi are suspected*.

5. Scrub and don gloves. A drape and mask are not required. Insert the lid speculum but do not further manipulate the lashes. Wash away excess povidone-iodine with saline.

6. *Aqueous sampling* (may be done with patient at the slit lamp or lying down). Using a 1 mL syringe (not an insulin syringe) with an orange 25-gauge needle, aspirate 0.1–0.2 mL of aqueous via a limbal paracentesis. A larger needle may be used if a lot of pus is present. Place the needle into the sheath left resting on a flat surface, without touching the tip of the needle (be mindful of needle-stick). Label and leave to one side.

7. *Vitreous sampling* (do in a sterile environment with the patient lying flat). Use a 5 mL syringe and blue 23-gauge needle and insert 4 mm (phakic) or 3.5 mm (pseudophakic/aphakic eyes) behind the limbus into the midvitreous cavity. Aspirate 0.2–0.4 mL. If the tap is dry, carefully move the needle within the vitreous cavity. If still dry, try a larger 21-gauge needle. Place the sheath on the needle as above. Label and leave to one side.

8. Inject the 0.2 mL of combined intravitreal antibiotics in the 1 mL syringe in a sterile manner and through the same area as the vitreous sampling. As the eye can be very soft, counter pressure helps get the needle through the sclera.

(Continued on next page)

Box 8.1: Aqueous and vitreous tap and intravitreal antibiotic injection—cont'd

9. Plate out immediately, as per local protocol, for example:

   a. Blood agar: place one drop from the syringe on an eccentric one-third of the plate and then streak with a loupe. Do not cut into the agar, as the organisms will not grow. Use a separate blood agar plate for aqueous and vitreous. Close with tape, and label.

   b. Robertson's cooked meat broth and brain heart infusion: put one drop in each bottle (avoid touching the rim). Close, mix, and label.

10. Send specimens immediately to the microbiology department for Gram (± Giemsa) stain, and then culture. If the laboratory is closed, incubate the plates and transfer at the first opportunity, but this may reduce the yield so avoid if possible.

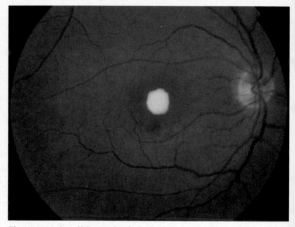

Fig. 8.23: Candida endophthalmitis extending from the retina into the vitreous.

and others are rare. Treatment is determined by the site of the lesion. Treat lesions confined to the choroid (outside the blood–retinal barrier) with intravenous amphotericin B. Lesions extending into the vitreous require planned vitrectomy within 2 days (so no need to take samples in casualty) with intraocular amphotericin B (10 μg), and fluconazole starting with 400 mg loading dose p.o. then 200 mg b.d. p.o. for 6 weeks (penetrates well into the eye). Alternatively, use oral voriconazole. For flat lesions in the retina give a trial of oral fluconazole.

Optometry and General Practice Guidelines

General Comments

Accurate diagnosis and assessment of patients with uveitis requires slit lamp examination. This is not usually available in general practice and topical steroids should not be initiated owing to their potential side effects including raised intraocular pressure, cataract, and exacerbation of dendritic corneal ulcers. All suspected intraocular inflammation should therefore be referred within 24 hours to an ophthalmologist.

Acute anterior uveitis accounts for 90% of all intraocular inflammation presenting to general practitioners but it accounts for a minority of patients with red eye.

General Practice

Photophobia and pain are the predominant complaints in patients with uveitis, with conjunctival injection centred primarily around the cornea (circumcorneal injection). It is usually possible to distinguish anterior uveitis from conjunctivitis from the history (p. 142).

Posterior uveitis is more difficult to diagnose from the history and is reliant upon proficient dilated fundoscopy. Symptoms of acute onset of floaters, with or without blurred vision, are far more likely to be related to posterior vitreous detachment than inflammation, but in either event urgent referral is required.

Optometrists

Optometrists who suspect anterior uveitis should take a careful history and look for anterior chamber cells. These are best seen against a dilated pupil, using a thin, maximally illuminated slit beam passed at 45° through the anterior chamber. Inflammatory cells can be seen to percolate upward in the back of the anterior chamber, and downwards immediately behind the cornea (see Fig. 8.1). Look for anterior vitreous activity using the same slit beam focused behind the lens. For patients with suspected posterior uveitis, look for vitreous haze, macular oedema, and perivascular infiltrates. Pars planitis may be difficult to detect without indentation. Any anterior or posterior segment inflammation requires same-day review by an ophthalmologist.

References

1. No authors listed. The Endophthalmitis Vitrectomy Study. Arch Ophthalmol 1995; 113:1479–1496.

Chapter 9
OCULAR ONCOLOGY

Conjunctival Tumours

Symptoms Non-specific symptoms include ocular pain, redness and discharge. Vision loss may occur from tumour growth covering the cornea or inducing astigmatism.

History and examination Ask about sun exposure. Perform detailed anterior segment slit lamp examination including the caruncle and conjunctival fornices by everting the upper eyelid. Palpate for enlarged preauricular or submandibular lymph nodes.

Differential diagnosis

The commoner lesions and their main features include:

- Nonpigmented tumours:

  1. *Papilloma* (Fig. 9.1):

     a. Benign.

     b. Pink fibrovascular fronds (pedunculated or flat).

     c. Viral aetiology.

     d. Symptomatic when large.

     e. Treat by delicate surgical excision, cryotherapy and topical therapy (interferon or mitomycin C).

  2. *Conjunctival intraepithelial neoplasia (CIN)* (Fig. 9.2):

     a. Benign (pre-malignant).

     b. Histologic grades (I–III) are based on the depth of conjunctival epithelial involvement.

     c. Fleshy, thickened, vascularized lesion located at the interpalpebral limbus with occasional corneal extension.

     d. Treat by excisional biopsy. Adjuvant cryotherapy and topical therapy (interferon or mitomycin C) may be used.

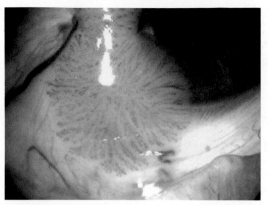

Fig. 9.1: Conjunctival papilloma.

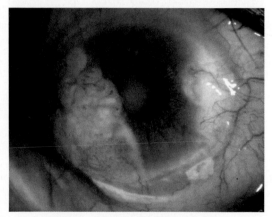

Fig. 9.2: Conjunctival intraepithelial neoplasia.

3. *Squamous cell carcinoma (SCC)* (Fig. 9.3):

   a. Malignant.

   b. Fleshy, pink, elevated masses with feeder vessels; can extend widely across the conjunctiva and invade deep into the orbit.

   c. Manage by excision with adjuvant cryotherapy, topical mitomycin C, or beta radiotherapy. Extensive local and

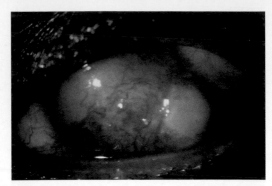

Fig. 9.3: Invasive squamous cell carcinoma.

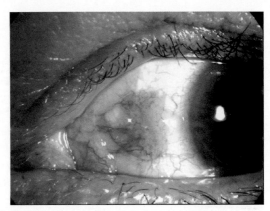

Fig. 9.4: Conjunctival naevus.

regional recurrence may require orbital exenteration with external beam radiotherapy.

■ Pigmented tumours:

1. *Naevus* (Fig. 9.4):

   a. Benign.

   b. Circumscribed, light brown, flat lesion in the interpalpebral zone and often with epithelial downgrowth cysts.

   c. Manage with photodocumentation and routine yearly observation if stable. Growing lesions and those that

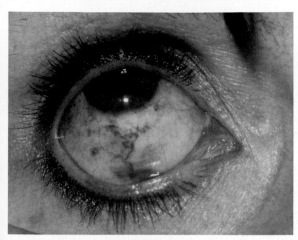

Fig. 9.5: Primary acquired melanosis.

develop prominent feeder vessels can be biopsied to rule out malignant melanoma.

2. *Primary acquired melanosis (PAM)* (Fig. 9.5):

   a. Benign (premalignant).

   b. Diffuse, patchy foci of increased conjunctival pigmentation. Sometimes extends to the eyelid skin and is occasionally nonpigmented. Acquired in middle-age and found in light-skinned patients.

   c. Manage by observation every 6 months with or without multiple incisional biopsies.

   d. Confirmed areas of PAM with atypia may be treated with cryotherapy although it is not certain whether freezing reduces a 50% risk of developing conjunctival melanoma.

   e. Dark-skinned patients may have diffuse racial pigmentation seen near the limbus, which is generally benign and does not require treatment or follow-up.

3. *Malignant melanoma (MM)* (Fig. 9.6):

   a. Malignant.

   b. May arise from a naevus, PAM, or *de novo*.

   c. Typically, darkly pigmented and focal, but variations include nonpigmented and diffuse forms. Feeder

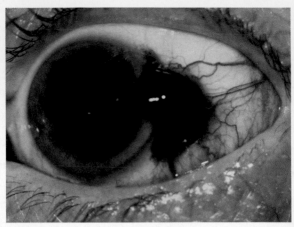

Fig. 9.6: Hyperpigmented conjunctival melanoma with sentinel vessels.

vessels may be present. Tumours arising in PAM may be multifocal and the eyelid skin may be affected.

d. Manage by wide, *en bloc* excision with lamellar dissection of the cornea and sclera at the cornoscleral limbus. Adjuvant cryotherapy or beta plaque radiotherapy may be applied to the tumour bed if there is doubt about the completeness of excision.

e. Careful follow-up is needed to identify new tumours arising in PAM and recurrences.

f. Extensive or recurrent lesions may require orbital exenteration.

g. Spread may occur to regional lymph nodes and is best managed by a combination of surgical excision of affected nodes and external beam radiotherapy. Metastatic disease can occur and may be fatal.

4. *Ocular melanocytosis* (Fig. 9.7):

a. Unilateral, congenital hyperpigmentation of the uveal tract extending to the episclera and presenting with increased iris pigmentation on the affected side and slate-grey discoloration of the sclera.

b. Termed oculodermal melanocytosis (*naevus of Ota*) if associated with ipsilateral periocular blue-grey

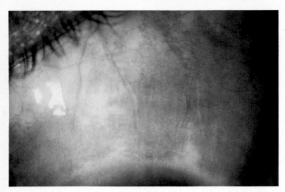

Fig. 9.7: Ocular melanocytosis.

skin discolouration, in V1 and V2 trigeminal distribution.

c. Patients have an increased risk of developing malignant choroidal melanoma and, rarely, primary orbital melanoma, so arrange yearly dilated fundus examination.

■ Vascular tumours:

1. *Pyogenic granuloma:*

   a. Benign fibrovascular tumour.

   b. Neither an infection nor a granuloma.

   c. Fleshy, thickened, red/pink-coloured lesions occurring near previous surgical sites.

   d. May respond to topical steroid therapy but may require local surgical excision with careful wound closure. An example is shown in Figure 1.27; (p. 38).

2. *Capillary haemangioma:*

   a. Benign.

   b. Circumscribed, red lesion found in infants.

   c. May enlarge over time, but usually undergoes spontaneous involution.

   d. Typically managed by observation, but local excision or intralesional steroid treatment may be used.

   e. For orbital and skin involvement, see pages 34 and 92.

3. *Kaposi's sarcoma:*

    a. Malignant.

    b. Bright red, solitary or multifocal mass associated with haemorrhage.

    c. May involve the eyelid skin. An example is shown in Figure 1.36.

    d. A characteristic lesion in AIDS.

    e. Treatment options include observation, low-dose radiotherapy, and excision. Intralesional interferon alpha2a chemotherapy is described. Generalized disease requires chemotherapy ± radiotherapy.

4. *Orbital varix and lymphangioma.* See pages 93 and 94.

- Lymphoid tumours:

    1. *Lymphoma* (Fig. 9.8):

        a. Malignant.

        b. Fleshy lesions with deep pink 'salmon patch' appearance.

        c. Most are extranodal marginal zone B-cell lymphomas of MALT type that develop *de novo* in conjunctiva and in which bilateral presentation and orbital involvement are common. Some develop in association with systemic lymphoma.

        d. Diagnosed by incisional biopsy followed by systemic evaluation.

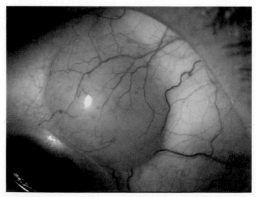

Fig. 9.8: Conjunctival lymphoma.

e. Disease localized to the conjunctiva and orbit is usually treated by external beam radiotherapy and the prognosis for the eye, for vision, and for life is generally good.

Investigations Baseline and serial photographs are useful to detect or monitor change. Excisional or incisional biopsy is performed to make a histological diagnosis. Orbital CT may be needed to determine tumour extension.

Treatment

- *Surgical excision*: may be part of the initial biopsy. Generally, wide surgical margins are preferred with primary closure of large defects. Techniques such as absolute alcohol epithelial debridement and lamellar corneoscleral–conjunctival resection may be used.

- *Surgical debulking*: is needed when, in established cases, tumour overgrowth limits the use of adjuvant treatments such as topical agents or cryotherapy, and for symptomatic relief.

- *Cryotherapy*: with a double or triple freeze-thaw technique is an important tool for local tumour control after biopsy.

- *Adjuvant treatments*: such as plaque radiotherapy, topical anticancer agents (interferon alpha or mitomycin C), and external beam radiotherapy may be used in selected cases.

- *Orbital exenteration*: is reserved for extensive invasion by malignant tumours such as SCC or MM.

Follow–up After diagnosis and treatment, premalignant and malignant conjunctival tumours require close and thorough follow-up every 3–4 months to exclude progression or recurrence.

Iris Melanoma

Background Iris melanomas account for 5–10% of all uveal tract melanomas. They are usually well differentiated and rarely metastasize. The mortality rate is around 5%, much lower than for ciliary body or choroidal melanomas.

Symptoms Visual changes occur with larger tumours that grow into the visual axis or induce a central cataract. There may be pain from elevated IOP associated with tumour pigment shedding, direct angle invasion, and anterior segment neovascularization. Tumours may also be asymptomatic.

Signs Iris melanomas are raised, replace the iris stroma, have variable pigmentation (though classically dark brown), and have visible intrinsic tumour vessels (Fig. 9.9). They usually arise from the pupillary margin, causing a peaked pupil or uveal ectropion. Focal cataract may be seen. Focal conjunctival and episcleral vascular dilation (sentinel vessels) are seen in the same quadrant as larger, more chronic malignant iris masses. Extraocular extension of a pigmented tumour through the sclera may occur.

History and examination Ask about visual symptoms, ocular surgery, cancer, or constitutional symptoms. Detailed ocular examination includes IOP, pre-and postdilation gonioscopy to determine angle and/or anterior ciliary body involvement, and dilated fundal examination. Transpupillary transillumination is used to determine the posterior extension of an iris tumour into the ciliary body.

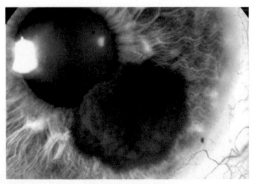

Fig. 9.9: Iris melanoma.

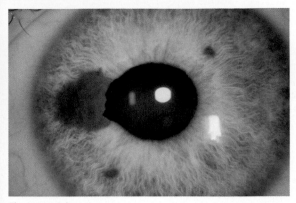

Fig. 9.10: Iris naevus.

Differential diagnosis

- Hyperpigmented lesions:

    1. *Iris naevus* (Fig. 9.10):

        a. Asymptomatic.

        b. Generally flat (<1 mm height) and pigmented.

        c. Sporadic, often present after the second decade, and rarely grow.

        d. Iris infiltration, sectorial cataract, or pupil distortion increase the suspicion of malignancy.

        e. Small, focal iris freckles may be associated with neurofibromatosis type I and the iridocorneal–endothelial (ICE or 'Cogan-Reese') syndrome. Review stable lesions yearly, but more frequently if suspicious.

- Hypopigmented lesions:

    1. *Iris metastasis:*

        a. Pink- or yellow-coloured, rapidly growing, uni- or multifocal lesion.

        b. Associated with pseudohypopyon, hyphaema, and elevated IOP.

        c. Many patients have a history of cancer (e.g. breast, lung), risk factors (e.g. smoking history, family history), or constitutional symptoms (e.g. weight loss, anorexia).

    d. Treat with chemotherapy for systemic tumour and external beam radiotherapy for the iris tumour.

2. *Iris cyst:*

    a. Cysts have an absence of internal reflectivity on ultrasound.

3. *Inflammatory nodules:*

    a. Koeppe (peripupillary) and Busacca (mid-iris) nodules are small grey/yellow nodules seen in granulomatous uveitis along with other signs of inflammation.

Investigations Colour photography for documentation and follow-up. Ultrasonography (A- and B-scan) to document size and internal reflectivity (usually low to moderate). Rarely, fluorescein angiography is needed. Incisional iris biopsy or fine needle biopsy may confirm the diagnosis prior to definitive treatment.

Treatment Treat elevated IOP but refractory glaucoma may indicate extensive ring involvement of the drainage angle by tumour that is better treated by enucleation. Occasionally, lesions may be observed if very small or if atypical/benign appearance. Local treatments such as tumour resection by sector iridectomy or combined iridocyclectomy for combined iris and localized ciliary body tumours may be performed with tumour-free margins. Primary radiation therapy with plaque (typically with the radioisotope ruthenium[106] in the UK) can be used for larger tumours unsuitable for local resection. Enucleation is reserved for:

■ Large iris masses infiltrating the angle and causing secondary glaucoma.

■ Diffuse ('ring') iris melanomas.

■ After failed local therapy.

■ Blind, painful eye from melanoma-induced glaucoma.

Follow-up Examine 4–6 monthly for tumour recurrence, including gonioscopy. Generally, there is a low metastatic potential.

Differential Diagnosis of Fundus Tumours

Choroidal naevus Typically asymptomatic, flat (<2 mm height), variably pigmented lesions with regular margins. Risk factors for transformation into a malignant choroidal melanoma include documented growth, height >2.0 mm, presence of orange pigment (lipofuscin), posterior location, and/or visual symptoms from macular involvement or associated serous retinal detachment (Fig. 9.11). Naevi with a low risk of malignant transformation are typically small (less than 6 mm basal dimension), flat (less than 1 mm height), and associated with drusen or RPE hyperpigmentation. Intermediate-risk naevi may be >2.0 mm in height and contain lipofuscin pigment granules. High-risk naevi have multiple risk factors, particularly documented growth and visual symptoms.

Photograph low-risk naevi for comparison and arrange annual review by an ophthalmologist or optometrist. Photograph intermediate-risk naevi and review every 4–6 months by an ophthalmologist for at least 1 year, then yearly. Promptly refer progressing, intermediate- and high-risk naevi to an ocular oncology centre.

Choroidal melanoma See page 404.

Congenital hypertrophy of the RPE (CHRPE) Asymptomatic, flat, dark black lesions with regular margins (Fig. 9.12). Usually unilateral, unifocal, and located in the peripheral retina. Solitary peripheral lesions require no follow-up. Central CHRPE may be followed serially to confirm that there is no growth, then discharged. Patients with adenomatous intestinal polyposis commonly have multiple bilateral CHRPE, so exclude a family history of bowel disease.

Subretinal haemorrhage Peripheral, domed, disciform, subretinal haemorrhage may resemble choroidal melanoma due to the variable pigmentation of blood elements (Fig. 9.13). Commonly caused by subretinal choroidal neovascularization (age-related, high myopia, inflammatory, post-traumatic) or retinal artery macroaneurysms. Subretinal haemorrhage resolves over time with reduction in the height of the lesion, unlike malignant tumours.

Choroidal detachment Particularly in hypotonous eyes or less commonly due to scleritis, carotid cavernous fistula, lymphoma, or uveal effusion syndrome (see Fig. 11.10). B-scan ultrasound is helpful if the diagnosis is uncertain.

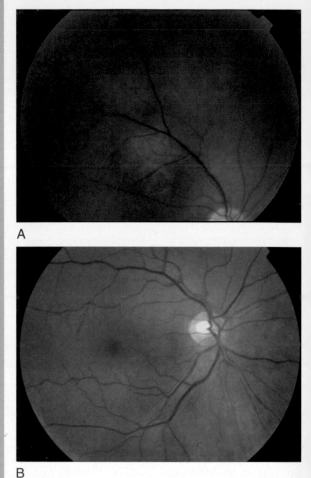

A

B

Fig. 9.11: High-risk **(A)** and low-risk **(B)** choroidal naevi.

Retinal capillary haemangioma A red nodular vascular tumour with dilated feeding arteriole and draining venule; may have secondary lipid exudates, subretinal fluid, or subretinal/preretinal fibrosis causing tractional retinal detachment (TRD) (Fig. 9.14). Arises in the first or second decades. Sporadic cases tend to be uniocular and unifocal with a less aggressive disease course. Inherited cases are associated with *von Hippel-Lindau* (VHL) syndrome, an autosomal dominant condition with associated

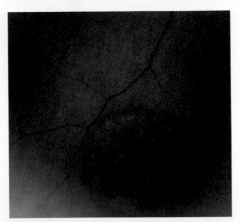

Fig. 9.12: Congenital hypertrophy of RPE.

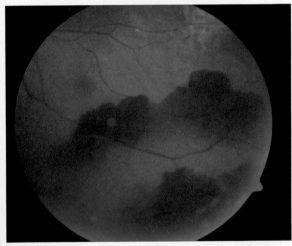

Fig. 9.13: Subretinal haemorrhage from a choroidal neovascular membrane.

cerebellar haemangioblastoma, phaeochromocytoma, and other visceral tumours. Use focal argon laser photocoagulation or external cryotherapy to treat small tumours. Vitreoretinal surgery may be needed to treat TRD. VHL patients are screened for new tumours every 4–6 months into the third decade, when the risk of new tumour formation declines.

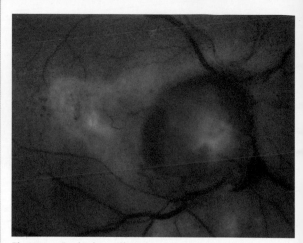

Fig. 9.14: Retinal capillary haemangioma.

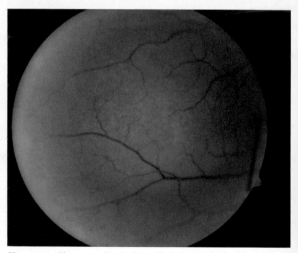

Fig. 9.15: Circumscribed choroidal haemangioma.

Choroidal haemangioma *Circumscribed choroidal haemangiomas* are low to medium elevated, orange-red coloured, round lesions (Fig. 9.15). They are associated with subretinal fluid or overlying intraretinal cysts. May be symptomatic, depending on their location. There is prominent vascular leakage on fluorescein angiography and high internal reflectivity with ultrasonography.

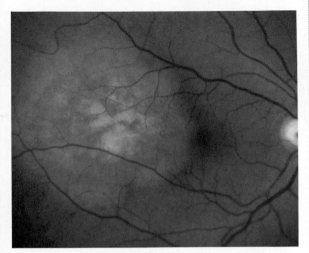

Fig. 9.16: Choroidal metastasis.

Lesions are treated with radiotherapy (plaque brachytherapy or external beam) or, if small, with verteporfin photodynamic therapy. *Diffuse choroidal haemangiomas* produce an extensive 'tomato ketchup'-red choroidal appearance. They are associated with Sturge-Weber syndrome with ipsilateral periocular cutaneous haemangiomas.

Choroidal metastasis Small, flat, pale/cream, multifocal, often bilateral, choroidal lesions with subretinal fluid accumulation (Fig. 9.16). Lesions that have regressed after chemotherapy often exhibit 'leopard spot' RPE pigment alterations. Patient may have a history of cancer (e.g. breast, lung), risk factors (e.g. smoking, family history), or constitutional symptoms (e.g. weight loss, anorexia). Systemic oncology evaluation is required if the diagnosis is suspected, particularly in patients without known cancer. Treatment of the systemic primary tumour is coupled with palliative external beam (primarily) or plaque radiotherapy to the involved eye.

Lymphoma See page 371.

Choroidal Melanoma

Background Choroidal melanoma (CM) is the most common primary malignant intraocular tumour. Patients are generally white, age 55–75, and have no known family history. Local tumour control can be achieved in >90% of cases. However, systemic metastasis occurs in 40% within 5 years of ocular treatment. Tumours are unilateral and rarely metastasize to the orbit or fellow eye.

Symptoms May present with vision loss, localized scotoma, metamorphopsia, and photopsia from the tumour and/or associated exudative retinal detachment. May be asymptomatic.

Signs Focal conjunctival and episcleral vascular dilation (sentinel vessels) are seen in the same quadrant as larger, more chronic ciliary body masses. Trans-scleral extension of the pigmented tumour occurs rarely. Posterior CMs are elevated, globular, tan to brown-coloured lesions (Fig. 9.17); occasionally CMs are pale (amelanotic melanoma) or minimally elevated while growing over a larger choroidal base (diffuse melanoma). Apical tumour growth through Bruchs' membrane results in the classic hyperpigmented 'mushroom' or 'collar-stud' appearance, but rarely in tumours <5 mm thick. Surface drusen and variable RPE hypertrophy suggest chronicity and inactivity, while the presence of subretinal fluid, exudative retinal detachment, and overlying orange lipofuscin

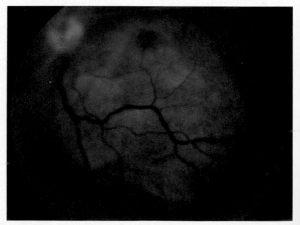

Fig. 9.17: Large choroidal melanoma.

pigment suggests tumour activity. Vitreous and subretinal haemorrhage may occur with larger tumours.

Classification Based on anatomic origin (ciliary body, and/or choroid), growth pattern (elevated versus diffuse), posterior location (macular, juxtapapillary, or peripapillary), and, most commonly, tumour size:

- *Small*: thickness <2 mm, basal diameter <8 mm.
- *Medium*: thickness 2.5–8 mm, basal diameter 8–16 mm.
- *Large*: thickness >8 mm, basal diameter >16 mm.

History and examination Ask about visual symptoms, ocular surgery, cancer, and constitutional symptoms. Detailed serial ocular examination includes IOP, gonioscopy to assess for angle invasion in anterior choroid/ciliary body tumours, and dilated fundoscopy with precise tumour drawing. Transpupillary transillumination delineates the extent of ciliary body involvement.

Differential diagnosis See page 399.

Investigations Arrange colour photography for documentation and follow-up. Use ultrasonography to document size (height with longitudinal and transverse basal dimensions; note any extrascleral extension), and internal reflectivity (usually low to moderate) (Fig. 9.18). The presence of internal blood flow

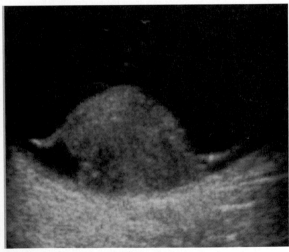

Fig. 9.18: B-mode ultrasound of choroidal melanoma with overlying retinal detachment (Courtesy of M. Restori).

helps to rule out nonmalignant disease such as disciform subretinal haemorrhage. Rarely, fluorescein angiography is required. Intraoperative trans-scleral choroidal biopsy may be used to confirm the diagnosis prior to treatment if the diagnosis is unclear. If melanoma is confirmed, investigate for metastases (liver function tests, liver ultrasound, chest X-ray) and if present, refer promptly to a medical oncologist.

Treatment Treatment options are based on the results of metastatic work-up, fellow eye status, patient age, preference, and health status. In general, do not perform ocular surgery in patients with confirmed metastatic disease unless for symptomatic relief (e.g. neovascular glaucoma).

Treatment options include:

■ *Observation*: typically for small melanomas with chronic appearance.

■ *Local therapy*:

1. Extrascleral plaque brachytherapy: typically with ruthenium[106] for tumours up to 7 mm in height, and/or

2. Local tumour resection: particularly for anterior, superonasal tumours with a small base and large height. Surgery requires specialized hypotensive anaesthesia.

3. Transpupillary thermotherapy: typically for a modest size tumour, continued or recurrent tumour growth following plaque brachytherapy in accessible, posteriorly located tumours, and for small melanomas close to the optic disc (on the nasal side) in an only or better eye.

■ *Enucleation*: typically for large or extensively recurrent tumours, or blind, painful eyes with melanoma-induced neovascular glaucoma.

Follow–up Lifelong. Examine tumours under observation 4–6 monthly, including serial ultrasounds. After local therapy, ophthalmic examination with photo documentation and ultrasound height assessment is performed initially every 4–6 months, then yearly if there is no growth. Advise patients to return immediately if their vision changes. Postenucleation sockets are followed if extraocular extension or orbital invasion is found. Request yearly liver function tests by the general practitioner to survey for metastatic disease.

Retinoblastoma

Background The most common malignant intraocular tumour in children. Cumulative incidence at 11 years old is 4.4/100 000 births in the UK. Most (82%) cases are diagnosed before age 3, with no sex or race predisposition. The majority of cases are unilateral.

Genetics Caused by mutation in the RB1 gene. A germline mutation is often associated with bilateral disease and autosomal dominant inheritance with almost complete penetrance (50% of offspring affected). Those with unilateral retinoblastoma are less likely to have a germline mutation or transmit the disease.

- 10% of cases have a family history (FH) of an inherited germline mutation; 75% of these develop bilateral tumours.

- 30% have a negative FH and develop bilateral tumours, 95% have new germline mutations.

- 60% have a negative FH and develop tumours unilaterally, <10% have new germline mutations.

- Siblings with negative FH have a small risk of disease, as some (<5%) carrier parents are unaffected due to germline mosaicism.

Clinical features Classically presents with leucocoria (55%) from a large retinal tumour mass (Fig. 9.19). Secondary strabismus (25%) with decreased visual function (8%), positive FH (10%) and rarely failure to feed due to ocular pain in infants may be reported. Extraocular, fungating tumours associated with extraocular extension are rare in developed nations. Preseptal/orbital cellulitis may occur. There may be elevated IOP (from secondary angle closure or direct tumour infiltration of the drainage angle), spontaneous hyphaema, conjunctival injection, buphthalmos, white/yellow tumour invasion into the anterior chamber or iris surface. A white/light yellow solid retinal mass is characteristic, with four growth patterns:

- *Endophytic*: into the vitreous cavity.

- *Exophytic*: into the subretinal space.

- *Combined* endo- and exophytic.

- *Diffuse*: minimally thickened, extensive tumour with retinal whitening.

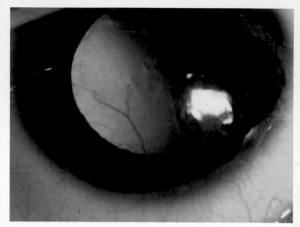

Fig. 9.19: Retinoblastoma (Courtesy DH Verity).

Exudative retinal detachment, vitreous haemorrhage, or vitreous opacity from vitreous seeding or posterior uveitis may occur.

Differential diagnosis A spontaneously regressed retinoblastoma (retinoma) may be seen as a white, calcified retinal mass, often with chronic RPE hyperpigmentation changes around the base.

History and examination Draw the family pedigree (p. 412). Detailed anterior segment examination includes IOP and dilated fundus examination. Infants typically require examination under general anaesthesia. Perform fundus examination of the immediate family members for spontaneously regressed retinoblastomas.

Investigations Arrange B-scan ultrasonography to document the presence and size of any mass lesion and any hyperechodensity within the tumour suggesting intralesional calcification (a typical finding). A CT scan of the orbits may be used to confirm the presence of intralesional calcification, extent of extraocular spread, and to exclude other diagnoses. CT is in declining use due to anxiety surrounding the risk of secondary paediatric cancers. MRI is used to determine extraocular or intracranial spread. Genetic testing of blood or tumour cells is used to differentiate germline mutations. Intraocular biopsies or other intraocular procedures *must not be performed* on eyes with suspected retinoblastoma.

Treatment

- ■ *Casualty*: Refer to specialty clinic that week for diagnosis.

- ■ *Clinic*: Refer to a designated treatment centre (in the UK: Barts & The Royal London Hospital, Moorfields Eye Hospital, Birmingham Children's Hospital). Treatment is customized for each child and eye with the primary goal of local tumour control and patient survival. The secondary goal is preservation of vision. Enucleation is used for advanced local tumours or after treatment failure. Local, globe-sparing treatment options include external cryotherapy, transpupillary thermotherapy, local (sub-Tenon's) chemotherapy, or plaque radiotherapy. Systemic chemotherapy may be used alone or with local treatments as primary or salvage therapy. External beam radiotherapy is currently used only as salvage therapy in children older than 1 year who have failed all other appropriate treatments, and who still have potential vision in their only or better eye.

Follow—up Regular review including examination under anaesthesia for recurrence/new tumours to age 7 by retinoblastoma centre then yearly by a local ophthalmologist. Arrange prompt neuroimaging in older bilateral retinoblastoma patients with new-onset CNS symptoms to look for ectopic intracranial retinoblastoma ('trilateral retinoblastoma'). The 5-year survival rate in the UK is >95%. The cumulative incidence of second primary neoplasms in heritable cases is ≈1%/year (typically osteosarcoma/soft-tissue sarcoma).

Optometry and General Practice Guidelines

General comments

Eye tumours are relatively rare, however eyelid tumours, particularly basal cell carcinoma, are not uncommon. Eyelid tumours are usually treated by oculoplastic surgeons rather than ocular oncologists and are covered in the oculoplastics chapter. The commonest referral to most ocular oncology services is a fundal naevus, to exclude (or treat) choroidal melanoma. Discriminating between naevi and melanomas can be difficult and many patients remain under regular review. The following factors suggest malignant potential: elevation, subretinal fluid, visual symptoms (blurred vision or distortion), yellow pigment (lipofuscin), and most importantly, documented growth. Low risk naevi do not routinely warrant hospital referral.

General practice

For general practitioners who are confident with an ophthalmoscope, fundal naevi may be a familiar finding, and assuming these are small, flat, discrete, and evenly pigmented, then arrange annual dilated optometry review, preferably by an optometrist with a fundus camera. If there are any worrying features refer to a general ophthalmologist.

Optometry

Benign appearing naevi are common: carefully document the clinical features and size in disc diameters, and if possible photograph the lesion. Arrange annual dilated fundus examination, and explain to the patient that they should ensure that this occurs if they change optometrists. Inform the patient's general practitioner. If there are visual symptoms, an increase in the size of the naevus or any suspicious features, then refer to a general ophthalmologist.

The following guide to referral urgency is not prescriptive, as clinical situations vary. Advice is based on clinical parameters rather than UK government guidelines on the referral of patients with suspected malignancy.

Urgent (within 2 weeks)

Soon (within 1 month)

Routine

Chapter 10

MEDICAL RETINA

Taking a Family History for Inherited Disease

Inherited disorders of the retina cover a broad phenotypic spectrum, ranging from retinitis pigmentosa to macular degenerations. The genetic mutation is known and testing is available for an increasing number of these disorders. Genetic counselling, accurate discussions about the disorder with patients, and the provision of low-vision support and social support are important.

If inherited disease is suspected, take a detailed family history. Tactfully ask about consanguinity ('did anyone marry or have children within the family') as this makes autosomal recessive inheritance more likely. Examine family members; carriers may show changes, others may have subclinical disease or features that help diagnose the proband (patient).

Draw a family tree as shown in Figure 10.1. Many inherited retinal diseases are mendelian, but non-mendelian (multifactorial), mitochondrial, and chromosomal inheritance occurs. Inheritance may be influenced by reduced penetrance (faulty gene but no disease) or variable expressivity (faulty gene produces variable disease severity). The following patterns of inheritance are well recognized.

Autosomal dominant

■ Affected individuals have an affected parent, but variable expression means they are sometimes asymptomatic.

■ The disease does not skip a generation, unless penetrance is incomplete.

■ Affected individuals have a 50% risk of having affected offspring.

■ Males and females are equally affected.

■ Look for male-to-male inheritance to exclude X-linked or mitochondrial inheritance.

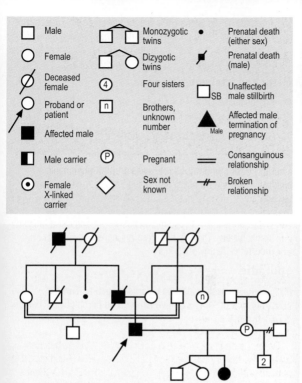

□	Male	Monozygotic twins	• Prenatal death (either sex)
○	Female	Dizygotic twins	⚑ Prenatal death (male)
⌀	Deceased female	④ Four sisters	□SB Unaffected male stillbirth
○ (arrow)	Proband or patient	n Brothers, unknown number	▲Male Affected male termination of pregnancy
■	Affected male	Ⓟ Pregnant	= Consanguinous relationship
◫	Male carrier	◇ Sex not known	─//─ Broken relationship
⊙	Female X-linked carrier		

Fig. 10.1: Drawing a family tree. Example shows autosomal dominant inheritance.

Autosomal recessive

- For rare genes, affected individuals are born of phenotypically normal parents and offspring are rarely affected, unless there is consanguinity.

- There is a 25% risk to each offspring of two carriers.

- Males and females are equally affected.

X-linked recessive

- Affected individuals are usually born of phenotypically normal parents.

- Affected males have unaffected sons, but all daughters are carriers.

■ A female carrier has a 50% risk of her son being affected or her daughter being a carrier. Carriers may show abnormal signs, such as the tapetal retinal reflex that occurs in X-linked retinitis pigmentosa.

Mitochondrial inheritance

■ Mitochondrial DNA is found in the egg but not sperm, so inheritance is maternal.

■ Children of affected males are unaffected.

■ Children of affected females all have the mutation, but the phenotype varies with the proportion of mitochondria with faulty genes.

Simplex

■ These are usually autosomal recessive but without a known family history. There is therefore an increased risk of recurrence in any offspring.

Sporadic

■ Originally used to describe disorders such as Down's syndrome (trisomy 21) in which there is no calculable risk of recurrence.

Fluorescein Angiography

Background The fluorophore, sodium fluorescein, is injected into an antecubital vein and circulates to the eye. A fundus camera fitted with an illumination source and barrier filter is then used to selectively photograph the retinal and choroidal circulation.

In health, fluorescein passes rapidly through the eye but the inner and outer blood–retinal–barriers prevent staining of the retinal substrate. Retinal vessels are clearly visible but an intact RPE reduces the apparent fluorescence of the choroid. Diseases that damage the ocular circulation, RPE, or blood–retinal–barrier can all potentially be detected angiographically.

Indications Retinal vascular disease; macular oedema; RPE disease; subretinal neovascularisation; choroidal ischaemia; iris angiography.

Method

1. Ask if fundus fluorescein angiography (FFA) would alter management and is it the most appropriate investigation. Would clinical examination, optical coherence tomography (OCT), autofluorescence imaging, or indocyanine green angiography be better?

2. Exclude contraindications, e.g., fluorescein, iodine, or shellfish allergy. For use in pregnancy see page 702.

3. Explain the risks (see below) and benefits. Obtain written consent.

4. Indicate to the photographer the area of interest and presumed diagnosis.

5. Insert a 23-gauge butterfly cannula into an antecubital vein. Some clinicians prefer to use a Venflon for more secure access. A dorsal hand vein may be used, but this increases the transit time and dilutes the bolus.

6. Inject 5 mL of 20% fluorescein over 4–6 seconds whilst looking for extravasation (swelling, pain, resistance to injection), then turn off the lights.

7. Retain i.v. access in case of anaphylaxis.

Adverse events

- *Yellowing of the skin and urine*: these last 24 hours and occur in all patients.

- *Nausea*: occurs in 5% (vomiting <1%) shortly after injection and resolves quickly. In those who experienced nausea with previous injections, consider warming the ampoule to body temperature, injecting more slowly, and giving promethazine (Phenergan) 30 mg p.o., 1 hour prior.

◼ *Extravasation*: if this occurs then stop injecting, elevate the arm, and apply an icepack for 10 minutes. Extravasation rarely causes periphlebitis, skin necrosis, and granulomas, but pain is common and may last a few hours.

◼ *Vasovagal syncope*: this is the commonest cause of collapse. Patients have a transient reduction in pulse rate, blood pressure and consciousness. Lie the patient flat, and elevate the lower limbs. Exclude other causes of collapse by history, examination, ECG, and blood glucose. Repeat observations in 1–2 hours, and discharge if well.

◼ *Skin rash and itch*: treat with oral antihistamines if itch alone or mild rash. Exclude anaphylaxis by auscultating the chest and checking respiratory rate, pulse, and blood pressure. If there is facial or other soft tissue swelling secure a 20-gauge Venflon or larger, give i.v. antihistamine (e.g. chlorpheniramine 10 mg over 1 minute), monitor extremely closely for bronchospasm or shock, and liaise immediately with physicians.

◼ *Anaphylaxis*: signs include reduced consciousness, pallor, facial swelling, tachycardia, hypotension, and bronchospasm. Provide *immediate emergency care as shown on page 687.*

Reading and reporting fluorescein angiograms
When asked to comment on angiograms, it is often better to start with a clear description, rather than a diagnosis. In general, most abnormalities are hyper- or hypofluorescent, and can be described with four terms: vascular filling defects, masking, leakage, and window defects.

◼ Hypofluorescence

1. *Vascular filling defect*: absent or obstructed retinal or choroidal vessels produce focal or diffuse hypofluorescence. Areas of capillary nonperfusion are suggested by leakage at the margin, and staining of the large vessel walls passing through the area, and telangiectasia (tiny, sacular vessel dilatations) (Fig. 10.2).

2. *Masking*: most commonly occurs when retinal haemorrhage, exudates, or other opacities block underlying retinal or choroidal fluorescence. Fundus

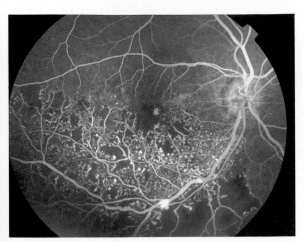

Fig. 10.2: Inferior retinal ischaemia from a branch retinal vein occlusion.

photographs may help discriminate vascular filling defects from masking (Fig. 10.3).

- Hyperfluorescence

    1. *Leakage*: produces hyperfluorescence that *increases in size and intensity* as leaking fluorescein accumulates in the extravascular space. If leaking fluorescein accumulates in a distinct anatomic space, such as under a pigment epithelial detachment, then the area of leakage may be well defined, but usually the margins blur as fluorescein diffuses through tissue (Fig. 10.4).

    2. *Window defect*: usually caused by focal RPE atrophy or a defect that increases the transmittance of choroidal fluorescence. Size remains the same as the RPE defect is constant, and early fluorescence fades as fluorescein leaves the choriocapillaris. Late staining of the sclera may leave some residual hyperfluorescence (Fig. 10.5).

A system for reporting angiograms is presented below, but always define the clinical question the angiogram was meant to answer.

1. If available check the name, date of birth, date of investigation, VA, and diagnosis on the request card. Ensure bright, even, back-illumination if viewing transparencies.

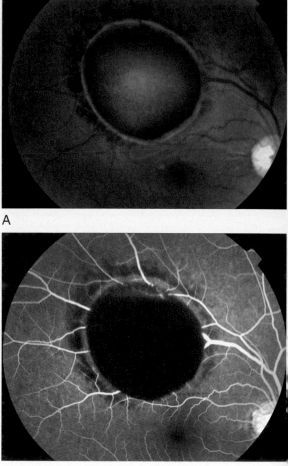

A

B

Fig. 10.3: Masking from a preretinal haemorrhage (Valsalva retinopathy).

2. View the colour fundus photographs alongside the angiogram.

3. Note if the image quality is poor and consider why, e.g. cataract.

4. Check the pre-injection image for autofluorescence from optic disc drusen.

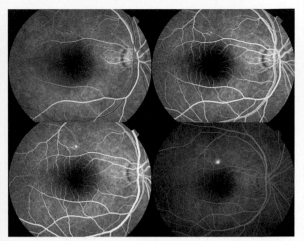

Fig. 10.4: Fluorescein leakage over time in central serous retinopathy.

5. Determine if the angiogram is a negative (filled vessels appear black) or positive.

6. Look at timing. Choroidal fluorescence appears at 10–15 seconds (arm to retina time). It is initially lobular but should be uniform after an additional 2 seconds (choroidal transit time). Retinal filling usually follows the start of choroidal filling. From the start of retinal filling to laminar flow in the veins takes about 10 seconds (retinal transit time).

   Causes of reduced choroidal or retinal flow include: tourniquet not released; low cardiac output in the elderly; pressure on the eye from holding eyelids open; ocular ischaemia from carotid or ophthalmic artery occlusion; giant cell arteritis; retinal vessel occlusion (choroidal times intact).

7. Look at vessel distribution and appearance. Do all the quadrants fill evenly or is there topographical variation? Look for tortuosity, telangiectasia, macroaneurysms (large arterial dilatations that may leak fluorescein), and segmentation (focal narrowing or disruption of the blood column). Exclude disc, retinal, or choroidal new vessels or other vascular changes such as diabetic IRMAs (*I*ntra*R*etinal *M*icrovascular *A*bnormalities). Look for patchy or diffuse areas of retinal capillary nonperfusion. Vascular staining is seen with ischaemia, vasculitis, and occlusion.

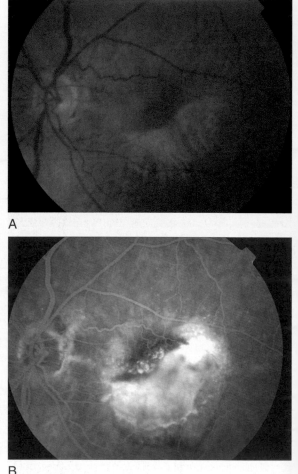

B

Fig. 10.5: Window defect from an RPE tear.

8. Look specifically at the macular using a 20 dioptre
   condensing lens (transparencies) or digital enlargement.
   Computer contrast enhancement may help.

   A. Measure the foveal avascular zone (FAZ). There is
      considerable variability in the size (650 micron average)
      but >1000 microns (two-thirds of a disc diameter)

suggests ischaemia. Drop-out of the fine, lacy capillaries at the FAZ margin may give a 'moth-eaten' appearance compared to normal. Check the notes for a corresponding reduction in VA (Fig. 10.6).

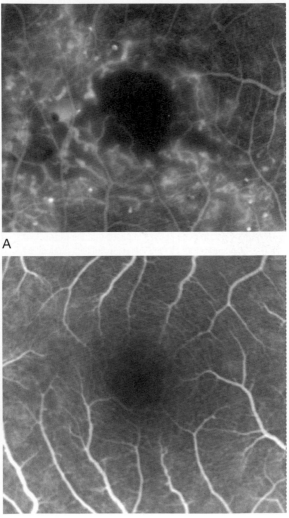

A

B

Fig. 10.6: Ischaemic foveal avascular zone **(A)** compared to normal **(B)**.

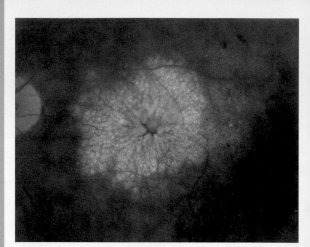

Fig. 10.7: Cystoid macular oedema.

    B. Look for macular oedema (hyperfluorescence that increases in size and intensity over time). Fluorescein may accumulate in cystic spaces and the radial arrangement of Henle's fibres sometimes produce a petaloid pattern (Fig. 10.7).

    C. Exclude choroidal neovascularization. These complexes occur most commonly in age-related macular degeneration and fill early from the choroidal circulation. A lacy network of new vessels suggests a 'classic membrane', whereas diffuse leakage suggests an 'occult membrane' (Fig. 10.8).

9. Look for fluorescein leakage at the optic disc. A small crescent of late staining at the disc margin is normal, but more than this may suggest disc new vessels or swelling. Disc drusen autofluoresce but do not leak (Fig. 10.9).

10. Answer any disease or patient-specific questions.

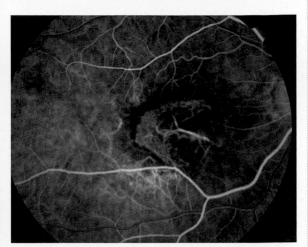

Fig. 10.8: Classic choroidal neovascularization.

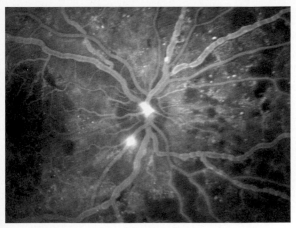

Fig. 10.9: Optic disc new vessels.

Indocyanine Green Angiography

Background Similar to fluorescein angiography except that indocyanine green (ICG) absorbs and emits in near infrared, and is albumin bound such that it does not leak freely from the choroidal capillaries. The use of infrared increases transmittance through the RPE, haemorrhage, and exudates, relative to fluorescein angiography. ICG can therefore image choroidal disease and haemorrhagic neovascularization. It is particularly helpful for idiopathic polypoidal choroidal vasculopathy (IPCV), acute multifocal placoid pigment epitheliopathy (AMPPE) (Fig. 10.10), and multiple evanescent white dot syndrome (MEWDS).

Method

■ ICG angiography can be performed just before or after fluorescein angiography but ask if it will alter management or if other tests would suffice.

■ *Exclude*: uraemia; liver disease; pregnancy; allergy to ICG, iodine, and seafood.

■ Obtain written consent.

■ Indicate to the photographer the area of interest and presumed diagnosis.

■ Dissolve 50 mg of ICG in the solvent provided.

■ Place an intravenous cannula in the antecubital fossa. Some clinicians use a 23-guage cannula, others prefer a Venflon for more secure access.

■ Inject as a rapid bolus but watch for extravasation.

■ Request late photographs, as some abnormalities are not evident for 20–30 minutes.

■ Retain i.v. access in case of anaphylaxis.

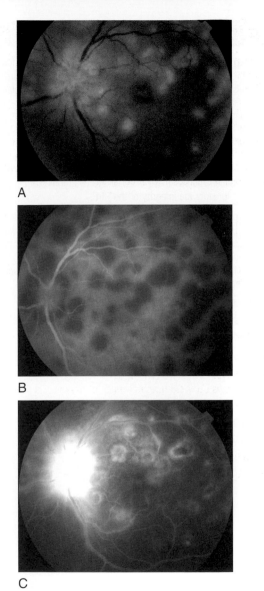

Fig. 10.10: AMPPE. Multiple areas of choriocapillary hypoperfusion are visible on the ICG **(B)** but not the fluorescein angiogram **(C)**.

Autofluorescence Imaging

Background Autofluorescence imaging detects the lipofuscin in the RPE as a measure of its metabolic activity. This in turn is driven by photoreceptor outer segment renewal and is a balance between accumulation and clearance. Lipofuscin increases progressively with age and is greatest at 10 degrees of eccentricity. The level of autofluorescence is raised if there is RPE dysfunction or increased metabolic load, and is decreased with photoreceptor cell loss. Various disorders give rise to characteristic changes, and this technique may be the only method of defining abnormalities such as those in bull's-eye dystrophies. It can also be used to verify the integrity of the RPE.

Methods Images can be obtained with an argon blue laser (488 nm) for excitation and a wide band-pass barrier filter with a wavelength cut off at 500–521 nm extending beyond 650 nm for the longer wavelengths. In most centres, a confocal laser ophthalmoscope is used which ensures that the autofluorescence recorded is derived from the ocular fundus (Fig. 10.11).

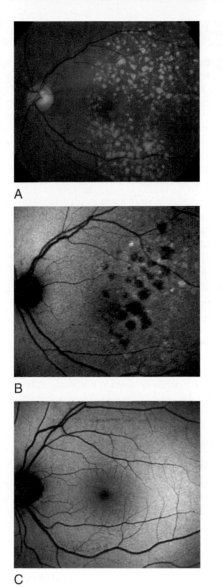

A

B

C

Fig. 10.11: Autofluorescence image of age-related macular degeneration with normal **(C)** for comparison.

Electrophysiology

Background Electrophysiology is an important diagnostic tool for many retinal, optic nerve, and functional eye diseases. Full electrodiagnostic testing is expensive, so ensure it is clinically indicated. Provide staff with a clinical summary including VA, refraction, history, the results of fundus examination and differential diagnosis.

■ Pattern electroretinogram (PERG)

1. *Indications*: disease of the macula or optic nerve.

2. *Method*: a recording electrode is placed on the cornea or conjunctiva (if using gold foil, anaesthetic is usually not required) and a reference electrode at the outer canthus. The standard stimulus is a high-contrast reversing checkerboard of low temporal frequency, and size 10 to 16 degrees. Defocus produces a poor waveform, so good refractive correction is important.

3. *Key points*: main measurements are P50 and N95. N95 arises in the retinal ganglion cells. P50 arises in part from the retinal ganglion cells and in part from other inner retinal neurones, but is driven by the macular photoreceptors and acts as an objective index of macular function. In the presence of an abnormal VEP (see below), an abnormal P50 localizes the disease to the macula and an abnormality confined to N95 localizes the disease to the optic nerve/retinal ganglion cells. The PERG is used in association with the (full-field) ERG to better characterize retinal function.

■ Full-field electroretinogram (ERG)

1. *Indications*: generalized retinal dysfunction.

2. *Method*: a recording electrode is placed on the ocular surface, a reference at the outer canthus, and ground on the forehead. Stimulus protocols are designed to discriminate rod and cone function: the rod-specific response is obtained under dark adaptation using a dim white flash and consists of a positive-going b-wave arising in the inner nuclear layer. A bright white flash then gives a mixed rod–cone response (dominated by rods) with a large negative-going a-wave, the first 10–12 ms of which reflects photoreceptor function; the oscillatory potentials (small wavelets superimposed on the ascending limb of the b-wave) arise from the amacrine cells but have limited

clinical value. After restoration of photopic conditions, cone function is recorded using both a 30 Hz flicker stimulus and single white flashes, both superimposed upon a rod-saturating background.

3. *Key points*: rod–cone dystrophies (e.g. retinitis pigmentosa) show severely decreased rod b-wave amplitude with reduction in the mixed-response a-wave confirming photoreceptor disease. Cone ERGs are less severely affected but characteristically show both delay and amplitude reduction. Cone–rod dystrophies show the cone ERGs to be more affected than the rod ERGs. Inner retinal dysfunction, such as X-linked retinoschisis or X-linked congenital stationary night blindness shows an electronegative ERG in which the rod-specific ERG is subnormal, but there is preservation of the photoreceptor-derived mixed response a-wave with selective b-wave reduction such that the a-wave is larger than the b-wave. This is known as a 'negative' ERG because the waveform is dominated by the negative a-wave, and indicates dysfunction post-transduction (Fig. 10.12).

■ Multifocal electroretinogram (mfERG)

1. *Indications*: assessing spatial function of central retinal cones.

2. *Method*: multiple hexagons are presented on a monitor which flash on and off according to a pseudorandom binary sequence. The waveforms are produced by mathematical calculation of the individual responses to each of the individual hexagons.

3. *Key points*: newer technique, highly dependent upon accurate fixation by the patient. May have some use in focal macular disease.

■ Electro-oculogram (EOG)

1. *Indications*: diagnosis of Best's vitelliform maculopathy (p. 503). Also useful in the diagnosis of AZOOR (acute zonal occult outer retinopathy).

2. *Method*: electrodes are placed at the lateral and medial canthi with a ground lead on the forehead. The cornea is positive relative to the retina so when the patient looks left to right between two fixed targets, a potential difference is recorded between the inner and outer canthal electrodes. The amplitude of the potential reaches a minimum under dark adaptation (the dark trough) and a maximum during restoration of photopic conditions (the light peak). The

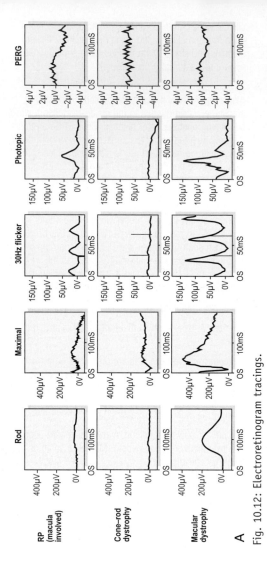

Fig. 10.12: Electroretinogram tracings.

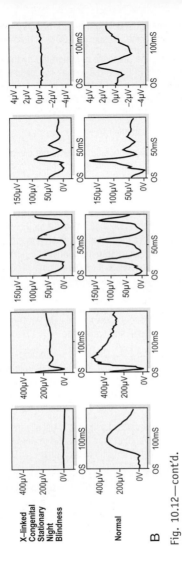

Fig. 10.12—cont'd.

ratio of the light peak to the dark trough is known as the Arden index, and is usually >180% in normals.

3. *Key points*: the response is generated by the interaction between the RPE and the retina. The degree of EOG light rise reduction is often related to the degree of rod ERG abnormality, but in Best's disease there is a normal ERG but severe reduction in the EOG light rise.

■ Visually-evoked potential (VEP)

1. *Indications*: these include: optic nerve disease; diagnosis of albinism; to assess visual potential in patients with media opacity; estimation of visual function in conjunction with ERG in infants and children; functional visual loss.

2. *Method*: active electrodes are placed in the occipital areas. The reference may be midfrontal, or the ipsilateral sylvian area. The stimulus is a flash and pattern. The waveform is recorded monocularly. The normal pattern reversal response has a prominent major positive component at ≈100 ms, the P100.

3. *Key points*:

   a. *Demyelination*: shows a delayed P100, with less effect on amplitude and waveform.

   b. *Albinism* is associated with misrouting of fibres in the optic chiasm so that there is a contralateral predominance in pattern appearance VEP such that the largest and earliest response from both right and left eyes occurs over the contralateral hemisphere.

   c. *Media opacities*: flash VEP is usually minimally affected, and so may be useful in detecting underlying maculopathy or optic neuropathy.

   d. *Cautionary note*: macular disease also causes VEP delay, and a delayed VEP in itself should never be assumed to reflect optic nerve disease unless there has been a measure of macular function obtained with mfERG or preferably PERG.

Recommended reading: Fishman GA, et al. Electrophysiologic testing in disorders of the retina, optic nerve, and visual pathway, 2nd edn. Ophthalmology monograph 2. San Francisco: AAO; 2001.

Retinal Laser Guidelines

General points

- The laser spot size is affected by lens selection. For example, selecting 100 μm on the laser produces the following spot size on the retina:

    1. Volk Area Centralis: 100 μm.

    2. Volk Transequator: 143 μm.

    3. Volk Quadraspheric: 200 μm.

- For macular treatment use an Area Centralis, for panretinal photocoagulation use a Transequator or Quadraspheric lens.

- Identify the foveal centre using fluorescein angiogram or clinical examination and a fixation target. Do not do this at the laser. In general, perform macular treatments with a 100–200 μm retinal spot size, 0.1–0.2 second duration, one spot size apart.

- In general, perform peripheral treatments with a 500 μm retinal spot size, 0.05–0.1 second, one spot size apart. Treatment is more uncomfortable in the far periphery, the horizontal meridia, and over previous laser scars or pigmentation.

- Shorter duration burns (0.05 sec) are more comfortable. Longer burns (0.1–0.2 sec) are more effective and less likely to rupture Bruch's membrane.

- Reduce power when treating pigmented fundi.

- Topical anaesthesia is usually adequate but some patients require peribulbar or sub-Tenon's anaesthetic for akinesia or analgesia, e.g. perifoveal treatment in a young, mobile patient.

- Some lasers offer both green or yellow laser light. Green light is attenuated by nuclear sclerosis, and power delivery may vary depending on the light path through the lens. Avoid green laser immediately after angiography as residual vitreous fluorescein provides troublesome fluorescence with green illumination. Green laser is also absorbed by luteal pigment when treating near the fovea. In these settings, yellow light is preferable.

For the treatment of retinal breaks (retinopexy), see page 526. Other common laser treatments are given below.

Macular Grid Laser

■ *Indications*: Macular oedema, particular in diabetics, or following branch retinal vein occlusion.

■ *Consent*: *Benefit* – improved visual prognosis. *Risks* – risks will vary with the indication for treatment but may include: blindness from foveal burn; paracentral scotoma; altered colour vision; re-treatment; subretinal neovascularization.

■ *Method*:

1. See General points, above.

2. Select an Area Centralis lens or equivalent and set the laser to 100 μm (100 μm retinal spot size), 0.05–0.2 seconds duration.

3. Test burn intensity and Bell's reflex (risk of foveal burn) using low-power burns (60 mW), near the temporal arcade.

4. Increase the power to give light-grey burns. More power will be needed in areas of oedema.

5. Avoid retinal haemorrhage, exudates, pigmentation, and scars. These produce variable laser absorption and more collateral damage. Avoid laser within the foveal avascular zone (FAZ).

6. Apply burns one burn width apart, over the area of oedema. A fluorescein angiogram may help define the area of leakage. For diffuse leakage, use a grid pattern (Fig. 10.13). For circinate leakage, treat locally.

7. For more specific protocols see the sections on individual diseases.

■ *Follow-up*: Usually 3–4 months.

Panretinal Photocoagulation (PRP)

■ *Indications*: Iris, retinal, or optic disc neovascularization secondary to retinal ischaemia, most commonly proliferative diabetic retinopathy or following retinal vein occlusion.

■ *Consent*: *Benefit* – reduced risk of visual loss but explain that PRP does not improve vision. *Risks* – reduced vision including blindness from foveal burn; reduced night vision; macular oedema; glare; reduced accommodation; re-treatment. Visual field loss may affect a patient's legal entitlement to drive.

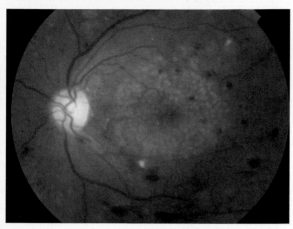

Fig. 10.13: Macular grid laser for diffuse macular oedema.

■ *Method*:

1. See General points, above.

2. Consider giving oral analgesics 30 minutes beforehand.

3. Set laser to 250 μm and use a Quadraspheric lens or equivalent (500 μm retinal spot size). Start with 60 mW and increase power to give moderate-intensity, grey-white burn.

4. If possible start inferiorly. Aim to cover the retina with evenly spaced burns, one burn width apart (Fig. 10.14).

5. Apply 2–3 treatment sessions of approximately 600 burns each, 1–2 weeks apart, aiming for a total of 1600 to 2000 burns. If there is iris neovascularization, full treatment should be completed within days.

6. Complete each quadrant in turn. This makes subsequent treatment easier and less painful.

7. Some clinicians avoid any treatment within the temporal arcades; others treat just within the arcades. Do not treat within two disc diameters of the foveal centre. Avoid vessels.

8. To preserve temporal visual field, avoid treating within 2–3 disc diameters nasal to the disc. Sometimes, this area is subsequently treated to control neovascularization.

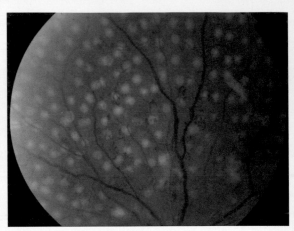

Fig. 10.14: Panretinal photocoagulation.

9. Neovascularization that fails to regress may have further 'fill-in PRP'. Refractory cases may require peripheral treatment with an indirect laser.

■ *Causes of pain during PRP*:

1. Inadequate anaesthesia.

2. High power or long duration burns.

3. Large number of burns.

4. Focused on the choroid rather than the retina.

5. Treatment over the long posterior ciliary nerves on the horizontal meridian.

6. Peripheral treatment.

7. Variable ocular pigmentation causing variable laser uptake.

8. Accidental treatment of previous laser burns.

If painful adjust laser parameters, arrange another treatment session or another method of anaesthesia. Consider indirect PRP under a block.

■ *Follow-up*: days to 2 weeks until PRP complete then 4–8 weeks depending on the underlying disease. Confirm that neovascularization has stopped with regression of the fine fronds of advancing new vessels. Larger new vessels often persist.

Laser for Macroaneurysm

■ *Indications*: Macular oedema or exudates caused by a leaking retinal arteriolar macroaneurysm.

■ *Consent*: *Benefit* – improve or stabilize vision. *Risks* – blindness from foveal burn; paracentral scotomas; altered colour vision; failure to prevent leakage; re-treatment; subretinal neovascularization. Offer a guarded prognosis if there is chronic (>3 months) macular oedema suggested by cyst formation, subfoveal pigmentation, fibrosis or exudates.

■ *Investigations*: Perform fluorescein angiography, as some macroaneurysms bleed then stop leaking.

■ *Method*:

1. See General points, above.

2. Set the laser to 200 μm and use an Area Centralis lens (200 μm retinal spot size). Start with 60 mW and increase the intensity to produce grey-white burns.

3. Treat around the macroaneurysm with a single confluent line.

4. If leakage persists, repeat the procedure and treat macroaneurysms directly.

5. Consider grid treatment (technique above) in areas of retinal telangiectasia with persistent oedema.

■ *Follow-up*: 2 weeks after first treatment for possible direct treatment, then 3 months to consider macular grid.

Laser for Choroidal Neovascularization

■ *Indications*: Extra- and juxtafoveal choroidal neovascularization secondary to age-related macular degeneration (AMD). If secondary to a presumed inflammatory cause, consider oral corticosteroid cover.

■ *Consent*: *Benefit* – for AMD, laser reduces the 3-year risk of severe visual loss from 63% to 45% (extrafoveal) or 58% to 49% (juxtafoveal), relative to the natural history. *Risk* – loss of vision including blindness from foveal or parafoveal burn, permanent paracentral scotoma, and re-treatment. Recurrence occurs in 50% and is often aggressive and subfoveal.

- *Method*:

  1. See General points, above. Do not perform this procedure unsupervised for the first time, as there is a high risk of foveal damage.

  2. Determine the angiographic limits of the lesion. Plan treatment by annotating digital images, or by projecting film in the laser room. For extrafoveal lesions treat 100–125 microns beyond the borders of the lesion. Laser juxtafoveal lesions if between 100 and 200 μm from fovea but do not treat beyond the edge of the lesion on the foveal side. If less than 100 μm treat as subfoveal and do not ablate with laser.

  3. Start by setting the laser to 100 μm and use an Area Centralis lens (100 μm retinal spot size).

  4. Use a long duration of 0.2–0.5 seconds depending on the patient's fixation stability.

  5. Outline the lesion including areas of contiguous haemorrhage.

  6. Fill in the lesion with dense, uniform, white, overlapping, 200 μm burns.

  7. Pay particular attention to the foveal border where recurrences usually occur.

- *Follow-up*: Repeat fluorescein angiography in 2 weeks. Retreat if persistent. Otherwise, review in 6 weeks to look for recurrence. Consider other treatments if the lesion becomes subfoveal.

Photodynamic Therapy (PDT)

- *Indications*: Current British (NICE) guidelines advise PDT funding for 100% classic subfoveal choroidal neovascular membranes with a VA of 6/60 or better. Predominantly classic (≥50%) is funded if part of a trial. Other indications may be considered on an individual case basis. Studies have shown benefit for purely occult membranes but these are not currently funded. Funding of PDT is complex, and changes, so consult local guidelines.

- *Contraindications*: Liver dysfunction, porphyria, sensitivity to verteporfin.

- *Consent*: *Benefit* – risk of moderate vision loss at 2 years is reduced from 69% to 41% (predominantly classic lesions).

Risks – transient or permanent loss of vision; acute vision loss occurs in 1–4%; photosensitivity (avoid sunlight for 48 hours, wear protective clothing and sunglasses); injection site complications; back pain; liver dysfunction; re-treatment; multiple fluorescein angiograms.

▨ *Method*:

1. Dilute verteporfin (6 mg/m^2 body surface area) in 5% dextrose.

2. Administer intravenously at 3 mL/min over 10 minutes, using a syringe pump and in-line filter.

3. Laser spot size = greatest linear dimension of the lesion angiographically (including contiguous blood, blocked fluorescence, or RPE detachment) + 1000 μm. This gives a 500 μm treatment margin around the lesion.

4. At 15 minutes postinfusion, centre the aiming beam over the lesion and activate the laser. The laser is a nonthermal diode and produces red light (689 nm) at an intensity of 800 J/sec or 600 mW/cm^2 for 83 s.

▨ *Follow-up*: 10–12 weeks, or earlier if the patient has symptoms. Re-treatment is often required.

Differential Diagnoses

Rubeosis iridis

- Retinal ischaemia, e.g. diabetes, retinal vein occlusion (Fig. 10.15), Eales' disease.

- Ocular ischaemic syndrome, e.g. atherosclerotic carotid artery disease.

- Intraocular inflammation, e.g. Fuchs' heterochromic iridocyclitis.

- Intraocular tumour, e.g. melanoma.

- Iris ischaemia (rare).

Retinal neovascularization

- Diabetes mellitus (Fig. 10.16).

- Retinal vein occlusion.

- Hypertension.

- Sickle cell retinopathy.

- Ocular ischaemic syndrome.

- Retinopathy of prematurity.

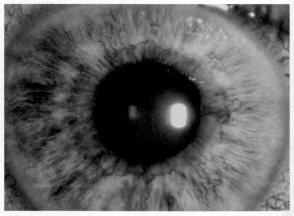

Fig. 10.15: Rubeosis iridis secondary to central retinal vein occlusion (Courtesy of DH Verity).

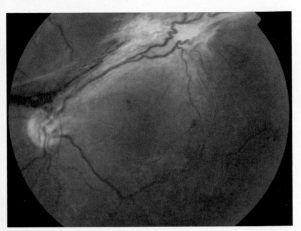

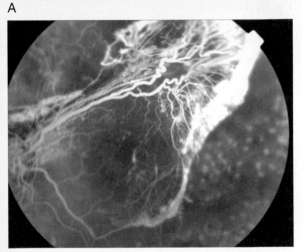

Fig. 10.16: Proliferative diabetic retinopathy.

- Familial exudative vitreoretinopathy.

- Norrie's disease.

- Eales' disease.

- Inflammation, e.g. vasculitis, posterior uveitis, pars planitis.

- Hyperviscosity syndromes.

- Chronic retinal detachment.

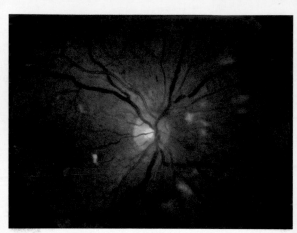

Fig. 10.17: Diabetic retinopathy.

- Radiation retinopathy.
- Talc emboli.

Intraretinal haemorrhage

- Diabetes mellitus (Fig. 10.17).
- Retinal vein occlusion.
- Hyperviscosity syndrome, anaemia, blood malignancy.
- Hypertension.
- Ocular ischaemic syndrome.
- Retinal arteriolar macroaneurysm.
- Subretinal disease, e.g. subretinal neovascularization, idiopathic polypoidal choroidal vasculopathy, lacquer cracks in myopic degeneration.
- Valsalva retinopathy (retinal haemorrhage caused by sudden increase in intra-abdominal pressure, e.g. coughing or vomiting. See Fig. 10.3.).
- Associated with retinal ischaemia, e.g. sickle retinopathy, Eales' disease.
- Retinal inflammation, e.g. Behçet's disease.
- Trauma.

- Associated with infection, e.g. HIV microangiopathy, Roth's spots.

Subretinal choroidal neovascularization

- Age-related macular degeneration.
- Postinflammatory or presumed postinflammatory, e.g. presumed ocular histoplasmosis syndrome, punctate inner choroidopathy, serpiginous retinopathy, birdshot chorioretinopathy.
- Myopic degeneration (Fig. 10.18).
- Trauma, e.g. choroidal rupture, photocoagulation.
- Dystrophic, e.g. Sorsby's fundus dystrophy; Best's and adult-vitelliform macular dystrophy.
- Optic nerve drusen.
- Angioid streaks – most commonly pseudoxanthoma elasticum.

Retinal telangiectasia

- Diabetes.
- Hypertension.
- Previous retinal vein occlusion.
- Sickle cell retinopathy.
- Idiopathic juxtafoveal telangiectasia (Fig. 10.19).
- Radiation retinopathy.
- Coats' disease.
- Incontinentia pigmenti.
- Fascioscapulohumeral dystrophy.

Retinal vascular tortuosity

- Polycythaemia.
- Leukaemia.
- Dysproteinaemia.
- Sickle cell disease.

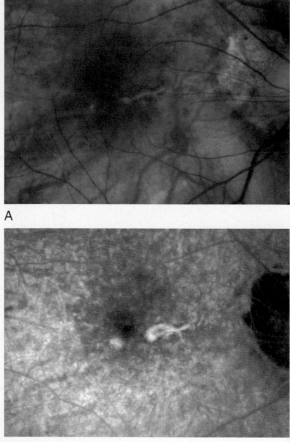

A

B

Fig. 10.18: Choroidal neovascularization associated with a lacquer crack and high myopia.

- Familial dysautonomia.
- Mucopolysaccharidosis VI.
- Fabry's disease.
- Hyperviscosity syndromes.
- Eales' disease.
- Racemose angioma (Fig. 10.20).

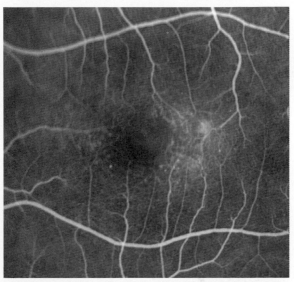

Fig. 10.19: Idiopathic juxtafoveal telangiectasia.

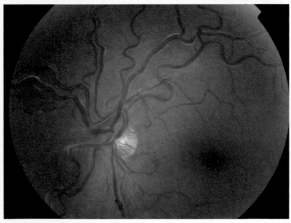

Fig. 10.20: Racemose angioma.

Retinal deposits

■ Exudates: diabetes, hypertension, macroaneurysm, retinal vein occlusion, vascular tumour, telangiectasia (Coats' disease).

- Drusen: age-related macular degeneration; basal laminar drusen; dominant dystrophies (Doyne's macular dystrophy/Mallatia Levantinese; Sorsby's dystrophy; North Carolina macular dystrophy).

- Crystals: juxtafoveal telangiectasia, talc, canthaxanthine, tamoxifen, Bietti's crystalline retinopathy.

- White dots: multiple evanescent white dot syndrome (MEWDS); birdshot chorioretinopathy; hereditary fundus albipunctatus.

- Flecks: Stargardt's/fundus flavimaculatus; pattern dystrophy.

- Yellow lesions: Best's macular dystrophy; pattern dystrophy (adult vitelliform macular dystrophy form); pigment epithelial detachment from central serous retinopathy; age-related macular degeneration; Harada's disease; metastasis.

Cherry-red spot at the macula

- Central retinal artery occlusion (Fig. 10.21).
- Sphingolipidoses, e.g. Tay-Sachs, Gaucher, and Niemann-Pick disease.
- Quinine toxicity.
- Traumatic retinal oedema.

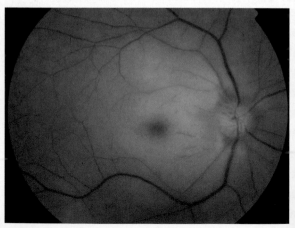

Fig. 10.21: Central retinal artery occlusion.

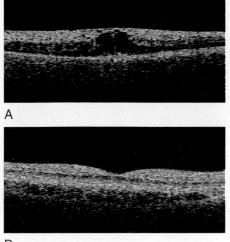

Fig. 10.22: Optical coherence tomography (OCT) of diabetic cystoid macular oedema **(A)**, compared to normal **(B)**.

- Ocular ischaemic syndrome.
- Macular hole with surrounding retinal detachment.

Macular oedema

- Diabetes mellitus (Fig. 10.22).
- Retinal vein occlusion.
- Pseudophakic (Irvine-Gass syndrome).
- Subretinal neovascularization.
- Uveitis/scleritis.
- Hypertension.
- Choroidal ischaemia.
- Retinitis pigmentosa.
- Vascular tumour, e.g. angioma.
- Nicotinic acid (no leakage on fluorescein angiography).
- Hereditary.
- Idiopathic.

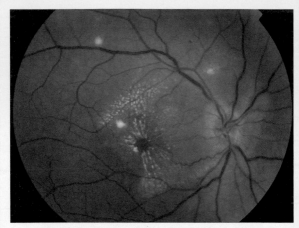

Fig. 10.23: Macular star from hypertensive retinopathy.

Macular star

- Hypertension (Fig. 10.23).

- Retinal vascular occlusion.

- Papilloedema.

- Inflammation: choroiditis; posterior scleritis; vasculitis; toxoplasmosis; chronic infection, e.g. syphilis.

- Idiopathic.

Macular atrophy

- Age-related macular degeneration (Fig. 10.24).

- Pathological myopia.

- Stargardt's disease.

- Cone dystrophy.

- Dominant retinal dystrophies, e.g. central areolar choroidal dystrophy.

- A3243G mitochondrial mutation (maternally inherited diabetes and deafness, MIDD).

- Best's vitelliform macular dystrophy.

- Pattern dystrophy, e.g. adult vitelliform macular dystrophy.

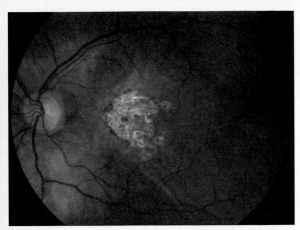

Fig. 10.24: Geographic atrophy from age-related macular degeneration.

- X-linked retinoschisis.

- North Carolina macular dystrophy.

- Toxic, e.g. chloroquine.

- Acquired, e.g. after pigment epithelium detachment, subretinal haemorrhage.

- Infectious, e.g. onchocerciasis.

- Solar retinopathy.

Bull's-eye maculopathy

- Macular, cone or cone/rod dystrophies, e.g. Stargardt's disease (Fig. 10.25).

- Drug toxicity, e.g. chloroquine.

- Batten's disease.

- Benign concentric annular macular dystrophy.

- Bardet-Biedl syndrome.

Angioid streaks

- Pseudoxanthoma elasticum (Fig. 10.26).

- Paget's disease.

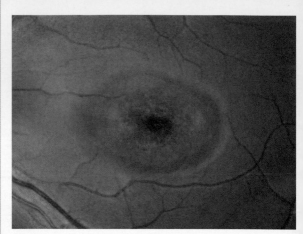

Fig. 10.25: Bull's-eye maculopathy from Stargardt's disease.

- Haemoglobinopathies, sickle cell disease.

- Ehlers-Danlos syndrome.

- Other rare associations, e.g. abetalipoproteinaemia.

Choroidal folds

- Idiopathic chorioretinal folds or hypermetropia (Fig. 10.27).

- Hypotony.

- Retrobulbar mass lesions.

- Thyroid eye disease.

- Scleral inflammation.

- Scleral buckle.

- Choroidal tumours.

- Choroidal neovascularization.

- Focal chorioretinal scars.

- Optic nerve head diseases associated with swelling.

- Papilloedema.

Pigmentary retinopathy

- See retinitis pigmentosa, page 496.

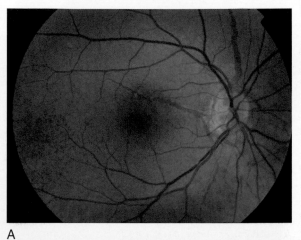

A

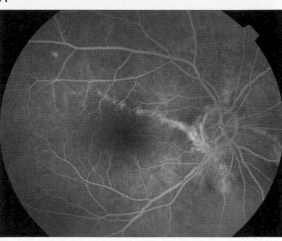

B

Fig. 10.26: Angiod streaks from pseudoxanthoma elasticum.

Vision loss with normal retina

■ Exclude subtle abnormalities:

1. Angioid streaks.

2. Choroidal folds.

3. Emboli.

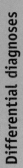
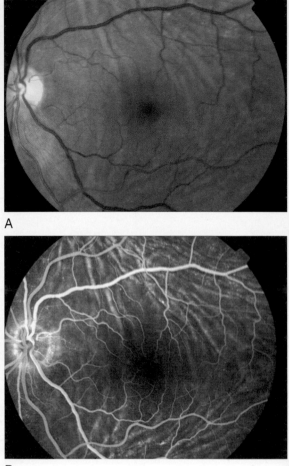

A

B

Fig. 10.27: Choroidal folds in a hypermetropic patient.

4. Pale disc.

5. Peripheral retinoschisis.

6. Albinism.

7. Cone dystrophy.

8. Autoimmune phenomena.

9. Old inflammatory lesions – acute zonal occult outer retinopathy (AZOOR).

10. History of malignancy – carcinoma-associated retinopathy (CAR), melanoma-associated retinopathy (MAR).

- Consider: previous arterial occlusion; optic nerve/visual pathway disease; amblyopia; functional vision loss; transient vision loss (disc oedema, CNS ischaemia, migraine, elevated IOP).

- For children, see page 579.

Age-related Macular Degeneration

Age-related macular degeneration (AMD) is a degenerative disorder affecting those over the age of 50 years. Features include drusen and RPE pigmentary abnormalities in the early stage, and geographic atrophy, choroidal neovascularization (CNV), pigment epithelial detachment (PED), and fibrous macular scarring in the late stages.

Early AMD

Symptoms Usually asymptomatic, but gradual central visual loss of night vision, prolonged after-images, or slight metamorphopsia may occur.

Signs Drusen of variable size and shape and macular RPE pigmentary abnormalities (hyperpigmentation or hypopigmentation) (Fig. 10.28).

Differential diagnosis Inherited dominant drusen; basal laminar-type drusen; drusen associated with choroidal nevus; other causes of retinal flecks such as Stargardt's dystrophy; pattern dystrophy; fundus albipunctate dystrophy; mesangiocapillary glomerulonephritis type II.

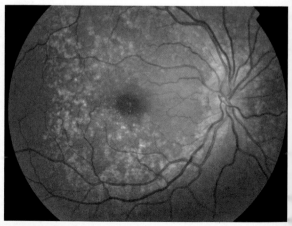

Fig. 10.28: Retinal drusen.

Investigations Fluorescein angiography only if CNV is suspected on clinical examination and/or Amsler grid testing. Autofluorescent imaging if available.

Treatment

- *Stop smoking.* Data from three epidemiologic studies showed that current smokers were at higher risk of incident AMD than both past smokers and those who never smoked.

- *Diet and antioxidant vitamin supplementation.* Some ophthalmologists recommend a diet rich in lutein and zeaxanthin (green leafy vegetables five or more times weekly) that has been shown to increase macular pigment density, but no robust clinical trial data exist. The age-related eye disease study group showed that an antioxidant vitamin combination (500 mg vitamin C, 400 IU vitamin E, 15 mg beta-carotene, 80 mg zinc, and 2 mg copper) has a moderate protective effect to the fellow eye of patients with vision loss in one eye from late AMD. Beta-carotene is contraindicated in smokers: there is also some concern on theoretical grounds in geographic atrophy although not all clinicians agree. Many ophthalmologists also place patients with bilateral intermediate and large drusen with no late AMD on vitamin supplementation, although the evidence is weaker.

Follow-up Regular ophthalmic review is not required, but provide an Amsler grid and instructions to return urgently should the patient develop new macular symptoms. Advise annual optometry review.

Geographic Atrophy

Symptoms In geographic atrophy (GA) there is a gradual loss of central vision or slight metamorphopsia. Extrafoveal atrophy may be asymptomatic.

Signs Sharply demarcated area(s) of GA that is pale relative to the surrounding retina, with increased visibility of underlying choroidal vessels. Intermediate or large drusen are present in most eyes surrounding the GA, unless the atrophy is very extensive (Fig. 10.29).

Differential diagnosis Stargardt's disease, Best's macular dystrophy, rod–cone dystrophies, Sorsby's dystrophy, chronic central serous retinopathy, basal laminar drusen, myopic macular degeneration, and chloroquine retinopathy.

Investigations Fluorescein angiography if exudative AMD (see below) is suspected on examination or Amsler grid testing.

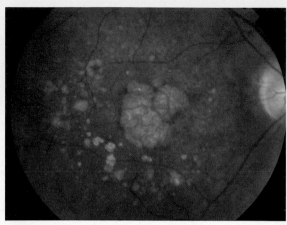

Fig. 10.29: Geographic macular atrophy.

Treatment See early AMD above. Arrange low-vision aids if necessary.

Follow-up Provide an Amsler grid and instructions to return urgently should they develop new macular symptoms. GA typically expands and this may reduce vision, as may the development of exudative AMD. Advise annual optometry review.

Exudative AMD

Symptoms Typically, rapid onset of visual loss, central blind spot or distortion. Uniocular, asymptomatic AMD may be picked up on routine eye testing.

Signs May appear as a greenish-grey lesion, often with sensory retinal detachment. There may be surrounding drusen, pigment change, subretinal haemorrhage and exudates. Classification is by angiography (see below).

Differential diagnosis

- CNV: other causes include myopia; angioid streaks; multifocal choroiditis; trauma; idiopathic; inherited dystrophies (Sorsby's).

- PED/serous detachments: other causes include central serous retinopathy; congenital optic nerve pit; macular hole with detachment; choroidal inflammatory disease; severe hypertension.

■ AMD variants: idiopathic polypoidal choroidal vasculopathy retinal angiomatous proliferation (Stage I; intraretinal neovascularization; progressing to Stage II; subretinal neovascularization; then Stage III; choroidal neovascularization with a retinal choroidal anastamosis).

Fluorescein angiography (FFA) Required to confirm the lesion type, plan treatment, and classify disease as follows.

■ *Classic CNV*: early well defined hyperfluorescence with late leak that obscures the boundaries (Fig. 10.30). May be 100% classic, predominantly classic (>50% of total lesion area), or minimally classic (<50%).

■ *Occult CNV*: hyperfluorescence is less well defined than classic lesions (Fig. 10.31). The following are 2 commonly described subtypes.

   1. *Fibrovascular PED*: an area of irregular RPE elevation that is less discrete than classic CNV in the transit phase and shows stippled hyperfluorescence in the midframes (1–2 minutes).

   2. *Late leakage of undetermined origin*: pooling of dye and specked hyperfluorescence that occurs in the late frames.

■ *Serous PED*: sharply demarcated area of uniform hyperfluorescence that develops rapidly under the dome of the PED and persists late with relatively sharp borders. May be associated with classic or occult membranes (Fig. 10.32).

■ *Disciform scar*: late staining of fibrosis, with no leak beyond borders unless residual active membrane exists (Fig. 10.33).

Treatment See early AMD above regarding antioxidant vitamins and smoking advice. Arrange low vision aids if necessary. If uniocular, warn patients of the risk to the fellow eye (10–15% per year). Provide an Amsler grid and instructions.

■ Laser
   Indications for argon laser treatment depends on the angiographic characteristics and lesion location. In general, treatment is most beneficial with classic lesions and if the patient is not hypertensive. Argon laser is most effective in treating extrafoveal lesions. The more accepted treatments are as follows, but indications change and research is rapidly evolving, so always consult current local or national guidelines.

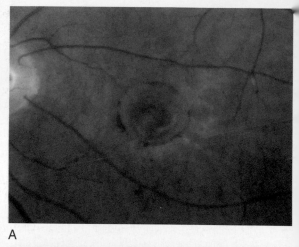

A

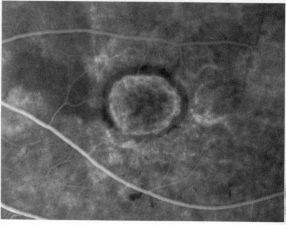

B

Fig. 10.30: Classic (100%) choroidal neovascular membrane **(A)** and early angiogram **(B)**.

1. Extrafoveal (>200 μm from foveal centre): laser.

2. Juxtafoveal (<200 μm from foveal centre): laser if between 100 and 200 μm from the fovea and no occult component, otherwise treat as subfoveal.

3. Subfoveal:

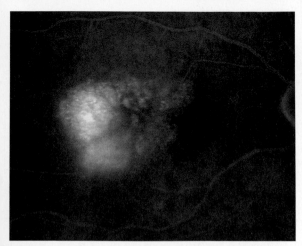

Fig. 10.31: Occult choroidal neovascular membrane.

    a. *Classic or predominantly classic* membrane: photodynamic therapy (PDT) and/or intravitreous VEGF inhibitors (see below).

    b. *Occult or minimally classic membranes*: PDT may help but funding is an issue in many countries, including the UK. Consider intravitreous VEGF inhibitors if available.

    For laser techniques including PDT, see page 437.

■ Intravitreous pegaptanib

1. *Indications*: Subfoveal CNV of all angiographic types and VA 6/60 or better, or as directed by local or national guidelines.

2. *Consent*: *Benefit* – reduces the risk of moderate visual loss from 70% to 55% (all lesion types; NNT 6.7). *Risks* – conjunctival haemorrhage, eye pain, vitreous floaters, traumatic cataract, retinal detachment (<1%), uveitis (<1%), endophthalmitis (<1%). The long-term safety is unknown.

3. *Method*: Pegaptanib (Macugen) is supplied in a single-use 1 mL glass syringe containing 0.3 mg in a 90 μL deliverable volume. Each syringe is fitted with a fixed 27-gauge needle. Inject via the pars plana (3.5 mm from the

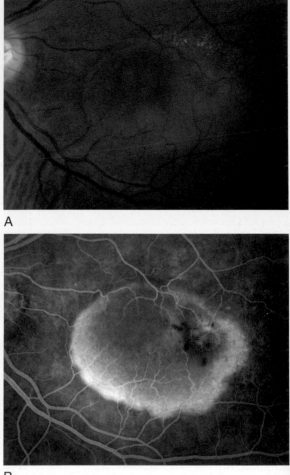

A

B

Fig. 10.32: Large pigment epithelial detachment.

limbus in aphakic or pseudophakic patients, and 4 mm in phakic patients), aiming the needle towards the optic disc to avoid the lens. Use strict aseptic conditions including povidone-iodine drops and a lid speculum.

4. *Follow-up*: Check IOP within 30 minutes. Review 2–7 days postinjection, then at 6 weeks to consider further

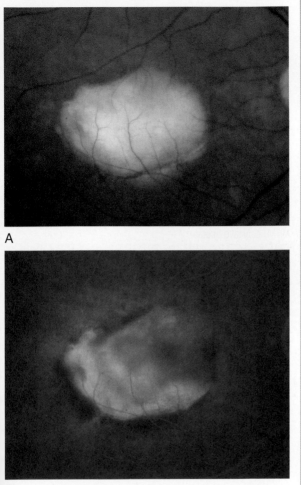

A

B

Fig. 10.33: Longstanding disciform scar. (Courtesy J Wong)

injections. Advise patients to immediately report any symptoms suggestive of endophthalmitis or retinal detachment.

- Intravitreous ranibizumab

1. *Indications*: Subfoveal CNV of all angiographic types.

2. *Consent*: *Benefit* – the MARINA phase III study of Lucentis for minimally classic/occult lesions showed 5% (treated) versus 38% (sham injection) moderate vision loss (>15 letters on ETDRS chart) at 1 year, giving an NNT of 3. The ANCHOR phase III study of predominantly classic lesions showed 4% (treated) versus 36% (PDT) moderate vision loss (NNT 3.1). *Risks* – similar to pegaptanib.

3. *Methods*: Pars plana intravitreal injection (see pegaptanib) monthly for 1 year. The PIER study compared Lucentis and sham injections, both given once per month for the first 3 months, thereafter, every 3 months. Treatment provided a 16 letter benefit compared to sham, but was less effective than monthly injections.

4. *Follow-up*: Check IOP within 30 minutes and review monthly. Advice is similar to that for pegaptanib.

■ Anecortave acetate

Administered every 6 months, in a posterior juxtascleral location using a blunt tipped curved cannula. Retaane (15 mg anecortave acetate suspension) has been approved for the treatment of subfoveal CNV with a classic component.

■ Ongoing clinical trials

Other treatment options include intravitreous steroids, several novel angiostatic agents (e.g. squalamine, bevacizumab [Avastin]) and surgical procedures such as macular translocation and autologous RPE transplantation.

Idiopathic Polypoidal Choroidal Vasculopathy

Background Idiopathic polypoidal choroidal vasculopathy (IPCV) is sometimes described as a subtype of exudative 'wet' age-related macular degeneration (AMD).

Clinical features Originally described as presenting in hypertensive, black women aged 40–60 years with exudative retinal elevation, haemorrhagic pigment epithelial detachments (PEDs), and hard exudates. Appears to be common in East Asians and occurs in Caucasians, although the case definition is less certain. Unlike AMD, it often occurs beyond the arcades or near the optic disc. It may have a similar presentation to central serous retinopathy.

Investigations Indocyanine green (ICG) angiography shows characteristic collections of dilated choroidal vessels with terminal dilatations (polyps). These leak in the later frames (Fig. 10.34).

Treatment IPCV may resolve spontaneously ($\approx$20%) but is often treated with focal laser to obliterate leaking dilatations (e.g. 200 mW, 200 micron spot size, 0.2 seconds), although the evidence for this is presently uncertain. It may not be possible to treat all lesions due to haemorrhage. Avoid laser to PEDs as this may cause an RPE tear.

Follow–up Six weeks after laser with repeat ICG.

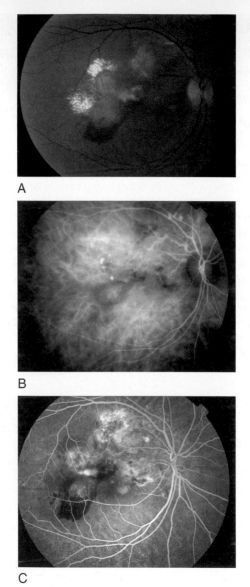

Fig. 10.34: Idiopathic polypoidal choroidal vasculopathy. The fundus shows haemorrhagic PED, hard exudates, and serous retinal elevation **(A)**. ICG **(B)** shows sacular vessel dilatations and leakage, not easily seen with fluorescein angiography **(C)**.

Diabetic Retinopathy

Background Diabetics can lose vision from macular oedema, macular ischaemia, vitreous haemorrhage, and tractional retinal detachment. The ophthalmologist has several tasks: confirm the diagnosis; classify its severity and monitor accordingly; offer advice; apply retinal laser as required; and treat associated eye disease such as cataract.

Key studies

- *Diabetic Retinopathy Study (DRS)*: defined high-risk proliferative diabetic retinopathy (PDR, criteria below) and risk of severe visual loss with different levels of retinopathy. Established that panretinal photocoagulation (PRP) more than halves the risk of severe visual loss in high-risk PDR.

- *Wisconsin Epidemiologic Study of Diabetic Retinopathy (WESDR)*: population-based study showed that glycosylated haemoglobin levels and duration of diabetes are risk factors for progression of retinopathy.

- *Early Treatment of Diabetic Retinopathy Study (ETDRS)*: defined clinically significant macular oedema (criteria below) and showed that laser treatment approximately halves the risk of moderate visual loss.

- *Diabetic Retinopathy Vitrectomy Study (DRVS)*: demonstrated that early vitrectomy for vitreous haemorrhage (within 3 months) improved visual prognosis in type 1 diabetes.

- *Diabetes Control and Complications Trial (DCCT)*: demonstrated that intensive insulin treatment reduced the risk of sustained progression of retinopathy in type 1 diabetes when compared to conventional insulin treatment.

- *United Kingdom Prospective Diabetes Study (UKPDS)*: showed that tight blood pressure and glycaemic control in type 2 diabetes reduced retinopathy progression and visual loss.

Classification of retinopathy

- *Mild non-proliferative diabetic retinopathy (NPDR)*: At least one microaneurysm.

- *Moderate non-proliferative diabetic retinopathy*: intraretinal haemorrhages or microaneurysms < ETDRS standard photograph 2a (Fig. 10.35) and/or cotton-wool spots, venous beading, intraretinal microvascular abnormalities (IRMA).

- *Severe nonproliferative diabetic retinopathy*: relies on the 4–2-1 rule, which requires one of the following:

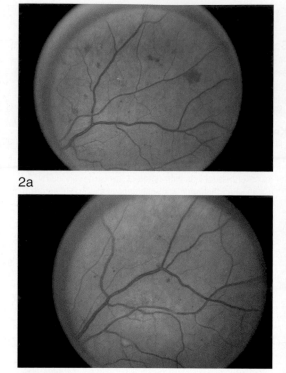

2a

6a

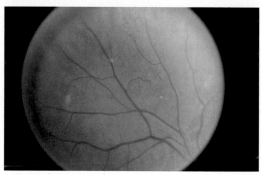

8a

Fig. 10.35: ETDRS standard photograph. 2a (retinal haemorhages), 6a (venous beading) and 8a (IRMAs). (Courtesy ETDRS Research Group.)

1. Intraretinal haemorrhages or microaneurysms in *four* quadrants.

2. Venous beading ≥ ETDRS photograph 6a (Fig. 10.35) in *two* quadrants.

3. IRMA≥ETDRS photograph 8a (Fig. 10.35) in *one* quadrant.

- *Very severe non-proliferative diabetic retinopathy*: at least two of the criteria for severe NPDR.

- *Non-high risk proliferative diabetic retinopathy*: new vessels on the disc (NVD) or elsewhere (NVE), but criteria not met for high-risk proliferative diabetic retinopathy (PDR) below.

- *High-risk proliferative diabetic retinopathy*: at least one of the following:

  1. NVD >$\frac{1}{3}$ disc area.

  2. NVD plus vitreous or preretinal haemorrhage.

  3. NVE >$\frac{1}{2}$ disc area plus preretinal or vitreous haemorrhage.

- *Advanced proliferative diabetic retinopathy*: tractional retinal detachment.

Macular exudates or thickening can occur with any severity of retinopathy. Treatment is advised if there is *clinically significant macular oedema (CSMO)* comprising at least one of the following:

- Thickening of the retina within 500 μm of the fovea.

- Hard exudates located within 500 μm of the fovea with adjacent retinal thickening.

- Retinal thickening at least one disc area in size, part of which is located within one disc diameter of the fovea.

History Ask about the duration and type of diabetes, blood sugar control, smoking and associated disease, especially hypertension and renal disease. Identify the clinicians monitoring the patient's diabetes.

Examination Examine the iris at high magnification for neovascularization (NVI). If present, or if IOP is elevated, perform gonioscopy to look for angle neovascularization (NVA). Perform careful fundus examination looking for atypical features. Exclude associated disease, especially posterior subcapsular cataracts. Classify severity.

Differential diagnosis

- *Nonproliferative diabetic retinopathy*: central or branch retinal vein occlusion; ocular ischaemic syndrome; hypertensive retinopathy; radiation retinopathy; leukaemia; anaemia; HIV microangiopathy.

■ *Proliferative diabetic retinopathy*: vascular obstruction; sickle cell retinopathy; ocular ischaemic syndrome; sarcoidosis; Eales' disease; tuberculosis; embolization from intravenous drug use.

Investigations Check blood pressure and fasting glucose if not diagnosed diabetic. Arrange fluorescein angiography if CSMO is present (to guide laser treatment) or if there is unexplained poor vision (to assess macular ischaemia). For interpretation of fluorescein angiograms, see page 415. Optical coherence tomography (OCT) may help confirm macular oedema.

Management Correspond with all relevant health workers to ensure glucose, blood pressure, and general health are well managed. Encourage smokers to stop and explain that poor glucose control threatens vision.

Ocular management depends on the findings:

■ Nonproliferative diabetic retinopathy.

   1. *Absent or mild*: refer to screening programme for annual review (1% risk of high-risk PDR in 1 year).

   2. *Moderate*: review 6–9 monthly (4% risk of high-risk PDR in 1 year).

   3. *Severe*: review 4–6 monthly (8% risk of high-risk PDR in 1 year).

   4. *Very severe*: review 3–4 monthly (17% risk of high-risk PDR in 1 year).

■ Proliferative retinopathy.

   1. *Non-high risk*: review in 2 months (50% risk of high-risk PDR in 1 year). Consider PRP if poor attendance or poor diabetic control.

   2. *High-risk or iris new vessels*: perform PRP within 1 week, preferably immediately. If there is coexisting CSMO, perform macular laser treatment first or at the same time. For laser technique, see page 433.

■ Vitreous haemorrhage.
   Treat mild vitreous haemorrhage as high-risk PDR. If the haemorrhage is dense enough to obscure the fundal view, perform B-scan ultrasound to exclude retinal detachment. Review monthly to monitor for iris new vessels or raised IOP.

Apply PRP as haemorrhage clears and the view improves.
Arrange vitreoretinal review if the haemorrhage persists for
1 month (type 1 diabetes), or 3–4 months (type 2)
(p. 534). Consider early referral if the other eye has poor
acuity.

■ Tractional retinal detachment.
If tractional retinal detachment threatens the macula, arrange
vitreoretinal review (p. 534). If not, review 2–3 monthly
depending on the retinopathy severity.

■ Maculopathy.

1. Not clinically significant: review in 4–6 months.

2. Clinically significant macular oedema (criteria above):
perform fluorescein angiography unless there is an
isolated circinate, and treat as per ETDRS:

    a. Focal laser to circinate ring.

    b. Modified grid to areas of macular thickening.

    c. Macular grid for diffuse thickening.

    d. Avoid laser treatment to the edge of, or within, the
    foveal avascular zone (FAZ).

For laser settings and example treatments, see page 433.
Consider earlier review for all categories if there is poor diabetic
or blood pressure control, or recent marked improvement in
diabetic control (can transiently worsen retinopathy).

Diabetic retinopathy and cataract surgery

■ Preoperative

1. Plan to operate early, before CSMO or high-risk PDR
develop.

2. If possible, treat CSMO and wait until resolved before
operating.

3. Treat high-risk PDR/NVI preoperatively if possible.

4. If there is no fundus view, perform B-scan ultrasound. If
tractional retinal detachment or vitreous haemorrhage is
present, refer for possible combined phaco-vitrectomy.

5. If there is high-risk PDR/NVI and it is not possible to
complete preoperative PRP, perform intraoperative indirect
PRP (allow extra time on the operating list).

6. Explain that there is a guarded prognosis if a dense
cataract prevents a good macular view, or if there is

advanced diabetic retinopathy or CSMO that cannot be treated preoperatively.

■ Intraoperative

1. Phacoemulsification technique is preferred.

2. Use a large-diameter optic, acrylic intraocular lens (to maximise retinal view postoperatively).

3. If intraoperative PRP is required, perform after crystalline lens removal and before intraocular lens insertion.

■ Postoperative

1. *Macular oedema*: examine the fundus within 1 week. If macular oedema is present it should be considered due to diabetes and treated as above. Macular oedema that develops after 1 week but before 6 months is probably pseudophakic and may resolve spontaneously. Manage expectantly for up to 1 year postoperatively.

2. *Progression of retinopathy*: increase frequency of review in eyes with severe NPDR or worse, as there is an increased risk of progression. Promptly treat high-risk PDR that occurs in the postoperative period.

Diabetic retinopathy and pregnancy

■ Ideally, patients should be reviewed preconception to assess baseline retinopathy.

■ Minimum review is at the end of the first trimester, weeks 20–24, then weeks 30–34.

■ Arrange more frequent review if there is severe retinopathy/ maculopathy or poor diabetic control.

■ Avoid fluorescein angiography if possible (p. 702).

■ Treat by laser as required.

Central Retinal Vein Occlusion

Background Central retinal vein occlusion (CRVO) typically occurs in patients over 45 years secondary to retinal vein thrombosis. Risk factors include diabetes, hypertension, hyperlipidaemia, and glaucoma. CRVO in those aged less than 45 years may suggest a clotting disorder.

Clinical features CRVO produces painless visual loss in one eye. Signs include: retinal haemorrhages in four quadrants (Fig. 10.36); dilated tortuous retinal veins; optic disc swelling; macular oedema; cotton-wool spots; neovascularization of the iris, angle, retina, or disc. Disc collateral vessels are a sign of resolution.

Classification

- Nonischaemic.

- Ischaemic.

    1. *Clinical examination*: RAPD, VA <6/60, multiple cotton-wool spots, dense midretinal haemorrhages, 'blood and thunder fundus'.

    2. *Fluorescein angiogram*: more than 10 disc areas of ischaemia.

History and examination Ask about glaucoma, systemic hypertension, raised lipids, diabetes or symptoms of diabetes (polyuria, polydipsia, weight loss). If younger than 45 years ask about thrombophilia: family history of thromboses aged <45 years; deep vein thrombosis; pulmonary emboli; thromboses in unusual sites, e.g. axillary vein; multiple miscarriages. Examine specifically for new vessels in the angle (undilated gonioscopy), iris, and optic nerve/retina. Examine both eyes for features of glaucoma. Perform digital ophthalmodynanometry to check for raised central retinal vein pressure. In normal eyes, the central retinal vein spontaneously pulses or can be made to 'wink' or collapse with minimal ocular pressure through the eyelids. In CRVO, the vein and artery 'wink' together or, in extreme cases, the artery is more easily compressed than the vein. The latter may also suggest reduced arterial pressure and ocular ischaemia, so compare with the fellow eye, assuming that is normal. Ocular ischaemia may present with loss of VA due to cilioretinal hypoperfusion.

Differential diagnosis Consider ocular ischaemic syndrome; diabetic retinopathy; optic disc swelling for other reasons; and radiation retinopathy.

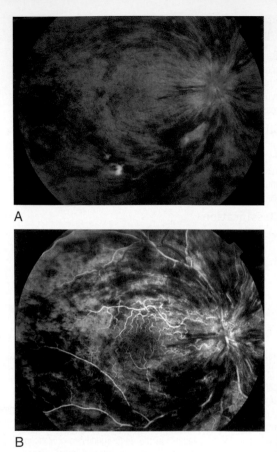

A

B

Fig. 10.36: Central retinal vein occlusion.

Investigations Check BP, FBC, ESR, lipids (thyroid function if abnormal), plasma protein electrophoresis, and thrombophilia screen if suspicious. Arrange fluorescein angiogram if ischaemia is suspected (see Classification above). Diabetic work-up varies from random or fasting glucose, to HbA1c, glucose tolerance test, and diabetologist review. Normal fasting glucose is ≤6.0 mmol; impaired fasting glycaemia 6.1–6.9 mmol; ≥7.0 mmol suggests diabetes, but repeat if there are no diabetic symptoms.

Treatment Liaise with the patient and the physician regarding low-dose aspirin and discontinuation of oral contraceptives. Treat glaucoma (cyclodiode is useful for neovascular glaucoma).

Arrange panretinal photocoagulation for neovascularization. Consider macular grid laser for patients <50 years with macular oedema and no angiographic evidence of macular ischaemia. Hypertension predisposes to recurrence, so involve the patient's general practitioner.

Alternative therapies Not proven but under review:

- *Laser*: chorioretinal anastomosis.

- *Surgical*: sheathotomy, radial optic neurotomy.

- *Medical*: haemodilution; tissue plasminogen activator; intravitreal steroids.

Follow–up Every 4 weeks for the first 3 months, then as clinically indicated. The Royal College of Ophthalmologists recommend follow-up for 2 years.

Recommended reading The Royal College of Ophthalmologists CRVO guidelines (contact details, p. 710).

Branch Retinal Vein Occlusion

Background Branch retinal vein occlusion (BRVO) occurs 2–3 times more commonly than central retinal vein occlusion (CRVO) but has similar risk factors. The main sequelae are macular oedema and vitreous haemorrhage from disc, and retinal new vessels. BRVO affecting the entire superior or inferior retina (hemicentral vein occlusion) has a higher risk of rubeosis and disc new vessels.

Symptoms Usually painless loss of vision in one eye but may be asymptomatic.

Signs Same as CRVO (see previous page) except for branch distribution (Fig. 10.37). Rubeosis is less common; macular oedema, disc and retinal new vessels, more so.

Classification

- *Ischaemic*: >5 disc areas of ischaemia on fluorescein angiography.

- *Nonischaemic*: <5 disc areas on angiography.

  1. With macular oedema.

  2. With macular ischaemia.

History and examination Similar to CRVO. Fully exclude systemic causes in patients with multiple BRVOs.

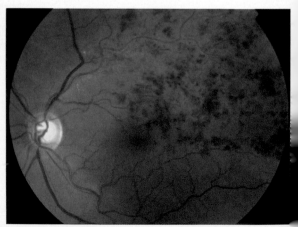

Fig. 10.37: Branch retinal vein occlusion.

Investigations Same as for CRVO.

Treatment Arrange macular laser at 3 months (p. 434) if there is no macular ischaemia and VA remains <6/12 from oedema. Treat neovasculization with scatter retinal laser.

Follow–up The Royal College of Ophthalmologists' (address, p. 710) recommend 3 monthly review for up to 2 years. Nonischaemic or treated BRVO may require less frequent review.

Central Retinal Artery Occlusion

Background Most commonly caused by atheroma, but also heart and carotid emboli, severely raised IOP, arteritis, or rarely vasospasm (retinal migraine).

Symptoms Sudden, painless, unilateral, often severe visual loss.

Signs Acute changes include retinal opacification, whitening, and oedema; cherry-red spot at the macula; RAPD; intra-arteriolar blood column segmentation (box-carring); possible cilioretinal artery sparing. An example is shown on page 446. Disc pallor occurs later.

History and examination Ask about transient ischaemic attacks, cerebrovascular accidents, symptoms of giant cell arteritis, or amaurosis fugax (retinal emboli causing transient uniocular visual obscuration lasting a few minutes). Auscultate the carotids for bruits using the stethoscope bell, check heart sounds for a valvular murmur, and radial pulse for atrial fibrillation. Look for intra-arteriolar calcific, cholesterol, or fibrinoplatelet emboli.

Differential diagnosis See the differential diagnosis of cherry-red spot at the macula (p. 446). Also consider giant cell arteritis, intraocular gentamicin toxicity, and acute ophthalmic artery occlusion.

Investigations Arrange BP; urgent ESR and CRP; blood sugar; FBC; lipids; ANA, rheumatoid factor, serum protein and haemoglobin electrophoresis; thrombophilia screen if suggested by history (p. 471); carotid artery Doppler; fluorescein angiogram and cardiac examination for embolic source. Investigations other than basic blood tests may be best undertaken by a physician.

Treatment If symptoms suggest occlusion for <24 hours duration, attempt to dislodge an embolus by:

- Firm ocular massage through closed eyelids for 15 minutes.

- Stat crushed acetazolamide 500 mg p.o., G. iopidine, and G. beta blocker.

- Offer anterior chamber paracentesis but explain that results are variable. If performed, prescribe G. chloramphenicol q.d.s. one week.

Follow−up Review initially in 2–4 weeks. Examine for iris neovascularization. Perform or review investigations and liaise with relevant clinicians. Advise immediate ophthalmic review if visual obscuration occurs in either eye. Local policies for carotid endarterectomy vary and depend on the degree of carotid occlusion, so discuss with a vascular surgeon.

Branch Retinal Artery Occlusion

Symptoms Unilateral, painless, sudden, visual field loss.

Signs Retinal swelling similar to central retinal artery occlusion (CRAO, previous page), except for branch distribution (Fig. 10.38). Emboli may be present.

Classification

- ▪ Single episode.
- ▪ Multiple episodes: consider systemic disease and urgent medical review.

History, examination, investigations See CRAO, above. Cilioretinal occlusion may occur in the presence of central retinal vein occlusion and is commonly missed. Exclude giant cell arteritis.

Treatment No therapy is of proven value.

Follow–up Initiate medical follow-up as indicated by the investigations. Evaluate for recurrences or new disease in 3–6 months. About 80% of symptomatic cases achieve VA of 6/12 or better.

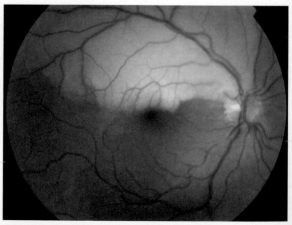

Fig. 10.38: Branch retinal artery occlusion.

Hypertensive Retinopathy

Symptoms Usually asymptomatic, but may have visual loss if there is optic disc swelling or macular oedema.

Signs These include venous deflection and narrowing at arteriovenous crossings; arteriolar narrowing and sclerosis producing altered light reflex (so-called copper and silver wiring); cotton-wool spots; lipid exudates with a macular star if severe (Fig. 10.39); retinal haemorrhage; macular oedema; macroaneurysms; focal choroidal infarctions that can produce acute, yellow, RPE spots; vitreous haemorrhage; retinal vascular occlusions; neovascularization. Retinal detachment, and later hyperpigmentation (Elschnig's spots) may occur in accelerated hypertension.

Classification

- Grade 0: normal.

- Grade 1: barely detectable arteriolar narrowing.

- Grade 2: obvious widespread plus focal arteriolar narrowing, ateriovenous crossing changes.

- Grade 3: retinal haemorrhages or exudates.

- Grade 4: disc swelling.

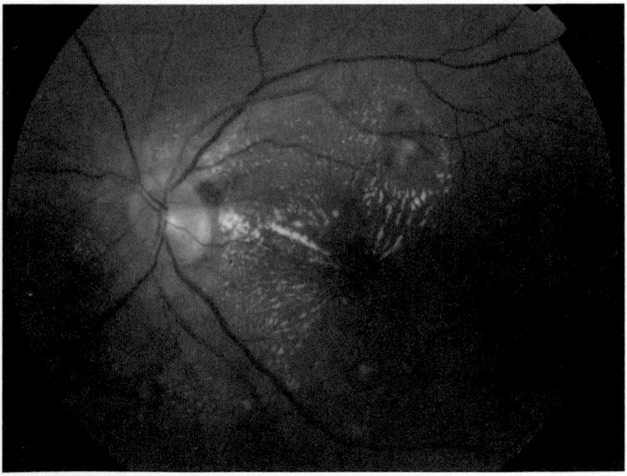

Fig. 10.39: Grade 3 hypertensive retinopathy with macular star.

History and examination Ask about known hypertension, diabetes, radiotherapy, or other systemic disease. Measure BP.

Differential diagnosis Consider diabetic retinopathy; collagen vascular disease; anaemia; retinal vein occlusion and radiation retinopathy.

Treatment Control of hypertension by a physician.

Follow—up Hypertensive retinopathy does not require regular ophthalmic review but concomitant disease may, e.g. retinal vein occlusion.

Macroaneurysm

Background An acquired dilation of the retinal arterioles, most common in late-middle-aged women. Associated with hypertension, embolic disease, and hyperlipidaemia.

Symptoms Blurred vision if the macula is involved.

Signs Arteriolar aneurysm, often with a large haemorrhage, exudation, and surrounding retinal oedema. Usually an isolated finding but bilateral in 10%.

Differential diagnosis Consider diabetic retinopathy; retinal telangiectasia; choroidal tumour; retinal capillary haemangioma; cavernous haemangioma; haemorrhagic age-related macular degeneration.

Investigations Haemorrhage produces masking on fluorescein angiography but otherwise early arterial filling is often seen. Late staining of the aneurysm may occur. Dilated leaking capillaries sometimes surround the aneurysm (Fig. 10.40). ICG may show flow in cases with haemorrhagic masking on FFA. Check BP, lipids, and glucose.

Treatment Many macroaneurysms thrombose and spontaneously involute. Laser photocoagulation may help patients with severe or persistent macular leakage and flow confirmed on angiography, but the evidence is uncertain and there are risks. The laser technique is described on page 437.

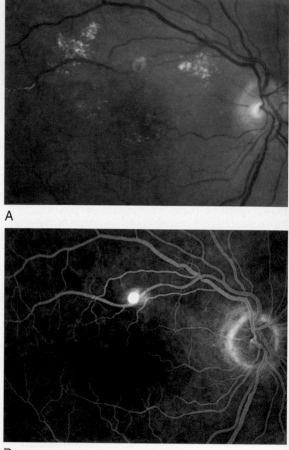

A

B

Fig. 10.40: Macroaneurysm with exudates **(A)**, and hyperfluorescence on angiography **(B)**.

Ocular Ischaemic Syndrome

Background Ocular ischaemia is most commonly secondary to carotid artery atherosclerosis, usually in patients aged >50 years. Less common causes include ophthalmic artery occlusion, carotid aneurysm, giant cell arteritis, and vasospasm.

Symptoms Visual loss (sometimes precipitated by bright light), pain (≈40%), and transient visual obscuration (10% have coexisting carotid emboli).

Signs

- Reduced VA

- *Anterior segment*: rubeosis iridis, elevated IOP, anterior chamber flare or cells, and cataract.

- *Posterior segment*: common features are retinal arterial attenuation, venous dilatation, retinal haemorrhages, disc neovascularization, and cherry-red spot at the macula. Others include retinal neovascularization, microaneurysms, cotton-wool spots, vitreous haemorrhage, and spontaneous arterial pulsations (spontaneous venous pulsations are normal).

History Ask about cardiovascular risk factors and features of giant cell arteritis.

Examination Check BP, blood sugar, and temporal arteries. Perform digital ophthalmodynamometry by lightly pressing on the upper lid whilst viewing the proximal retinal arteries; reduced perfusion pressure causes the arteries to pulsate.

Differential diagnosis For the causes of rubeosis iridis, retinal haemorrhages, neovascularization, and cherry-red spot at the macula, see pages 440–447. Specifically, consider retinal vein or artery occlusion, diabetic retinopathy, and giant cell arteritis.

Investigations Fluorescein angiography shows patchy choroidal filling and increased retinal and choroidal transit times (normal values, p. 419), vascular staining, and macular oedema in some cases. Carotid artery ultrasound usually shows >90% obstruction.

Management Discuss >60% carotid stenosis with a vascular surgeon. Note IOP may rise if subsequent endarterectomy improves ciliary body perfusion. Ask the patient's GP to manage any cardiovascular risk factors. Consider panretinal photocoagulation for disc, retinal, or iris new vessels. Inflammation is typically just mild flare and does not require treatment, but consider topical steroids if there are cells or discomfort. In eyes with visual potential, consider brimonidine as a first-line treatment of raised IOP due to its possible neuroprotective effect. Cyclodiode is sometimes required if topical therapy fails.

Juxtafoveal Telangiectasia (Parafoveal Telangiectasia)

Background A condition in which the parafoveal capillaries have irregular, sacular dilatations, and very occasionally capillary obliteration. Typically presents at age 40–60 years. Also called parafoveal telangiectasia.

Classification Classified into four groups (Table 10.1). Group 2 is the most common and is characterised by 'right-angle' capillaries, opaque perifoveal retina, inner retinal crystals, and RPE hyperpigmentation that may simulate adult Best's disease.

Examination Full ocular examination including retinal periphery. Check BP.

Differential diagnosis See page 443.

Investigations

- *Fluorescein angiography*: Features include: telangiectatic vessels; outer retinal hyperfluorescence; RPE hyperpigmentation that may mask choroidal fluorescence. An example is shown on page 445 (Fig. 10.19). Choroidal neovascular membranes sometimes occur in Group 2.

- *Blood glucose*: reported associated with diabetes and the features may appear similar.

- *Electrophysiology*: if Best's disease is suspected.

Treatment Laser is not proven and is only considered in cases with visually significant exudates and oedema that can be treated without applying laser to the foveal avascular zone. This is more likely to help in Group 1 disease.

Juxtafoveal telangiectasia (parafoveal telangiectasia)

Table 10.1: Classification of juxtafoveal telangiectasia (parafoveal telangiectasia)

Classification	Description	Usual site of perifoveal telangiectasia	Typical clinical features
Group 1A	Unilateral congenital	Temporal	Macular oedema and exudates may significantly reduce acuity
Group 1B	Unilateral idiopathic	Limited to edge of the foveal avascular zone	Limited leakage with good acuity
Group 2	Bilateral acquired	Temporal or more extensive	Mild macular oedema. Acuity mildly reduced.
Group 3	Bilateral idiopathic with capillary obliteration	Entire perifoveal region	Enlarged foveal avascular zone with severe visual loss

Sickle Cell Retinopathy

Background Different mutations in the beta-haemoglobin gene produce either HbC or HbS, and subsequently homozygous HbSS (sickle cell disease), HbSC (sickle cell haemoglobin C disease), and HbAS (sickle trait). Patients with HbSC are at higher risk of eye disease than those with HbSS.

Clinical features

▪ *Conjunctiva*: dark-red, comma-shaped vessels particularly in the inferior bulbar conjunctiva.

▪ *Iris*: focal iris atrophy and neovascularization.

▪ *Angle*: sickled red blood cells in the anterior chamber can elevate the IOP. Many clinicians avoid or minimize the use of mannitol or acetazolamide in sickle patients, particularly those with intraocular haemorrhage, as this may theoretically increase sickling via dehydration and acidosis. Despite the theoretical risk, there are very few clinical reports of acetazolamide producing a sickle crisis.

▪ *Retina*:

1. Angiod streaks.

2. Focal collections of superficial or pretinal haemorrhage that are initially bright red but degrade to form a 'salmon-patch haemorrhage'. Residual haemosiderin may produce refractile bodies (iridescent spots) and secondary RPE migration may leave intraretinal pigment (Fig. 10.41).

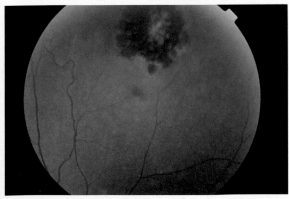

Fig. 10.41: Black sunburst (intraretinal pigment) in sickle cell retinopathy.

3. *Vessels*: increased tortuosity, silver wiring, central and branch retinal artery occlusion, microhaemorrhages, peripheral ischaemia and vascular loops, enlargement of the foveal avascular zone, macular ischaemia and thinning. Retinopathy is classified as:

   a. Stage I: peripheral ischaemia.

   b. Stage II: peripheral anastomoses that do not leak fluorescein.

   c. Stage III: sea fan peripheral neovascularization that leaks fluorescein (Fig. 10.42).

   d. Stage IV: vitreous haemorrhage.

   e. Stage V: tractional and/or rhegmatogenous retinal detachment.

■ *Choroid*: vaso-occlusion that may produce secondary RPE and outer retinal damage.

Differential diagnosis For causes of neovascularization, see page 440.

Investigations Test sickle status, if this is not known. Consider fluorescein angiography and angioscopy if retinal neovascularization is suspected. Angioscopy utilizes intravenous fluorescein and an ophtalmoscope with a blue filter to detect peripheral leakage not visible on a fundus camera.

Treatment Although some clinicians advocate scatter photocoagulation (0.2 seconds, 500 μm spot size, grey-white burns, one burn width apart) in the area of nonperfusion for problematic stage III disease, this is rarely required, as many sea fans autoinfarct.

Follow–up The value of regular review in those who are asymptomatic is doubtful. Vitreous haemorrhage requires 2–4 weekly retinal ultrasounds if the fundus view cannot exclude retinal detachment. Refer for possible vitrectomy if there is nonclearing vitreous haemorrhage (within 3–6 months), tractional macular elevation (within 1 month), or rhegmatogenous retinal detachment (same day).

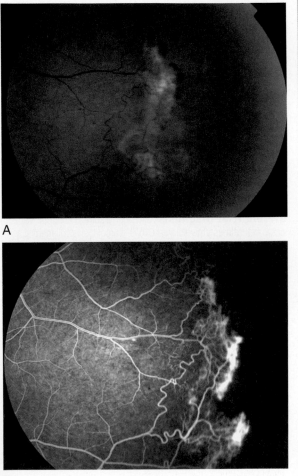

A

B
Fig. 10.42: Stage III sickle cell retinopathy.

Eales' Disease

Background Rare, idiopathic, occlusive, peripheral vasculitis typically affecting healthy adults aged 20–30 years. More common in India and the Middle East.

Clinical features Common retinal features are vascular sheathing (venous > arterial), haemorrhage, peripheral ischaemia (collaterals, neovascularization, vascular tortuosity, sclerosed vessels), and vitreous haemorrhage. Rubeotic glaucoma, disc new vessels, macular oedema, branch retinal vein occlusion (BRVO), macular holes, and tractional or rhegmatogenous retinal detachment may occur. Vitritis and anterior uveitis are mild or absent. The disease is usually bilateral although often asymmetric at presentation (Fig. 10.43).

Differential diagnosis Consider diabetic retinopathy, sickle cell retinopathy, isolated BRVO, sarcoidosis, collagen vascular diseases, and Coats' disease.

Investigation Fluorescein angiography shows vascular staining and leakage. Other tests are chosen as indicated to exclude other disease, e.g. glucose, sickle testing, ANA, sACE, CXR.

Treatment Scatter photocoagulation in areas of ischaemia may lead to regression of neovascularization. Refer nonclearing vitreous haemorrhage or retinal detachment for possible vitrectomy.

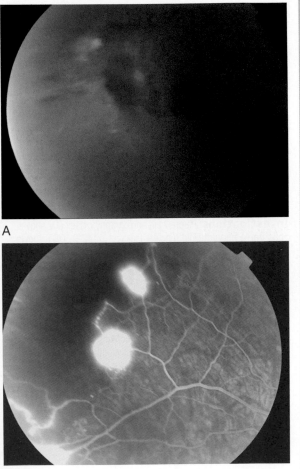

A

B
Fig. 10.43: Eales' disease.

Pseudophakic Macular Oedema (Irvine-gass Syndrome)

Background Macular oedema occurring 1–12 months after cataract extraction. Thought to be caused by inflammation, although anterior chamber activity is typically mild or absent. More common if surgery is complicated by vitreous loss (10–20% versus 1%).

Symptoms Initially good VA, then gradual central blurring.

Signs Macular oedema, often cystic.

History and examination Exclude diabetes, uveitis, retinitis pigmentosa, vitreous traction, and retained vitreous lens material as contributory factors.

Investigations Fluorescein angiography classically shows optic nerve and petalloid macular leakage (p. 422). OCT shows macular thickening (p. 447).

Management The evidence base is poor but consider G. ketorolac (Acular) 0.5% and G. dexamethasone 0.1%, both q.d.s. for 2 months then taper over 1 month. Reinstate if the oedema recurs when treatment is discontinued. If oedema persists after 3 months, add acetazolamide 250 mg s.r. b.d. or triamcinolone (Kenalog) 40 mg as a sub-Tenon's injection (avoid if steroid responder). Trials of intravitreal triamcinolone are in progress. Surgically relieve any anterior or posterior chamber vitreous traction.

Follow–up Two monthly whilst on treatment.

Central Serous Retinopathy

Symptoms Patients with central serous retinopathy (CSR) may complain of blurred central vision, slow recovery from bright light, scotomata and distortion. Symptoms are usually unilateral. The typical patient is male, 30–50 years old, with a type A personality.

Signs These include serous detachment of the sensory retina in the macular area, sometimes with pigment epithelial detachment (Fig. 10.44). Detachment may be difficult to detect in chronic disease.

Classification Acute, chronic, and recurrent.

History and examination Ask about previous episodes, refractive change (increased hyperopia from retinal elevation) and risk factors (pregnancy; local or systemic corticosteroid use; hypertension; emotional stress; allergic respiratory disease). An Amsler grid appears distorted. Previous episodes may leave bilateral atrophic RPE changes in either eye and in chronic disease VA may be poor. Choroidal neovascularization occurs in 3–4%.

Differential diagnosis Consider idiopathic polypoidal choroidal vasculopathy (IPCV), pigment epithelial detachment, optic disc pit, peripheral choroidal tumour, rhegmatogenous retinal detachment, age-related macular degeneration, choroidal inflammation, and idiopathic choroidal effusion.

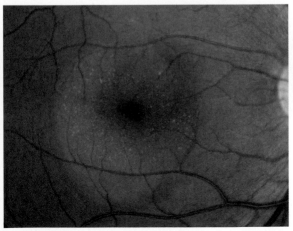

Fig. 10.44: Central serous retinopathy.

Investigations Fluorescein angiography shows 'smoke-stack' (Fig. 10.45) or more commonly 'ink-blot' leakage (Fig. 10.4); test refraction; measure ocular length (A-scan ultrasound); consider cortisol level in some cases. In chronic CSR, angiography

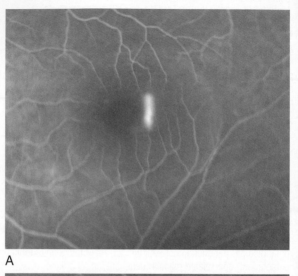

A

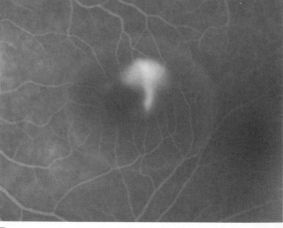

B

Fig. 10.45: Central serous retinopathy with a 'smoke-stack' seen in an early **(A)** and later **(B)** fluorescein angiogram.

shows diffuse hyperfluorescence. If the diagnosis is in doubt, ICG angiography may help by showing choroidal hyperfluorescence at a site of normality on fluorescein angiography, and also excludes IPCV.

Treatment Most acute cases resolve spontaneously within 4 months, so observe. Approximately 85% of acute cases retain 6/6 VA, but 30–50% recur. Recurrent or chronic cases have a worse prognosis. Advise against corticosteroid use if possible. Argon laser treatment of a single leaking focus reduces the interval to recovery but does not change the long-term visual prognosis and may risk choroidal neovascularization. Chronic CSR has been treated with macular grid laser and photodynamic therapy although the benefit is unproven at present.

Follow-up 3–6 monthly until resolved.

Retinitis Pigmentosa

Background Retinitis pigmentosa (RP) is a group of rod–cone dystrophies with heterogeneous modes of inheritance and variable clinical phenotypes, age of onset and severity. Key features are night-blindness (nyctalopia), visual field loss, and bone-spicule retinal pigmentation.

Classification

■ By inheritance.

1. Autosomal recessive (AR): 60% of cases.

2. Autosomal dominant (AD): 10–25% of cases.

3. X-linked (XL): 5–18% of cases.

■ By phenotype: e.g. sector RP, paravenous, adult onset.

History Ask about: nyctalopia; VA; glare; field loss; visual requirements (driving); consanguinity and associated systemic disorders, especially congenital deafness (Usher's syndrome), anosmia (Refsum's syndrome), and polydactyly (Bardet-Biedl syndrome).

Examination Exclude associated changes: myopia; cataracts; glaucoma; vitreous cells; macular oedema; cellophane maculopathy; peripheral telangiectasia. Localized loss of the red colour of the fundus occurs in early disease. Bone-spicules occur in well-established disease. Unlike most fundal pigment changes, they are intraretinal; confirm that they obscure the underlying retinal vessels. Also note their topographical distribution or photograph. Advanced disease shows retinal vessel attenuation, RPE atrophy, and disc pallor (Fig. 10.46).

Examine family members to determine the inheritance pattern. Draw a family pedigree (p. 412). Consider AR inheritance if both parents are normal, more than one sibling is affected (particularly a female), or there is consanguinity. X-linked female carriers may show bone-spicules, altered (tapetal) retinal reflex, and ERG changes. Isolated cases (simplex or sporadic RP) occur in approximately 40% but many are probably unconfirmed AR.

Differential diagnosis consider glaucoma with normal RPE pigmentary changes; normal reticular changes; syphilis; rubella; drug toxicity; cancer associated retinopathy; trauma; congenital hypertrophy of the RPE (CHRPE); 'bear-track' RPE hypertrophy; diffuse unilateral subacute neuroretinitis; female choroideremia carriers. White RPE changes can occur or even

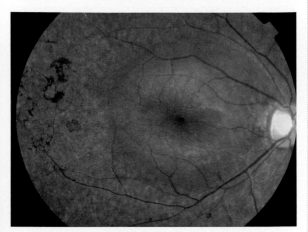

Fig. 10.46: Retinitis pigmentosa.

predominate (retinitis punctata albescens), appearing similar to fundus albipunctatus, a less progressive condition sometimes classified under RP or congenital stationary night blindness.

Rare metabolic disorders with pigmentary retinopathy include:

- *Bardet-Biedl syndrome*: AR cone–rod dystrophy with corneal thinning (uncommon), polydactyly, hypogonadism, obesity, cognitive deficiency, and renal disease.

- *Bassen-Kornzweig syndrome* (abetalipoproteinaemia, acanthocytosis): presents in infancy with altered fat and vitamin A metabolism with strabismus, neuromuscular disturbance, ataxia, and fat intolerance.

- *Batten's disease* (neuronal ceroid lipofuscinosis, 'amaurotic idiocy'): AR or AD disease with lipopigment accumulation in neural tissue. Produces bull's-eye maculopathy with global loss of ERG responses, negative ERG, mental deterioration, ataxia, seizures, and early death.

- *Gyrate atrophy*: see page 501.

- *Homocystinuria*: an AR deficiency of homocysteine breakdown with myopia, ectopia lentis, glaucoma, optic atrophy, CNS and vascular disease.

- *Kearns-Sayre syndrome*: a mitochondrial DNA deletion with progressive external ophthalmoplegia before age 20 years, short stature, heart block, neuromuscular weakness, ataxia, deafness, cognitive deficiency, diabetes, and

hypoparathyroidism. Regular cardiac review is
recommended.

■ *Oxalosis*: A metabolic AR disorder that produces oxalate
deposition with optic atrophy, RPE changes, retinal vascular
obstruction, renal, bone, and vascular disease.

■ *Refsum's disease*: AR elevation of phytanic acid with cataract,
anosmia, ectopia lentis, glaucoma, polyneuritis, and ataxia.

Investigations

■ *Electroretinography*: usually shows a markedly reduced or
extinguished response. Scotopic amplitudes ≥100 mV suggest
a better prognosis.

■ *Goldmann visual field test*: initial field loss is variable, but
classically bilateral, symmetric, and midperipheral, with central
vision preserved until late.

■ *Estermann driving fields*: for legal requirements see page 688.

■ *Fluorescein angiography*: avoid if possible, as extremely
uncomfortable.

■ *OCT*: may confirm macular oedema.

■ *Fundus autofluorescence*: quantifies macular atrophy if it is
clinically uncertain.

■ *Syphilis serology*: in doubtful cases.

■ *Genetic testing*: is available for a growing number of inherited
diseases.

Management RP requires specialized support. Advise drivers
of their obligation to inform the licensing authority (p. 710).
Consider:

■ Low-vision aids and sunglasses.

■ Blind or partial sight registration.

■ Cataract surgery. Use low illumination and an IOL with a low
risk of posterior capsular opacification and phimosis.

■ Acetazolamide sometimes reduces macular oedema. Try
250 mg modified release once daily for 2 weeks and increase
to 250 mg b.d. if no improvement. Discontinue treatment if
there is still no effect after a further 2 weeks.

■ Counselling, once the diagnosis and likely inheritance pattern
have been established. Misinformation may profoundly affect
work and family planning, so involve experienced staff. In
general, those with sector RP maintain good VA, and AD RP

has a better prognosis than AR or XL RP. For patient information see, http://www.rcophth.ac.uk/scientific/publications.html

- Provide contact details of support groups, e.g. British RP Society (p. 710).

- The future role of gene therapy and retinal/RPE transplantation is uncertain.

- Arrange yearly review.

Cone Dystrophy

Classification

■ *Stationary*: may show only subtle alteration in colour vision, anomalous trichromacy, or rod monochromacy.

■ *Progressive*: includes several conditions: blue cone monochromacy; pure cone degeneration; cone–rod degenerations; benign concentric annular dystrophy; cone dystrophy with supernormal ERG.

■ *Systemic disease*: may coexist with several systemic disorders, including many of the metabolic diseases associated with retinitis pigmentosa (p. 496).

■ *Toxic*: chloroquine, digoxin.

History and examination Ask about VA, colour vision, and problems with bright light. Some forms show mendelian inheritance (usually autosomal recessive), so examine family members and draw a family pedigree (p. 412). Check colour vision with Ishihara plates and, if abnormal, consider Farnsworth-Munsell 100-hue test. Fundoscopy may be normal, but the characteristic finding is macular atrophy or bull's-eye maculopathy (p. 450).

Investigations Electrophysiology shows cone dysfunction with absent or mild rod involvement.

Management Offer counselling with senior staff, low-vision aids, sunglasses or tinted contact lenses, and blind or partial sight registration, as appropriate. No treatment exists at present.

Follow–up Yearly if patient wishes.

Gyrate Atrophy

Background An autosomal recessive defect of the mitochondrial enzyme ornithine aminotransferase produces hyperornithaemia. Extraocular features tend to be absent or subtle.

Symptoms Typically, night blindness (nyctalopia) occurs in childhood or teens, with loss of visual field and central acuity in later life.

Signs Chorioretinal atrophy with a scalloped border (Fig. 10.47).

History and examination Draw a family pedigree (p. 412). Exclude associated high myopia and presenile cataract.

Differential diagnosis Consider choroideremia, high myopia, and thioridazine retinopathy.

Investigations Measure serum ornithine, monocular and Estermann driving fields. The ERG and EOG are both abnormal. Fluorescein angiography is not required but shows hyperfluorescence in the affected areas, with leakage at the borders of unaffected retina.

Management Offer counselling with a senior clinician, yearly review, low-vision aids, and blind or partial sight registration as required. Pyridoxine (vitamin B_6) supplementation and reduced dietary protein may lower serum ornithine levels. The impact on visual function is not certain.

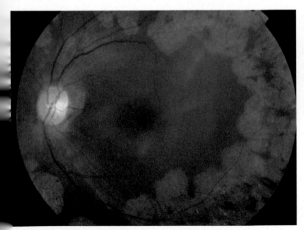

Fig. 10.47: Gyrate atrophy.

Choroideremia

Background X-linked chorioretinal degeneration due to mutations in geranylgeranyl transferase Rab escort protein I.

Symptoms Night blindness (nyctalopia) and visual field loss in young males.

Signs Midperipheral atrophy of the RPE and choriocapillaris with resulting prominence of the choroidal vessels and sclera. Retinal blood vessels are less affected than in retinitis pigmentosa (Fig. 10.48).

History and examination Examine family members and draw a family pedigree (p. 412). Female carriers are generally asymptomatic, but almost invariably show regional irregular fundal pigmentation and patchy RPE atrophy in later life.

Differential diagnosis Consider retinitis pigmentosa, gyrate atrophy, albinism and thioridazine retinopathy.

Investigations Arrange Estermann driving fields if relevant. Fluorescein angiography is rarely needed, but shows reduced background fluorescence and prominent choroidal vessels caused by RPE and choriocapillaris atrophy. Electrophysiology may initially be normal, but marked abnormalities usually develop.

Management Offer genetic counselling with an experienced clinician, annual review, low-vision aids and blind or partial sight registration. No treatment is currently available. The condition is usually slowly progressive with late macular involvement.

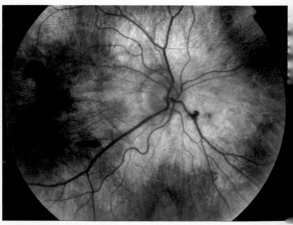

Fig. 10.48: Choroideremia.

Best's Disease

Background Autosomal dominant macular dystrophy due to mutations in the UMOZ gene.

Symptoms May be asymptomatic or present in childhood or teens with poor central acuity.

Signs The macula may appear normal or show variable, evolving vitelliform changes described as egg-yolk, scrambled egg, pseudohypopyon, and then atrophy (Fig. 10.49). Choroidal neovascularization sometimes occurs.

History and examination Examine family members and draw a family pedigree (p. 412). Inheritance has variable penetrance, so affected relatives may be asymptomatic and have subtle signs, although the electro-oculogram (EOG) abnormality is seen in all those with the mutant gene.

Differential diagnosis Consider central serous retinopathy, pigment epithelial detachment, toxoplasma, and other causes of macular atrophy (p. 448).

Investigations Reduced light-induced rise of the EOG is diagnostic. Fluorescein angiography shows hypofluorescence initially (blockage from vitelliform material), and hyperfluorescence if RPE atrophy occurs. Testing for the affected Bestrophin gene is

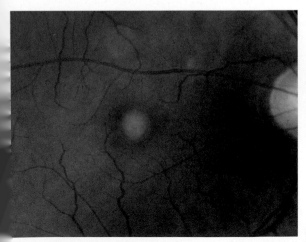

Fig. 10.49: Best's disease.

now possible. Consider fundus autofluorescence if available. This shows decreased signal from the pale material.

Management Offer genetic counselling with a senior clinician and annual review. No treatment exists at present.

Pattern Dystrophy

Background An autosomal dominant macular disease.

Symptoms May have paracentral distortion, loss of VA or may be asymptomatic.

Signs The macula may show a pale subretinal or pigmented deposit at the fovea or in a linear distribution (Fig. 10.50). With time, central atrophy may occur. Choroidal neovascularization is rare.

History and examination Examine family members and draw a family pedigree (p. 412). Although autosomal dominant, there is variable expression and incomplete penetrance, so affected relatives may be asymptomatic and signs subtle.

Differential diagnosis Consider central serous retinopathy, Best's disease and age-related macular degeneration.

Investigations Autofluorescence imaging (if available) is helpful and shows hyper-autofluorescence of the fundal lesions. Genetic testing is possible (RDS gene).

Management Offer genetic counselling with a senior clinician and annual review. No treatment exists at present.

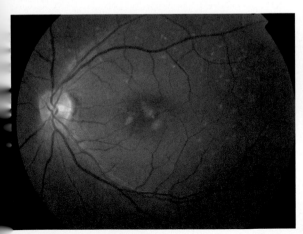

Fig. 10.50: Pattern dystrophy.

Stargardt's Disease

Background A common autosomal recessive (AR) disease with yellow RPE flecks (fundus flavimaculatus) plus macular atrophy due to mutations in the ABCA4 gene. The carrier rate is high so children may be affected (pseudo-dominance).

Symptoms Poor central vision in childhood or teens is most common, but patients may present later in life.

Signs May be normal initially, but the macula develops 'beaten-bronze' appearance or expanding atrophy, surrounded by yellow flecks. 'Salt-and-pepper' peripheral pigmentation may occur later (Fig. 10.51).

Differential diagnosis Exclude other causes of macular atrophy (p. 448), especially cone dystrophy. The yellow flecks have a more patterned appearance than drusen. Unlike retinitis punctata albescens, the visual field, vessels, and discs are minimally affected. Fundus albipunctatus is an AR disease with nyctalopia and smaller white dots throughout the fundus. VA is normal.

Investigations The pattern electroretinogram (PERG) is abnormal in all cases, the full field ERG is abnormal in 15%, and the electro-oculogram in 2.5%. Fluorescein angiography classically shows a dark choroid with hyperfluorescent flecks, but not always. Fundus autofluorescence helps quantify

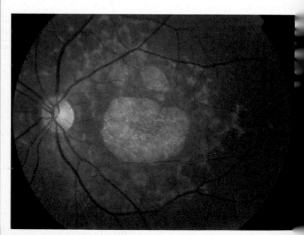

Fig. 10.51: Stargart's disease.

RPE damage. The yellow flecks are hyper-autofluorescent. Genetic testing is possible but not widely available.

Management Offer counselling with senior staff, blind or partial sight registration, low-vision aids, and annual review. There is no treatment.

North Carolina Macular Dystrophy

Background An autosomal dominant macular dystrophy with variable expressivity. The gene locus is known.

Symptoms May be asymptomatic or present in childhood with poor central acuity.

Signs The macula characteristically shows well-defined atrophy centred on the fovea with hyperpigmented edges, often with remarkably good VA (Fig. 10.52). In some patients changes are limited to fine, densely packed, drusen-like deposits in the central 3 degrees.

History and examination Examine family members and draw a family pedigree (p. 412). Although autosomal dominant, affected relatives may be asymptomatic and signs subtle.

Differential diagnosis Consider macular dystrophies with atrophy.

Investigations Colour photography.

Management Offer genetic counselling with a senior clinician, annual review, and low-vision aids. No treatment exists at present.

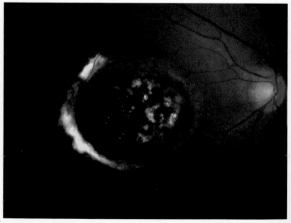

Fig. 10.52: North Carolina Macular Dystrophy.

Albinism

Background A genetic disorder of melanin production.

Classification

- Ocular.
- Oculocutaneous.
  1. Tyrosinase-negative.
  2. Tyrosinase-positive.
- Albinoidism.

Symptoms Photophobia and blurred vision.

Signs Although highly variable, signs are generally most severe in tyrosinase-negative individuals, intermediate in tyrosinase-positive and ocular cases, and mildest in albinoidism. Features include VA loss, nystagmus, strabismus, refractive errors, iris transillumination, pale fundus, foveal and optic nerve hypoplasia, and misrouting of fibres in the optic chiasm. Skin pigmentation is variable in ocular albinism.

History and examination Draw a family tree (p. 412) and examine family members. Ocular albinism is commonly X-linked but sometimes autosomal recessive. Female carriers may show mild iris and characteristic fundus changes (Fig. 10.53). Oculocutaneous cases are usually autosomal recessive. In tyrosinase-positive patients ask about recurrent infections (Chediak-Higashi syndrome) and bleeding/bruising problems (Hermanski-Pudlak syndrome).

Investigations Consider electrophysiology (p. 428), neuroimaging, tyrosinase testing, FBC, and coagulation. Prenatal (intrauterine) testing is possible.

Management Arrange genetic counselling with an experienced clinician, and low-vision aids if required. Albinos have an increased risk of basal and squamous cell carcinomas, so refer to dermatology if suspected. Refer patients with immunocompromise or bleeding diathesis to haematology.

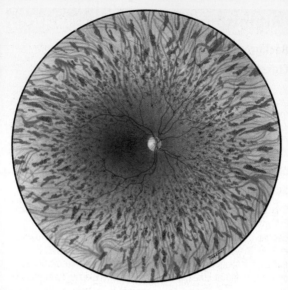

Fig. 10.53: Albinism-female carrier (Courtesy of
P Leaver/PM Sullivan. Artwork T. Tarrant).

Syphilis

Background A sexually transmitted infection caused by the spirochaete *Treponema pallidum*. Mother-to-child transmission can also result in congenital infection.

Classification and systemic features

- *Primary*: genital ulcer (chancre).

- *Secondary*: lymphadenopathy, rash, mucous membrane lesions, meningitis.

- *Latent*: no clinical manifestation. May last for many years.

- *Tertiary*: cardiovascular disease (aortitis, aortic regurgitation, angina), neurosyphilis (myelopathy, mental changes), systemic gummata (fibrous deposits).

Signs Ocular disease may occur at any stage. Primary infection may rarely present with a chancre on the eyelid. Signs of secondary and tertiary infection include oculomotor palsies, madarosis (loss of eyelashes), conjunctivitis, interstitial keratitis, episcleritis, scleritis, glaucoma, Argyll Robertson pupil (light-near dissociation), field loss, uveitis, chorioretinitis, choroidal ischaemia, periarteritis, neuroretinitis, and optic neuritis. Late changes may mimic retinitis pigmentosa with paravascular retinal pigment, vascular attenuation, and pale discs. Congenital syphilis classically produces interstitial keratitis and pigmentary retinopathy.

Investigations

- *VDRL*: this measures antiphospolipid antibody levels and is not specific to syphilis. Never use VDRL as the sole screening test as false positives occur in a variety of conditions including connective tissue diseases and pregnancy. VDRL is valuable for monitoring treatment as the titres are high in active disease and fall with effective therapy.

- *FTA-ABS, MHA-TP or TPHA*: these tests all measure specific antitreponemal antibody levels and in most patients they remain positive for life, even after effective therapy. Other treponemes (including yaws) give positive results, as occasionally do other spirochaetes (Lyme disease).

Management Refer to an infectious disease consultant for systemic treatment (often high-dose penicillin). In many countries, syphilis is a notifiable disease. In at-risk individuals, consider referral for HIV testing, as this may coexist. Topical steroids may be required for ocular inflammation. Only consider systemic steroids after full investigation and treatment of any underlying infection.

Solar Retinopathy

Background Foveal phototoxicity secondary to sun-gazing.

History Ask about predisposing factors, such as recreational drug use, mydriatic or photosensitizing medications, e.g. tetracycline, use of condensing lenses, e.g. telescopes, and viewing a solar eclipse.

Symptoms Blurred vision, scotoma, chromatopsia, metamorphopsia and afterimage.

Signs VA is usually 6/12 to 1/60 acutely with reduced near acuity and Amsler grid changes. Fundoscopy reveals a uni- or bilateral yellowish foveal lesion, sometimes with a grey annulus (Fig. 10.54). This fades over a week, leaving a small, well-defined, deep red spot which persists for life, or rarely mild RPE changes. Recovery of VA is usual. A national UK survey following a solar eclipse suggested most cases resolve.

Differential diagnosis Consider Best's disease, cone dystrophy; light-damage from an operating microscope, central serous retinopathy, age-related macular degeneration, and toxic retinopathy. For other causes of macular atrophy see page 448.

Investigations Fluorescein angiography is often normal.

Treatment Systemic steroids and antioxidants (ginko glycosides) have been used, but the evidence is not clear.

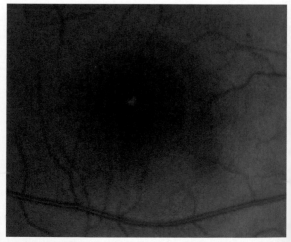

Fig. 10.54: Solar retinopathy.

Toxic Retinopathies

Chloroquine and hydroxychoroquine

Symptoms Blurred vision, abnormal colour vision and scotomas.

Signs

- *Reversible*: whorl-like corneal epithelial changes (verticillata) and abnormal foveal reflex.

- *Irreversible*: fine granular macula appearance (Fig. 10.55). 'Bull's-eye' maculopathy is the only sign associated with impaired VA and central visual field disturbance.

History and examination Determine the dose and duration of treatment. Test near and distance acuity, macular function (Amsler grid), colour vision, and visual field. Use a red pin to detect central scotoma or colour desaturation. Examine the cornea on a slit lamp for verticillata and perform dilated fundoscopy.

Differential diagnosis

- *Granular macular changes*: age-related macular degeneration (AMD).

- *'Bull's-eye' maculopathy*: retinal dystrophies such as cone dystrophy, Stargardt's disease, and benign concentric annular macular dystrophy can usually by differentiated by drug and family history and electrodiagnostic testing. Consider also AMD, and lipofuscinosis (usually presents in childhood).

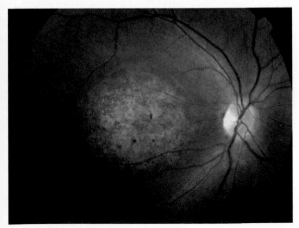

Fig. 10.55: Chloroquine retinopathy.

Treatment Stop medication if toxicity develops.

Follow–up For routine screening in cases without macular damage, arrange the following follow up:

- *Chloroquine*: 6–12 months depending on local protocol.

- *Hydroxychloroquine*: toxicity is rare at normal doses not exceeding 6.5 mg/kg/day unless there is impaired renal/hepatic function. Patients should be monitored yearly by a physician or optometrist who should enquire about visual symptoms, and recheck near and distance VA. Arrange ophthalmology review if a baseline assessment by the physician/optometrist is abnormal, or if the patient develops change in acuity or blurred vision (as assessed by reading chart) whilst on treatment.

Desferrioxamine (Deferoxamine)

Symptoms Decreased vision, scotomata, nyctalopia, photopsia, metamorphopsia, and hearing loss. Acute toxicity occurs typically 7–10 days post-i.v. infusion.

Signs May appear normal early in the course of the disease despite positive symptoms. Signs are usually bilateral, including irregular outer retina/RPE pigmentation, RPE hypopigmentation, and granularity (late phase). May involve just the macula or the entire retina. Disc swelling and optic atrophy are reported.

Investigations Arrange visual fields. Fluorescein angiography shows a variable mottled appearance with blocked fluorescence in the transit phase and late hyperfluorescence, even in the presence of a normal-appearing retina. Electroretinogram, electro-oculogram, and visually evoked potential may all be affected.

Treatment Discontinue deferoxamine if possible.

Follow–up Visual recovery is possible over 3–4 months. Damage may be more common in the presence of an abnormal blood–retina barrier, e.g. diabetes.

Phenothiazines (thioridazine and chlorpromazine)

Symptoms Blurred vision, abnormal colour vision (brownish tinge), nyctalopia in the acute form, typically 2–8 weeks after excessive ingestion. The chronic form leads to progressive vision loss and nyctalopia.

Signs

- *Thioridazine*: the fundus may be normal initially, then develop fine to coarse pigmentary retinopathy, usually uniformly in the macula to midperipheral retina (Fig. 10.56). Late stages show nummular area of atrophy and severe diffuse outer retinal degeneration.

- *Chlorpromazine*: mild pigmentary retinal changes, cataract, and corneal deposits.

Differential diagnosis

- *Late atrophy*: gyrate atrophy, Bietti's crystalline dystrophy, syphilis, and choroideremia.

- *Pigmentary retinopathy*: retinitis pigmentosa (p. 496).

Investigation Fluorescein angiography may be helpful in detecting mild RPE abnormalities. The electroretinogram is abnormal.

Treatment Discontinue medication but liaise with psychiatrists.

Follow-up If the thioridazine dosage exceeds 800 mg/day or chlorpromazine dosage exceeds 2400 mg/day, review 6 monthly, otherwise screening is not required.

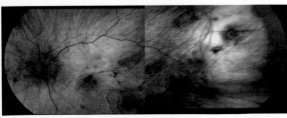

Fig. 10.56: Thioridazine toxicity.

Optometry and General Practice Guidelines

General comments

The most urgent retinal referral is central retinal artery occlusion. It is sometimes possible to dislodge the embolus, but as the period of retinal ischaemia extends, the visual prognosis declines. Visual symptoms are often acute and severe, with patients classically describing a curtain coming over the vision. There may be a history of cardiovascular risk factors. Also consider retinal detachment (p. 556).

Any history of acutely blurred or distorted central vision is worrying. For example, the choroidal neovascularization (CNV) associated with 'wet' age-related macular degeneration (AMD) often produces distortion occurring over a few days, whereas atrophic 'dry' AMD typically has a more insidious onset. The former may require urgent treatment; the latter can be referred routinely.

Beware the absence of acute symptoms in those with good vision in the fellow eye; they may be unaware of monocular blurred vision. Conversely, many patients experience a chronic decline in monocular vision as an acute symptom, when for some reason the better eye is covered. A careful history may help.

Optometrists

Dilate and carefully examine patients with suspected AMD. Any macular elevation or haemorrhage suggests a CNV, so refer to hospital that day. CNV occasionally occur in patients under 50 years, but there is often other eye disease, e.g. high myopia. In younger patients consider central serous retinopathy. Retinal elevation (sometimes subtle) may cause a small hypermetropic shift, so VA may improve with a +1 dioptre add.

General practice

Dilated fundoscopy by an optometrist will uncover many retinal diseases and is a useful means of triage for all except the most urgent referrals. Serious drug-induced toxic maculopathies are relatively uncommon, but, if referring, detail the drug dose and duration. Hydroxychloroquine is much safer than chloroquine (p. 513). Monitor cardiovascular risk factors in patients diagnosed with retinal artery or vein occlusion. Studies show that smokers are more likely to get sight-threatening AMD, and diabetics with poor glucose control are more likely to lose vision. Encourage near relatives to accompany patients referred to hospital with suspected inherited disease, e.g. retinitis pigmentosa.

The following guidelines for hospital referral urgency are not prescriptive, as clinical situation vary. In particular, macular disease with an uncertain diagnosis should be referred urgently.

Immediate

Same day

Urgent (within 1 week)

Soon (within 1 month)

Routine

Chapter 11
SURGICAL RETINA

Indirect Ophthalmoscopy

Indirect ophthalmoscopy takes time to master.

1. Explain the procedure to the patient.

2. Ensure the patient is lying supine on a single pillow, eyes well dilated. Provide enough space to move to either side and behind the patient's head. Instil local anaesthetic in both eyes. Turn off the room lights.

3. Put on the indirect headpiece and adjust the tension band so that it will not move when your head is tilted. Adjust the interpupillary distance to give a single image.

4. View the red reflex then interpose a 20 D lens into the light path. Some lenses have a white circular marking on the metal frame. This side of the lens should face the patient. When learning, and for difficult examinations such as children or those with small pupils, a 28 D lens is easier to use but provides lower magnification. Move the lens sideways and anteroposteriorly until the fundal details appear.

5. To increase patient compliance and comfort, start with a peripheral fundal examination using a dim light – avoid bright illumination of the posterior pole.

6. Develop a routine for peripheral fundal examination, e.g. start at 6 o'clock and move clockwise 360°; this makes it easier to remember the position of retinal features. Ask the patient to look in the appropriate direction, for example, towards their feet for inferior peripheral examination. Tilting your head to the side facilitates a more peripheral view.

7. Two indenters are commonly used: Schokett and T-bar. Use a cotton-bud if neither is available. Gently indent the patient's eyelids immediately above the upper tarsus, or below the lower tarsus, until a retinal elevation is visible. Move the indent back and forward and view the retina as it rolls over the apex of the indent. This dynamic examination may open small breaks and the tangential view may reveal small operculated

tears. It is sometimes necessary to gently indent directly on the ocular surface to view the retina at 3 and 9 o'clock.

8. Draw the findings. The image is inverted, so it is helpful to draw the disc and fovea then rotate the paper 180°, and draw as seen. Some surgeons use colour to show the attached (red) and detached (blue) retina (see Fig. 11.6).

Posterior Vitreous Detachment

Background Spontaneous posterior vitreous detachment (PVD) is extremely common, but PVD may also follow eye surgery, trauma, uveitis, or laser. In the majority of cases it causes no serious problem. In others it causes troublesome floaters or retinal tears that can lead to retinal detachment.

Symptoms Photopsia (flashes) commonly in the temporal field, and floaters. Vitreous haemorrhage may reduce VA.

Examination Maximally dilate both eyes. PVD can be difficult to detect but biomicroscopy may show a '*Weiss ring*' of thickened vitreous cortex avulsed from the optic disc (Fig. 11.1). The space behind a PVD is usually optically clear, unlike the condensed vitreous. The detached vitreous face is sometimes visible without a lens, using a slit beam focused in the midvitreous cavity. This fine, crumpled membrane slopes away when viewed top to bottom, and swirls with eye movement. In eyes with no previous surgery check for *Shafer's sign*. Using a bright, thin, slit beam focused into the anterior vitreous (no lens), ask the patient to look up-down-straight ahead. If fine, pigmented cells (tobacco dust) are visible the test is positive (Fig. 11.2). Repeat looking left-right-straight ahead. The test may help exclude a break; only 8% of eyes with retinal breaks are Shafer negative. If positive, arrange urgent vitreoretinal review, even if no break is found.

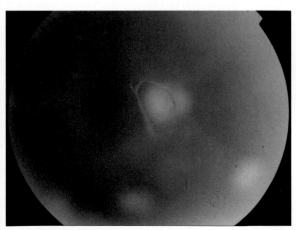

Fig. 11.1: Weiss ring.

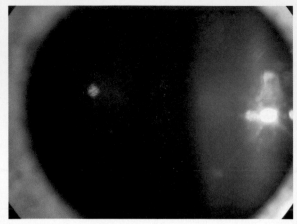

Fig. 11.2: Anterior vitreous pigment cells (tobacco dust).

Document 360° indented, indirect ophthalmoscopy. Examination with a three-mirror is easier but may miss peripheral breaks. It is only appropriate if the attending clinician is not confident with indentation.

Investigations Ultrasound if the fundal view is inadequate to exclude a retinal break.

Management PVD does not usually require treatment. Advise patients that floaters will tend to become less troublesome and may ultimately disappear. Very occasionally, persistent floaters are treated with vitrectomy.

Follow−up Discharge with a documented *retinal detachment warning*: if the patient notices any sudden change or worsening of floaters, flashes, or any visual field defect they should return immediately. Provide a patient advice sheet.

Retinal Degenerations and Tears

Peripheral retinal degenerations

Background There are several peripheral vitreoretinal degenerations. Some predispose to retinal detachment (RD).

Classification

- *Lattice*: retinal thinning associated with overlying vitreous liquefaction, retinal vascular sclerosis, and abnormally strong vitreoretinal adhesion (Fig. 11.3).

- *Nonlattice*: several peripheral degenerations such as white-without-pressure, snail-track, microcystoid, reticular, and pavingstone.

Management

- *Lattice*: there are three common situations: lattice alone, atrophic round holes in lattice, and lattice associated retinal tears. Retinopexy may be appropriate to reduce the risk of RD (Table 11.1).

- *Nonlattice*: prophylactic treatment is not usually required. Provide all patients with a retinal detachment warning ([RDW] p. 522).

Table 11.1: Treatment of retinal degenerations and tears				
Group	PVD	Incomplete or no PVD	Risk factors such as fellow eye RD	Subretinal fluid*
Lattice degeneration	–	–	±	++
Round holes in lattice	–	–	±	++
Acute flap-shaped tears with or without lattice	+	++	++	++
Fully operculated round hole	–	–	±	++

++, treat virtually all; +, treat most; ±, variable or contentious; –, seldom treat. PVD, posterior vitreous detachment.
*Obtain a same-day vitreoretinal consult as surgery may be indicated

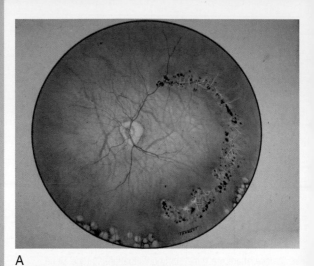

A

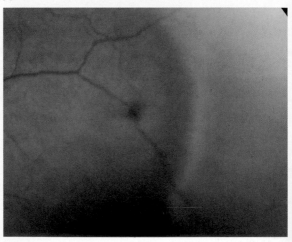

B

Fig. 11.3: **(A)** Lattice degeneration temporally with peripheral paving stone degeneration inferiorly. **(B)** White without pressure. **(C)** Microcystoid. **(D)** Reticular degeneration (Courtesy of P Leaver/PM Sullivan. Artwork T Tarrant).

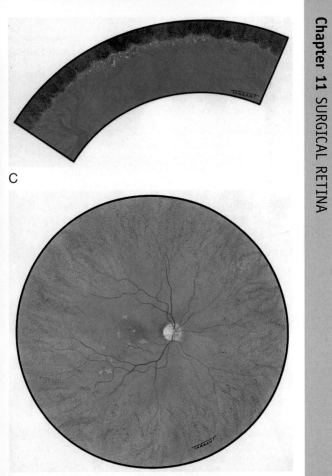

C

D
Fig. 11.3—cont'd.

Retinal breaks

Background Full-thickness defects that usually occur following posterior vitreous detachment (PVD). Their configuration influences the likelihood of subsequent retinal detachment (RD).

Symptoms, signs, and investigations Similar to PVD except Shafer's sign is usually positive (p. 521).

Management See Table 11.1. This outline will be modified by factors such as the break size and position, other ocular disease, patient/clinician preference, and increased pigmentation under break (indicates RPE hyperplasia and chronicity). Provide an RDW.

Retinopexy Two options exist: laser or cryotherapy (Fig. 11.4). If possible, select laser as it is less destructive. Laser safety training is often mandatory. For techniques see Box 11.1 and 11.2.

Consent

- *Benefit*: reduced risk of RD and visual loss.

- *Risk*: failure to prevent RD, re-treatment, visual field defect, accidental macular treatment and visual loss, subsequent distortion from epiretinal membranes (can also occur with untreated retinal breaks).

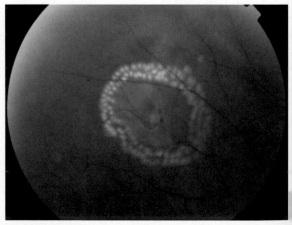

Fig. 11.4: Retinal U-tear with a thin collar of subretinal fluid and fresh laser retinopexy.

Box 11.1: Laser retinopexy

1. Obtain written consent. Warn the patient that they will feel the laser pulse, but try not to move:

2. Connect the argon laser to either the slit lamp or indirect output.

3. Once warmed up, fire a test shot against a nonreflective object.

4. Ensure patient is maximally dilated, in a darkened room, with topical anaesthesia in both eyes. Others in the room require protective goggles.

   Slit-lamp: select the lens that gives the best view, e.g. transequator contact lens or three-mirror. Noncontact lenses (e.g. 90 D) may be used, but require more power and don't stabilize the eye. Select 200 microns spot size; 0.1 seconds.

   Indirect ophthalmoscope with 20 D lens: good for peripheral breaks and allows indentation. Spot size varies with focusing.

5. Adjust the aiming beam brightness.

6. Confirm landmarks to prevent accidental macular burns.

7. Laser power will vary with media clarity, fundus pigmentation, and machine. Start low and gradually increase to produce a definite white spot.

8. Encircle the break and any subretinal fluid with two rows of semi-confluent spots (Fig. 11.4).

9. Occasionally periocular LA is needed if patients cannot tolerate laser treatment.

Box 11.2: Cryotherapy

1. Explain the procedure and obtain written consent.

2. Anaesthetic requirements vary from topical, subconjunctival injection at the cryo-site, to peribulbar. Fellow eye topical anaesthesia may help keep lids open.

3. Most machines require gas purging, e.g. set the temperature to −25°C, depress footpedal for 10 seconds, wait 1 minute, and repeat.

4. Cryoprobes are notoriously unreliable, so check. Set the treatment temperature (typically −85°C), dip into sterile water, depress the footpedal for 10 seconds, lift out. A 5 mm ice-ball should have formed. Release pedal. Within 2 seconds it should be possible to free the ice-ball from tip.

Box 11.2: Cryotherapy—cont'd

5. The handle is usually marked to manually orient the probe, as the tip is not visible during treatment.

6. *Beware*: it is possible to indent the break with the probe handle whilst the tip is accidentally treating the macula. Avoid treating the ciliary body (painful).

7. View the fundus with the indirect ophthalmoscope and a 20D lens.

8. Indent the break with the probe tip, and plan treatment.

9. The break margin requires treatment but not the central defect.

10. Larger breaks may require treatment in more than one site, but avoid unnecessary treatment to reduce the risk of epiretinal membranes.

11. Depress the footpedal until the treatment area freezes, then release.

12. Wait until fully thawed before moving the probe to another site to avoid scleral/choroidal damage.

13. Wait 1 minute after the last treatment before turning off machine. This allows gas to escape

14. Provide analgesia.

Follow-up Two weeks. If an RPE reaction fully encircles the break, discharge with an RDW for annual dilated optometry review. Review those with subretinal fluid within 2 days, then as required.

Rhegmatogenous Retinal Detachment

Background Usually occurs secondary to retinal tears (*rhegma*). These are most commonly caused when the posterior vitreous face separates from the internal limiting membrane and vitreoretinal adhesions tear the retina. Syneretic vitreous fluid passes through these tears, detaching the retina from the RPE. More common in high myopes.

Symptoms Flashing lights in the temporal field, floaters, field loss, variable loss of VA.

Signs Bullous RD is easily detected (Fig. 11.5) but the only sign of shallow elevation may be loss of choroidal markings and subtle elevation. RD may be associated with an RAPD, low IOP, vitreous haemorrhage, and tobacco dust (p. 521). Chronic detachments often have thinned retina, RPE pigmentation at the border of attached and detached retina ('high-water mark', example p. 552), and may have retinal telangiectasia or retinal scarring (proliferative vitreoretinopathy, PVR). There is sometimes a mild anterior uveitis or raised IOP.

Examination Record VA, RAPD, lens status (clear, cataractous, pseudoaphakic or aphakic), and presence of posterior

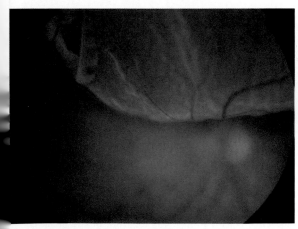

Fig. 11.5: Superior bulous retinal detachment with a superotemporal U-tear.

vitreous detachment (PVD, p. 521). Draw the extent of the RD noting macular involvement, breaks, and lattice degeneration. Check the periphery of both eyes using an indirect ophthalmoscope, 20D lens (or equivalent), and 360° indentation. Finding breaks can be difficult but their position is suggested by Lincoff's Rules (see Fig. 11.6). Trauma may cause tears at the anterior retinal border that are hard to detect (see Retinal dialysis; p. 552). Grade any proliferative vitreoretinopathy (PVR) as A (increased vitreous haze and pigment), B (inner retinal fibrosis), and C (full-thickness retinal folds), and note if anterior (A) or posterior (P), and extent in clock hours, e.g. PVR CA2, CP6.

Investigations If there is significant media opacity, perform same-day ultrasound.

Differential diagnosis Consider PVD, serous RD (no breaks with shifting subretinal fluid), and tractional RD (usually caused by fibrosis from severe diabetic retinopathy or PVR). *Retinoschisis* occurs secondary to an intraretinal split that produces an appearance similar to RD. It is often bilateral and symmetric, is more common in hypermetropes, tends not to

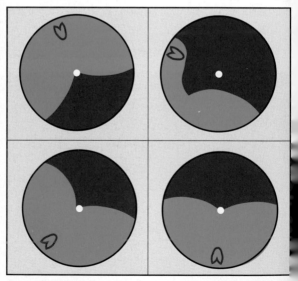

Fig. 11.6: Lincoff's rules. The location of the break is suggested by the configuration of retinal detachment. Detached retina is shown in blue.

produce a 'high-water mark', and unlike RD produces an absolute rather than partial scotoma. The elevated inner retinal layer appears thin and atrophic. Retinoschisis is extremely uncommon in myopes.

Management Refer for same-day vitreoretinal opinion. Aim to repair most sight-threatening macula-on RDs within 24 hours and macula-off RDs less urgently, but as soon as possible. Three surgical options exist:

▪ *Pneumatic retinopexy*: suitable only for a minority of straightforward cases with superior breaks. A vitreous injection of expansile gas produces a flotation force that tamponades retinal breaks and flattens the retina. Cryotherapy or laser retinopexy creates an adhesive scar between the break and RPE, preventing vitreous fluid moving into the subretinal space.

▪ *Conventional (cryobuckle) surgery*: a silicone explant is sutured externally to the sclera, indenting the RPE toward the retina. This relieves vitreoretinal traction and promotes re-attachment. Surgery may be augmented by trans-scleral drainage of subretinal fluid. Retinopexy is applied to seal the break. Gas is sometimes injected.

▪ *Vitrectomy*: an endoscopic light, vitreous infusion cannula, and vitrector are inserted through three 20 or 23-gauge ports at the pars plana. The vitrector is used to remove the vitreous, relieving any vitreoretinal traction. Retinopexy is by trans-scleral cryotherapy or endoscopic laser. A slowly absorbing gas (sulphur hexafluoride [SF_6] or octafluoropropane [C_3F_8]) tamponades the retina, or silicone oil in complex cases.

Consent In a national audit, 81% of primary RDs required only one operation but subspecialists achieved 87% success. The final re-attachment rate is >95% with two or more operations. The VA following macula-off RD varies widely, but some reduction is to be expected. Macula-on RDs usually retain good acuity although epiretinal membranes may occur in 4–8% of cases. Severe loss of vision can occur from haemorrhage and infection (<1%). Prophylactic retinopexy may be required in the fellow eye (see Table 11.1).

▪ *Pneumatic retinopexy*: lower success rate than other options but simpler procedure. The consequences of gas injection are similar to vitrectomy.

▪ *Cryobuckle*: Risks include diplopia (≈3%); myopic shift; postoperative discomfort (common).

■ *Vitrectomy*: markedly impaired vision until gas absorbs in 1 week (air), 2 weeks (SF_6), or 2 months (C_3F_8). Patients must not fly during this period as gas expansion may dangerously elevate IOP. Patients should advise anaesthetists that they have gas in their eye, as inhaled nitrous oxide may also elevate IOP. Most patients require 10 days of head posturing to float the gas bubble onto the breaks. Postoperative IOP elevation is normal and may require treatment. Silicone oil is removed later if the retina is secure, typically at 3–6 months. Silicone may lead to chronic IOP elevation and corneal changes. See the general risks of vitrectomy below.

■ *Risks of vitrectomy*: Patients undergoing vitrectomy should be aware of the following risks: general progressive nuclear sclerosis (81% at 6 months, 98% at 1 year); iatrogenic retinal breaks (≈5%) that require retinopexy/gas injection and may lead to RD; choroidal haemorrhage (<1%); endophthalmitis (<1%). Intravitreal gas injection may be required.

For patient information see http://www.rcophth.ac.uk/scientific/publications.html

Postoperative care Patients are usually discharged at the first postoperative day, or treated as day cases. Confirm the retina is attached. The RPE pump will often remove shallow residual subretinal fluid. All patients require a retinal detachment warning (p. 522) and G. chloramphenicol 0.5% q.d.s. 2 weeks, G. atropine 1% b.d. 2 weeks, and G. dexamethasone 0.1% q.d.s. 2 weeks, then tail off over 3 weeks.

■ *Pneumatic retinopexy*: check for inferior secondary retinal breaks caused by gas-induced vitreous traction. Advice is as for vitrectomy, but more frequent follow-up is required initially, e.g. day 1, 3, and 7.

■ *Cryobuckle*: check there is an adequate indent directly under the breaks and consider anterior segment ischaemia (uncommon) if there is raised IOP, anterior uveitis, and pain. Routine follow-up is day 1, 10, 30, then optometrist yearly.

■ *Vitrectomy*: the gas fill should be at least 70% of the vitreous cavity, especially if there are inferior breaks. Advise on head posturing, e.g. right cheek to pillow for a right eye RD with nasal breaks. Posture 50 minutes per hour for 10 days and be active for the 10 minute rest period to avoid deep vein thrombosis. Transient, fine, crystal-like lines on the posterior lens surface are common ('gas cataract'). Inadvertent lens touch by endoscopic instrumentation produces a focal, linear opacity. Measure IOP.

1. If <25 mmHg, discharge and review in 10 days.

2. If >25 mmHg add G. betablocker b.d. (unless contraindicated) and review in 10 days.

3. If >30 mmHg add G. betablocker b.d., G. apraclonidine 0.5% t.d.s., acetazolamide 250 mg s.r. b.d. p.o. and review in 5–7 days.

4. If >35 mmHg give stat acetazolamide 500 mg p.o., G. betablocker, G. apraclonidine and recheck IOP in 2 hours. Send home when IOP <30 mmHg on G. betablocker b.d., G. apraclonidine 0.5% t.d.s., acetazolamide 250 mg s.r. b.d. p.o.. Review in 5–7 days. If IOP fails to respond, consider gas overfill (look for absent gas-fluid meniscus inferiorly). Remove gas if necessary.

For routine vitrectomy see day 1, 10, 30, 60, then optometrist yearly.

Diabetic Vitreoretinal Surgery

Persistent vitreous haemorrhage

Background The fragile new vessels that define proliferative diabetic retinopathy may bleed into the vitreous cavity, reducing VA, and preventing treatment with panretinal photocoagulation (PRP). As 20% of haemorrhages clear within 1 year, surgical timing is crucial: operate early and expose some patients to unnecessary surgical risks; operate late and delay PRP and visual recovery.

Key study *Diabetic Retinopathy Vitrectomy Study*[1] For type 1 diabetics, early vitrectomy (1–6 versus 12 months) increased the chance of VA ≥6/12 at 2 years. Not significant for type 2, but none had intraoperative PRP and 30% had lensectomy. Surgical technique has improved.

History Determine age, if type 1 or 2 diabetes, duration of visual loss, total number of PRP burns and surgical risk factors.

Examination Note VA, IOP, rubeosis, lens status, RAPD, density of vitreous haemorrhage, retinopathy and fellow eye disease.

Investigations Arrange ultrasound to show vitreous or retinal detachment. Repeat every 2 months if the fundal view remains inadequate.

Treatment Vitrectomy timing:

- Type 1 diabetics at 3 months.

- Type 2 at 4–6 months.

Consider earlier surgery if rubeosis, raised IOP, incomplete PRP, or poor fellow eye VA. Simultaneous vitrectomy and cataract surgery is often required but avoid cataract surgery if possible, as diabetics may get posterior synechiae from increased post operative inflammation after combined surgery.

Consent

- *Benefit*: improve and stabilize vision. VA ≥6/12 in 36% of type 1 diabetics, 16% of type 2 diabetics.[1]

- *Risk*: rapid visual loss including NPL. Haemorrhage may recur but resolves more quickly in vitrectomized eyes. See Risks of vitrectomy (p. 532) and PRP (p. 434).

Recurrent vitreous haemorrhage

May occur despite adequate PRP, if inactive new vessels have ongoing vitreous traction. Vitrectomy can relieve vascular traction if haemorrhages are frequent and slow to clear.

Tractional retinal detachment

Background Proliferative fibrovascular membranes may cause tractional retinal detachments. Consider surgery if they involve or threaten the fovea.

Examination Note VA, IOP, rubeosis, RAPD, lens status, presence of posterior vitreous detachment, extent of PRP and membranes, retinal breaks, and fellow eye disease.

Treatment Vitrectomy and membrane removal by delamination (horizontal dissection between the membrane and retina), segmentation (vertical membrane division to relieve tangential traction), or *en bloc*. PRP is often required.

Consent

- *Benefit*: improve or stabilize vision in approximately 75%. VA ≥6/60 in 50–60% Complete retinal re-attachment, 80–85% (one operation).

- *Risk*: see Risks of vitrectomy (p. 532) and PRP (p.434). Retinal breaks during membrane dissection cause retinal detachment in 5–15%. Recurrent vitreous haemorrhage occurs in approximately 10%. Gas injection may be required at the time of surgery, to reduce the risk of retinal breaks causing retinal detachment.

Epiretinal Membrane

Background Thin preretinal membrane formed by fibroblastic cells. Most often idiopathic but may be secondary to retinal breaks, inflammation, diabetes, vitreous haemorrhage, retinal vascular occlusion, trauma, or any other disease that stimulates fibrosis. Sometimes called cellophane maculopathy, or preretinal gliosis. Macular pucker occurs when membrane contraction causes full-thickness retinal folds.

Symptoms Most patients are asymptomatic but the commonest symptom is distortion. VA reduction is usually mild (≥6/9 in two-thirds of cases) and nonprogressive.

Signs Typically cellophane-like, preretinal membrane causing fine wrinkles of the macula (Fig. 11.7). Thicker membranes are often associated with other disease. Bilateral in 25%. RPE changes and macular oedema may occur, and may indicate a worse surgical prognosis. Most have posterior vitreous detachment; if not, question the diagnosis.

History and examination Assess subjective severity and visual requirements. Record: near and distance VA, Amsler grid, lens status, vitreous attachment, retinal periphery and fellow eye disease.

Investigations Fluorescein angiography is not routinely required but may show vessel distortion and leakage. Optical

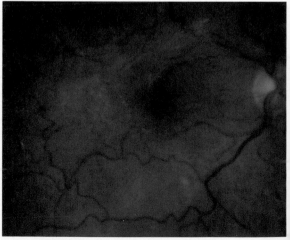

Fig. 11.7: Epiretinal membrane (Courtesy M Michaelides).

coherence tomography (OCT) can help exclude suspected vitreomacular traction syndrome.

Management

- *Casualty*: routine clinic referral.

- *Clinic*: discuss vitrectomy and membrane peel. The aim is to reduce distortion and improve VA.

Consent VA improves ≥2 lines in 74%, with 24% unchanged and 2% worse. Most patients report some improvement in metamorphopsia but few achieve entirely normal vision. Without surgery, VA is generally stable. Occasionally (<1%) the membrane separates spontaneously and VA improves. Explain the risks of vitrectomy (p. 532). Complications are reported to occur in 8% of cases.

Follow-up

- *No surgery*: discharge for annual optometrist review.

- *Postoperative*: G. chloramphenicol 0.5% q.d.s. 2 weeks, G. atropine 1% b.d. 2 weeks, G dexamethasone 0.1% q.d.s. 2 weeks then tail off over 3 weeks. Review subjective change in distortion, near and distance VA, lens opacity, residual membrane or wrinkling, and retinal periphery at day 1, 10, 30, 90, then discharge for annual dilated optometrist review. Membranes recur in 7%.

Vitreomacular Traction Syndrome

Background Partial vitreous detachment occurs but with points of residual attachment. These produce vitreomacular traction at one or more sites, and often also at the optic disc. This causes secondary macular oedema that may be aggravated by coexisting epiretinal membranes in 50% of cases.

Symptoms Blurred vision, metamorphopsia, photopsia, micropsia, and monocular diplopia.

History and examination Determine the duration and exact nature of symptoms and test with an Amsler grid. Use high-power macular lenses or a contact lens as vitreomacular traction can be hard to detect. Note any points of vitreous attachment. Exclude peripheral breaks that may be associated with epiretinal membranes.

Differential diagnosis Consider isolated epiretinal membrane, full- or partial-thickness macular hole, and other causes of macular oedema (p. 447).

Investigations Optical coherence tomography (OCT) is extremely helpful and shows vitreous attachment, foveal elevation, and macular oedema (Fig. 11.8). Fluorescein angiography is not routinely required but shows diffuse and extensive leakage and optic disc staining.

Treatment Spontaneous vitreous separation occurs in 11% but without treatment 64% lose 2 lines of VA over ≈6 years. Vitrectomy reduces retinal thickening in most cases and VA improves 2 lines or more in 44–75%, but falls by 2 lines in 0–15%. Firm vitreoretinal adhesion coupled with macular oedema can result in macular hole formation during surgery.

Follow–up As for epiretinal membrane surgery (see previous page).

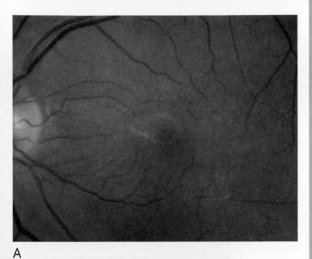

A

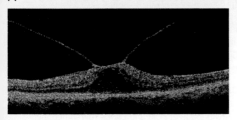

B

Fig. 11.8: Vitreomacular traction syndrome seen in **(A)** colour photograph and **(B)** on OCT.

Macular Hole

Background A full-thickness retinal defect centred on the fovea. Commonest in late-middle-aged women. Usually idiopathic but may occur in high myopes, following trauma, or prolonged cystoid macular oedema.

Symptoms Reduced VA, distortion or incidental finding.

Signs

- *Stage I*: yellow spot with loss of normal foveolar depression.

- *Stage II*: round or curvilear full-thickness retinal defect (<350 μm).

- *Stage III*: full-thickness macular hole (FTMH). A pre-foveal operculum is common.

- *Stage IV*: FTMH with complete posterior vitreous detachment (Fig. 11.9). Associated findings include a grey cuff of subretinal fluid surrounding the hole, fine yellow-white deposits in the base of the hole, underlying RPE atrophy and occasionally retinal detachment in high myopes. VA is typically 6/24–6/60. Approximately 30% also have an epiretinal membranes (p. 536).

History and examination Record: duration and severity of symptoms, near and distance VA, lens and refractive status, vitreous attachment, stage of hole and check retinal periphery. Perform Watzke-Allen test using a macular lens: shine a narrow slit of light vertically across the hole; ask, 'Is the line of light continuous, narrowed, or broken?' If significantly narrowed (>50%) or broken, the test is positive, suggesting a FTMH rather than pseudo- or lamellar hole. Repeat in the horizontal meridian.

Differential diagnosis *Partial-thickness (lamellar) holes* tend not to have cuff of fluid around the hole or RPE changes but they may progress to FTMH. *Pseudohole* an epiretinal membrane or macular cysts create the appearance of a FTMH.

Investigations Not routinely required.

- *B-scan ultrasonography*: may show posterior vitreous detachment if not visible clinically.

- *Fluorescein angiography*: RPE atrophy may give central hyperfluorescence with the cuff of subretinal fluid producing a hypofluorescent annulus.

- *Ocular coherence tomography*: if available, may confirm uncertain cases.

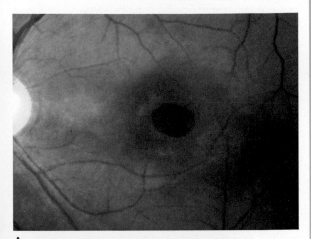

A

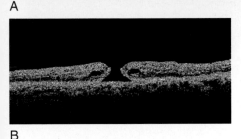

B

Fig. 11.9: **(A, B)** Stage IV macular holes.

Management

■ *Casualty*: routine clinic referral.

■ *Clinic*: studies suggest stage I holes do not benefit from vitrectomy and gas injection but consider for stage II–IV holes of up to 9–12 months duration. Surgical success probably reduces the longer the hole has been present, but the duration may not be known and surgery is done as the only way to possibly improve vision. To maximize gas tamponade many, but not all, recommend face-down posturing for 50 minutes in every hour, for 7–14 days. Many peel the internal limiting membrane and some use adjuncts such as serum or autologous platelets. Spontaneous hole closure occurs in 12% but VA tends to remain unchanged.

541

Consent Stage III and IV: approximately 80% anatomic closure; 70% get 2 line VA improvement, 10% no change, 10% lose VA. Explain the risks of vitrectomy and gas injection (p. 532). Failed primary surgery may warrant re-operation.

Follow-up

■ *No surgery*: discharge for annual optometrist review.

■ *Postoperative*: G. Chloramphenicol 0.5% q.d.s. 2 weeks; G. Atropine 1% b.d. 2 weeks; G. Dexamethasone 0.1% q.d.s. two weeks, then tail off over three weeks. Inspect for raised IOP, retinal breaks, visual and anatomic outcome, and cataract, at day 1, 7, 30, and 90, then discharge for annual optometrist review. The risk of contralateral FTMH is approximately 10–20%, but is unlikely if the vitreous is detached. Provide an Amsler grid.

Vitreous Haemorrhage

Background Vitreous haemorrhage is a sign, not a diagnosis, so it is important to determine the cause.

History Ask about floaters, photopsia, duration of reduced acuity, diabetes, sickle cell disease, cardiovascular risk factors (risk of vein occlusion), anticoagulants, eye or head trauma, headache, and previous eye disease.

Examination Note VA, rubeosis, anterior chamber red blood cells, IOP, whether phakic, pseudophakic, or aphakic, posterior vitreous detachment (PVD), haemorrhage location and density. Fundoscopy may be easier using a 28 D lens (or equivalent). Dilate and examine the fellow eye, as this may assist diagnosis, e.g. diabetic retinopathy, age-related macular degeneration (AMD).

Differential diagnosis Consider PVD, retinal tears, neovascular AMD with break-through bleeding, neovascularization from central or branch retinal vein occlusion, sickle cell retinopathy, and trauma. Intracranial haemorrhage may be associated with retinal or vitreous haemorrhage (Terson's syndrome), particularly in patients with raised intracranial pressure and coma. Vitreous haemorrhage alone seldom produces an RAPD or NPL.

Investigations Request B-scan ultrasound if the fundal view is poor. Look specifically for retinal breaks, retinal or vitreous detachment, and macular elevation (disciform lesions).

Management For PVD see page 521, retinal tears page 526, nonclearing diabetic vitreous haemorrhage page 534, vein occlusion page 471, AMD page 454, sickle cell retinopathy page 487, and trauma page 551.

Follow-up In those not undergoing vitrectomy to clear the haemorrhage, repeat the ultrasound examination at 2 weeks then at intervals until the fundal view improves. The interval depends on the cause – PVD related haemorrhage carries a high risk of retinal tears and requires frequent scans ($\approx$2 weekly), whereas diabetic vitreous haemorrhage is less likely to be associated with rhegmatogenous retinal detachment. Watch for raised IOP and ghost cell glaucoma. Haemorrhage tends to clear more quickly in those with anterior chamber red blood cells, aphakia, and previous vitrectomy. Haemorrhage from AMD and central retinal vein occlusion carry a poor prognosis.

Uveal Effusion Syndrome

Background Idiopathic choroidal effusions secondary to reduced trans-scleral outflow, typically in middle-aged men. Hypermetropic or nanophthalmic eyes are predisposed.

Clinical features Spontaneous onset of choroidal effusions (Fig. 11.10) with shifting subretinal fluid, often with a chronic relapsing–remitting course. IOP is normal and there is no vitritis. Macular involvement may reduce VA.

Differential diagnosis

- *Rhegmatogenous retinal detachment*: look for retinal breaks and an absence of shifting fluid.

- *Serous retinal detachment*: shifting subretinal fluid may occur in uveal effusion syndrome but look for signs suggesting other causes, e.g. scleritis, retinal vasculitis, vitritis, or disc swelling.

- *Ocular hypotony*: choroidal effusions settle as the IOP normalizes.

- *Choroidal mass*: visible on examination or with ultrasound.

Investigation Look for scleritis and choroidal mass using B-scan ultrasound. Measure axial length and refraction. Fluorescein angiography may rule out other diseases and has

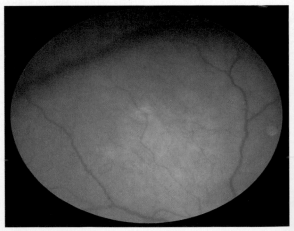

Fig. 11.10: Uveal effusion syndrome.

been reported to show choroidal leakage that is also seen with indocyanine green.

Treatment There are reports of improvement with NSAIDs but this may be coincidental. Subscleral sclerectomy is often effective.

Hereditary Vitreoretinal Degenerations

If a hereditary degeneration is suspected, ask to examine the relatives. Genetic testing is available for the conditions listed below.

Stickler's syndrome

An autosomal dominant vitreoretinal degeneration, also known as hereditary progressive arthro-ophthalmopathy. Caused by a mutation of the gene coding type II or XI collagen, and classified as type 1 or 2, respectively. Associated with abnormalities of the ears (sensorineural and conductive deafness), face (cleft palate, flat midface), joints (premature arthropathy, laxity), and bones (spondyloepiphyseal dysplasia). Ocular involvement includes congenital high myopia (average −5.00 D), angle anomalies and glaucoma, presenile wedge-shaped cataracts, and congenital vitreous abnormalities (type 1 membranous, or type 2 beaded condensations). Patients are at very high risk of retinal detachment, irrespective of whether they exhibit typical paravascular pigmented lattice (Fig. 11.11). Some, but not all clinicians arrange regular review so that prophylactic retinopexy can be applied as required.

Familial exudative vitreoretinopathy

Familial exudative vitreoretinopathy (FEVR) is usually autosomal dominant (chromosome 11), but occasionally X-linked recessive and sporadic. It produces a fundus appearance similar to retinopathy of prematurity (Fig. 11.12). Three stages are based on the severity of the retinal features: (1) peripheral nonperfusion, especially temporally; (2) localized tractional retinal detachment, exudation, and neovascularization, and (3) more extensive tractional, exudative and rhegmatogenous detachments. Fluorescein angiography shows areas of nonperfusion and leakage. Most cases are mild but often progressive, so observation is required. Some require retinal photocoagulation to reduce the ischaemic stimulus, or retinal detachment surgery.

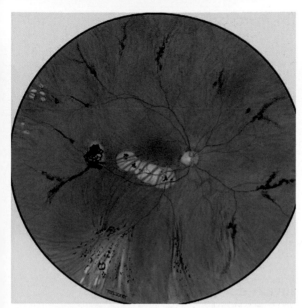

Fig. 11.11: Stickler's syndrome (Courtesy of P Leaver/PM Sullivan, artwork T Tarrant).

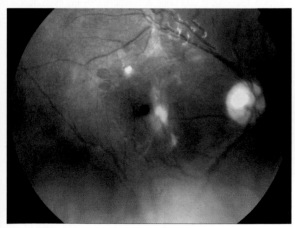

Fig. 11.12: Familial exudative vitreoretinopathy.

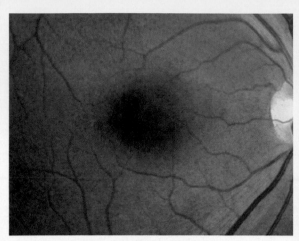

Fig. 11.13: Juvenile X-linked retinoschisis.

Juvenile X-linked retinoschisis

An X-linked retinal dystrophy with secondary vitreous changes and variable phenotypic expression. Caused by a defect of the gene coding a protein (retinoschisin) thought to influence cellular adhesion. Presents in childhood with reduced VA and cystic foveal cavities that coalesce to produce schisis of the nerve fibre layer (Fig. 11.13). Peripheral retinoschisis may also occur, as may neovascularization, vitreous haemorrhage and retinal detachment. ERG shows reduced B wave amplitude, and OCT shows schitic separation of the retinal layers, sometimes in more than one plane. Treatment may include amblyopia therapy, panretinal photocoagulation for new vessels, and retinal detachment surgery.[2]

Marfan's Syndrome

Background An autosomal dominant connective tissue disorder.

Systemic features These include tall, thin stature, long limbs and fingers (arachnodactyly), joint laxity, scoliosis, pectus excavatum, high arched palate, aortic dilatation, mitral valve prolapse, and hernias.

Ocular features Look for myopia, corneal abnormalities (including keratoconus), angle anomalies, ectopia lentis (Fig. 11.14), and retinal detachment.

Differential diagnosis of ectopia lentis:

- *Trauma.*

- *Homocystinuria*: an inborn error of metabolism with marfanoid appearance, fair complexion, osteoporosis, mental deficiency, circulatory insufficiency and thromboembolic events (sometimes precipitated by general anaesthesia). Heterozygotes have hyperhomocysteinaemia with an increased risk of premature (age <50 years) retinal vein, and retinal artery occlusion.

- *Weil-Marchesani syndrome*: short stature, reduced joint mobility, myopia, microsperophakia, and pupil block from displaced lenses.

- *Rare causes*: sulphite oxidase deficiency, hyperlysinaemia, Ehlers-Danlos syndrome, pseudoexfoliation syndrome, high myopia, congenital glaucoma, retinitis pigmentosa, aniridia, hypermature cataract, and intraocular tumour.

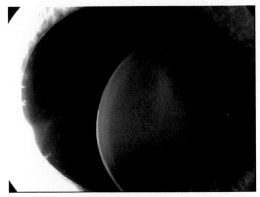

Fig. 11.14: Ectopia lentis in Marfan's syndrome.

Investigations Genetic testing of the affected fibrillin gene is available.

Management Arrange genetic counselling with an experienced clinician and cardiology review. Lens instability may lead to prolapse into the anterior chamber with pupil block, elevated IOP, and corneal decompensation requiring emergency lens removal. Zonular deficiency makes routine cataract surgery difficult, so consider vitreolensectomy with an anterior chamber or sutured posterior chamber IOL, or aphakia and contact lens correction.

Posterior Segment Trauma

Blunt or penetrating ocular trauma can produce various injuries due to ocular penetration, tissue compression, shearing, and tensile strain. If the injury results from an alleged assault or workplace injury, make detailed notes documenting the timing and circumstances of injury: measure or preferably photograph all injuries, and consider an orbital X-ray. Label injuries correctly: cut (clean edges); laceration (ragged wound); penetration (full-thickness defect); perforation (entry and exit wound). Consider tetanus prophylaxis and extraocular injury. For eyelid injury see page 50; cornea, page 205; angle recession, page 313; uveitis, page 353 and optic neuropathy, page 661. Exclude the following posterior segment injuries.

Commotio retinae

Photoreceptor damage produces a white retinal sheen immediately after injury (Fig. 11.15). VA is unaffected unless the macula is involved. No treatment is required. Provide a retinal detachment warning (p. 522) and review in 1–2 weeks.

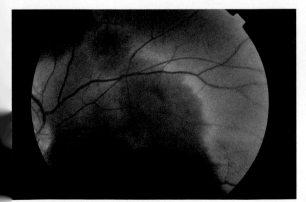

Fig. 11.15: Retinal commotio.

Retinal breaks

More common in the inferotemporal and superonasal quadrants. Look for Shafer's sign (p. 521). Some traumatic breaks do not require retinopexy as the healing response produces a chorioretinal adhesion. Provide a retinal detachment warning and review in 1 week. Head injury without direct ocular trauma seldom produces retinal breaks.

Retinal dialysis

These very peripheral retinal tears may progress to retinal detachment and are easily missed. Perform indented fundoscopy or three-mirror examination unless penetrating injury is suspected. Retinal detachment surgery is usually required (cryobuckle) if retinal detachment is present, so keep nil by mouth and arrange same-day vitreoretinal review (Fig. 11.16).

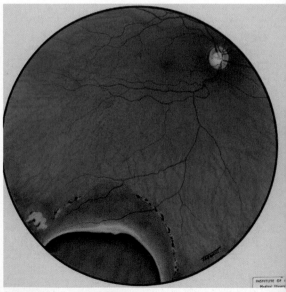

Fig. 11.16: Retinal dialysis with a 'high-water mark' indication long duration (Courtesy of P Leaver/PM Sullivan; artwork T Tarrant).

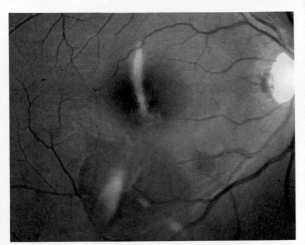

Fig. 11.17: Choroidal rupture with foveal involvement.

Choroidal rupture

Rupture and retraction of the choroid–Bruch's–RPE complex allows the underlying sclera to be seen as a white streak (Fig. 11.17). Alternatively, it may be obscured by subretinal haemorrhage. If there is submacular haemorrhage, discuss urgently with a vitreoretinal surgeon, as some advocate drainage. Otherwise, manage conservatively with review in 2–3 weeks.

Ruptured globe

Ruptured sclera is easily missed if haemorrhagic chemosis obscures the view or the injury is posterior. Ask about the mechanism of injury, and previous eye disease or surgery. Gently examine for hypotony, deep or collapsed AC, hyphaema, corneal or lens injury, uveal or vitreous prolapse, vitreous haemorrhage, reduced ocular motility, and VA. Normal IOP does not exclude the diagnosis but normal fundal examination makes posterior scleral rupture from blunt trauma unlikely. If intraocular haemorrhage obscures the view and the index of suspicion is low, ultrasound (USS) may help rule out lens dislocation, retinal detachment, vitreous haemorrhage, and posterior scleral rupture. Avoid USS if penetration is thought likely, as transducer pressure during examination may extrude intraocular tissue (consider CT instead). Request plain X-rays if metal orbital or intraocular foreign body

Box 11.3: Primary repair of ruptured globe

1. Explain the procedure and the uncertain, usually guarded prognosis. Subsequent surgery is often required to improve vision or remove the eye. Primary evisceration or enucleation is rarely necessary and only after review by two consultants.

2. Warn the anaesthetist that surgery sometimes takes several hours.

3. Gently insert a lid speculum.

4. Perform a 360° conjunctival peritomy and carefully examine the sclera back to the four vortex veins. Blunt injury often produces rupture at the limbus, under the recti, or through old surgical wounds. This tends to be limited to one wound, but this may be extensive.

5. Consider slinging the recti with 2/0 silk sutures to help position the eye. Recti may need to be temporarily disinserted to access underlying wounds. Measure the muscle's distance from the limbus before removing and pre-place a double-armed 5/0 Vicryl suture at the anterior muscle border. Reattach after scleral repair.

6. Gently lift prolapsed, nonviable uveal tissue, vitreous, or blood with a dry cellulose sponge and trim flush with the sclera using fine scissors. Avoid excessive vitreous traction. Alternatively, use a vitrector at high cut rate, e.g. 300 cuts/min.

7. Remove any IOFBs visible at the wound opening.

8. Close corneal wounds with interrupted, simple, 10/0 Nylon sutures. Bury knots. It can be difficult to rotate sutures in hypotonous eyes, so start the first bite within the wound margin so that the knot ties within the wound. Close sclera with 8/0 Nylon sutures, conjunctiva with 7/0 Vicryl.

9. It may not be possible to suture very posterior wounds, but these often seal spontaneously after 10 days.

10. Cadaveric sclera is occasionally required to replace missing tissue. Silicone explants can be used if none is available.

11. Once closed, reinflate the eye with intraocular saline and revise any leaking wounds. Cyanoacrylate glue can seal small leaks; dry tissue before applying.

12. Once the globe is secure, examine for conjunctival foreign bodies and eyelid injury.

13. Gently inject subconjunctival antibiotic unless there are open posterior wounds.

(IOFB) are possible, but if revealed, use CT to localize. MRI is unsafe with metal FBs. Examination under anaesthesia with conjunctival recession is sometimes required, so keep nil by mouth except for prophylactic ciprofloxacin 750 mg b.d. p.o.. Guard the eye with a plastic shield preoperatively. For repair of ruptured globe, see Box 11.3.

Follow up Day 1 postoperatively, exclude endophthalmitis, retinal detachment, and hypotony. Later complications include phthisis, proliferative vitreoretinopathy with retinal detachment, tissue downgrowth and sympathetic ophthalmia. Rx G. dexamethasone 0.1% 1 hourly by day, Oc. betamethasone nocte, G. ofloxacin 2 hourly, G. atropine 1% o.d. Continue oral antibiotics for 10 days. Review in 1 week. Explain the symptoms of retinal detachment (p. 529) and sympathetic ophthalmia (p. 354).Do not enucleate seeing eyes (even faint perception of light) in an attempt to prevent sympathetic ophthalmia in the undamaged eye, as the visual prognosis is hard to predict and enucleation is not proven to reduce the risk of sympathetic ophthalmia.

Intraocular foreign body

Intraocular foreign body is most commonly caused by metal hammering metal. Signs are similar to penetrating injuries (see Ruptured Globe above) but endophthalmitis is more common (≈10%). The decision whether to remove as a primary procedure or subsequently depends on the IOFB size and material, visual potential, surgeon, and patient preference. Discuss with a vitreoretinal surgeon. Endophthalmitis, organic or reactive metal IOFBs (iron/copper) usually require primary removal. Surgery usually involves a three-port pars plana vitrectomy with removal through a sclerotomy. Sometimes a magnet is used to retrieve ferrous IOFBs via a sclerotomy, with or without vitrectomy. Document the IOFB size and send for culture. Pre- and postoperative management is similar to ruptured globe, but explain the risks of vitrectomy (p. 532). Gas tamponade may be required, so flying may be contraindicated for several weeks.

Optometry and General Practice Guidelines

General comments

Many patients have a few longstanding vitreous floaters or the occasional flash of light (photopsia), and do not require ophthalmology review. Clues to significant vitreoretinal traction are a sudden increase in the number of floaters or change in the nature of the photopsia, especially flashes of light in the temporal field. Risk factors for retinal detachment (RD) include high myopia, trauma, and previous RD in either eye. In the context of photopsia and floaters, a field defect suggests retinal detachment and blurred vision suggests macular detachment or vitreous haemorrhage. Any of these features warrant same-day ophthalmology review. The commonest differential of photopsia is migraine. Any patient with flashes or floaters should be given a retinal detachment warning.

Optometrists

- Acute onset or suddenly changed symptoms of flashes and/or floaters in one eye should be treated as an RD until proven otherwise. Same-day ophthalmology review is required regardless of findings, so dilated fundoscopy by an optometrist is not therefore required. Anxious patients can be reassured that >90% of cases will not have RD.

- Longstanding floaters, or the occasional flash of light should be investigated by the optometrist. Maximal dilation is necessary to view the extreme periphery, therefore use a combination of tropicamide 1%, and phenylephrine 2.5% (after excluding narrow angles, drop allergies, a history of unstable cardiac disease or iris clip intraocular lenses). Warn not to drive until the drops have worn off. Refer abnormalities as detailed below.

General practice

The optometry guidelines also apply, except that many general practitioners will not feel as confident with ophthalmoscopy. If so, then refer chronic mild floaters for routine hospital review. If there are any acute symptoms or features suggesting significant vitreoretinal traction (see above), arrange same-day ophthalmology review.

No referral is required for posterior vitreous detachment or lattice degeneration if these occur in isolation. The following guide to referral urgency is not prescriptive, as clinical situations vary.

Immediate

Same day

Routine

References

1. The Diabetic Retinopathy Vitrectomy Study Research Group. Early vitrectomy for severe vitreous hemorrhage in diabetic retinopathy. Two-year results of a randomized trial. Diabetic Retinopathy Vitrectomy Study report 2. Arch Ophthalmol 1985; 103:1644–1652.
2. Thanks to Martin Snead of Adenbrooke's Hospital, Cambridge, for critique.

Chapter 12

PAEDIATRICS

History and Examination

Basics Before each consultation, read the notes and decide what questions need to be answered: perform the key parts of the examination first in uncooperative children. Be flexible; for example, it may sometimes be better to examine a child before taking a history. Children (and their carers) are often anxious and it helps to perform the examination in a child-friendly setting, without wearing a white coat. Speak and move gently, and explain what you are going to do. Consider examining the child's carer or toy first and warn that drops sting. Fundoscopy, retinoscopy, and portable slit lamp examination can sometimes be carried out with the child asleep.

History Note the presenting complaint and birth, family, social, and drug/allergy history. If relevant, draw a family tree (p. 412). Ask if the child attends any other clinics. Ask about hearing and normal developmental milestones.

Vision assessment Acuity develops throughout infancy and does not reach normal adult levels until about the age of 2 years. It may not be possible to obtain accurate acuity assessment of each eye separately until 3–4 years of age.

An age-appropriate vision test should be performed. Log MAR tests are preferable. Check the eye suspected of being the worst first. Observe the child's response to occlusion. If an eye is densely amblyopic, covering the good eye causes distress.

In an infant with suspected blindness, test the blink response to threat and bright light and see if the child fixes and follows a silent stimulus. Do a spinning baby test. The normal response is tonic deviation of the eyes in the direction of rotation with reflex saccadic movement in the opposite direction. Severe visual impairment due to higher visual pathway damage produces prolonged nystagmus on cessation of rotation (normally only 1–2 beats). Oculomotor apraxia produces tonic deviation without saccades, and characteristic head thrusts are used to break fixation.

Examination Observe the child's visual attention, alertness, and the presence of any facial abnormality or head posture.

Significant field defects can usually be detected by holding an interesting target straight ahead and then moving a toy in the periphery and seeing if the child looks towards this.

With a torch, examine the conjunctiva, corneal clarity, and pupil reactions. Examine the anterior segment in more detail with a portable slit lamp or direct ophthalmoscope using plus lenses. Infants can be examined on the normal slit lamp by holding them in a prone position when they will extend their neck and can be 'flown' into the chin rest.

Look for nystagmus and examine ocular movements. If a squint is suspected, perform cover–uncover, and alternate cover tests to look for manifest and latent deviation, respectively. Examine the pupil response to light and exclude a relative afferent pupil defect (RAPD).

Perform cycloplegic refraction and fundal examination to exclude refractive errors, media opacities, and fundus abnormalities. Document if examination is difficult or incomplete. Use G. cyclopentolate 0.5% under 6 months of age and 1% if older. Some add G. phenylephrine 2.5% in dark eyes or if dilatation is poor.

If adequate cycloplegia is not achieved then use Oc atropine 1% b.d. for 3 days prior to, but excluding, the day of examination to avoid corneal smearing. Atropine drops can be substituted if ointment is unavailable. These do not smear the cornea and can be used on the day of examination, but systemic absorption is higher.

Using a 'nonstinging' anaesthetic eyedrop (e.g. proxymetacaine) before dilating drops may reduce discomfort, lacrimation, and future anxiety about eyedrops.

Check the red reflex then start fundoscopy using an indirect ophthalmoscope and a 28 D or 30 D lens (or equivalent), and then a direct ophthalmoscope or higher magnification lens for a more detailed disc examination. Reducing the illumination improves cooperation. In older children, slit lamp biomicroscopy should be possible.

If glaucoma is suspected, check the IOP with an air puff tonometer or Tonopen in younger children who cannot be checked with applanation tonometry.

If cooperation is lost

■ *Casualty*: in an emergency situation it is important to obtain as full an examination as possible. Record any relevant tests that were not completed. Explain to the carer what needs to be done and why. Swaddle the child in a blanket then complete the fundus and anterior segment examination.

■ *Clinic*: consider ending the consultation and re-booking. Rarely, examination under anaesthetic is required.

Prescribing Glasses

Background Most infants have 1–3 dioptres (D) of hypermetropia, often with a degree of astigmatism. The hypermetropic refractive error usually emmetropizes by the age of 6–7 years. There is some evidence that fully correcting hypermetropia in a child may reduce emmetropization, so small degrees are not usually corrected and large degrees are usually undercorrected. Anisometropia is a risk factor for the development of amblyopia.

The following are *guidelines* for the prescription of glasses in children, as situations vary.

Hypermetropia If a child has >4 D of hypermetropia, correct two-thirds of the spherical equivalent, with full correction of any associated astigmatism. Correcting hypermetropia may improve reading in some children with normal distance acuity. Fully correct hypermetropia if the child has a convergent squint.

Myopia Correct myopia if there is reduced vision, which is likely to occur with myopia of −0.5 D or more. Correcting even small degrees of myopia in a child with intermittent exotropia may substantially improve control of the squint.

Anisometropia Fully correct more than 1 D of anisometropia after age 3 years. Higher degrees will need correcting at younger ages. If there is one nearly emmetropic eye and the fellow is amblyopic and hypermetropic, fully correct the amblyopic eye. If both eyes are hypermetropic with similar vision, give an equal correction to each eye, maintaining the interocular difference, e.g. for +6 D OD and +3 D OS give +4 D OD and +1 D OS.

Astigmatism Correct 1.50 D or more of astigmatism. Consider correcting smaller degrees in older children if it improves their acuity. Astigmatism is often overestimated in children, secondary to off-axis retinoscopy.

Bifocals Bifocals may be a useful alternative to surgery in children with convergence excess esotropia. They may also be useful in some children, such as those with Down's syndrome, who may have poor accommodation.

Leucocoria

Leucocoria is a white pupil (Fig. 12.1). It is a serious sign that requires urgent referral and assessment. The more common causes include:

- Infantile cataract: see next page.
- Coats' disease: page 564.
- Persistent hyperplastic primary vitreous: page 565.
- Toxocariasis: page 565.
- Retinoblastoma: page 407.

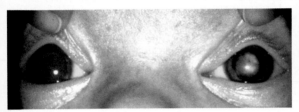

Fig. 12.1: Leucocoria in the left eye due to congenital cataract.

Infantile Cataract

Background Bilateral or unilateral lens opacity is historically termed congenital cataract if presumed present at birth. The cumulative incidence by 1 year is 2.5 cases per 10 000 births in the UK. It is bilateral in 66%, with 55% being isolated cataract and 45% associated with other ocular or systemic disorders. Inherited cataract (usually autosomal dominant) accounts for 56% of bilateral lens opacities. Associated ocular anomalies are more common with unilateral cataract, particularly persistent hyperplastic primary vitreous (PHPV), whilst systemic disease usually produces bilateral cataract, with prenatal infection and Down's syndrome being the commonest.

History and examination Ask the parents about the pregnancy and family history. Check the pupils for an afferent defect. A portable slit lamp makes cataract assessment easier and helps exclude associated anterior segment dysgenesis. The quality of the retinal image on direct or indirect ophthalmoscopy is another measure of severity; if the posterior pole cannot be easily seen visual deprivation is expected. Common cataract morphologies are nuclear, lamellar, anterior polar, posterior subcapsular, posterior with lenticonus, and total lens involvement. Examine the parents, as they may have unrecognized cataract. Other signs include delayed visual development, strabismus, and nystagmus.

Differential diagnosis Consider other causes of leucocoria (see previous page)

Investigations *B-scan ultrasonography* to assess posterior structures and the globe size (including interocular asymmetry), and biometry if required. *Paediatric assessment* to exclude systemic causes and associations. Routine investigations include TORCH screen (maternal infection), urinary reducing sugars (galactosaemia), and urinary amino acids (Lowe's syndrome). *Electrodiagnostic testing* may be indicated if retinal dysfunction is suspected.

Treatment

- ■ *Casualty*: refer to a specialty clinic the same week, as visually significant unilateral or bilateral cataracts are ideally removed within 6 weeks of birth, to avoid deprivational amblyopia.

- ■ *Clinic*: the decision to operate is made by the parents, after discussion with a surgeon experienced in infant cataract surgery. Bilateral cataracts detected early are treated by lensectomy and anterior vitrectomy, with the resulting aphakia treated with glasses or contact lenses. Unilateral cataract is managed the same way but with a contact lens, rather than glasses, postoperatively. Intraocular lens implants can be used from 4 months of age, but are associated with an increased complication rate, and posterior capsular thickening will require YAG or surgical capsulotomy. Lens implantation before age 4 months is possible, but controversial. The lens power depends on the age of the child, with infants and younger children left hyperopic to allow for later 'myopic shift' as the eye grows.

Consent Warn the parents that paediatric cataract surgery is not the same as adult surgery and that the visual result is less predictable. Considerable parental input is required after surgery. The major complications are glaucoma, amblyopia, and strabismus. Aphakic glaucoma is a significant complication, particularly for children undergoing early surgery when the risk can be up to 50%. It would appear to reduce when surgery is performed later, even by waiting until over 4 weeks of age. Strabismus and amblyopia occur in virtually all cases of unilateral cataract, whether treated or not. Amblyopia is also common with bilateral cataracts. In children undergoing lens implantation, primary posterior capsulorrhexis or later capsulotomy will be required. After unilateral surgery, failure to patch the nonaffected eye is the leading cause of poor vision. Also, discuss the more general risks of cataract surgery.

Follow–up Even if no surgery is undertaken, clinic review is required to ensure that the good eye develops normally, and to review the cataractous eye. Long-term, regular follow-up after surgery is mandatory to monitor for complications. Children should be seen at 1 day, then 1, 2, and 4 weeks after surgery, and regularly thereafter. Refract at the second postoperative visit and prescribe contact lenses or glasses initially for near vision (give the retinoscopy with no subtraction for working distance). Refraction should be regularly updated, and glasses or contact lenses altered accordingly, with bifocal or varifocal correction from about 2 years of age. Check IOP at every visit. Increased corneal thickness may give falsely elevated IOP readings and examination under anaesthesia may be required. Patching will be required for amblyopia. Postoperative therapy includes topical antibiotic, steroid and mydriatic.

Coats' Disease

The main features are unilateral, idiopathic retinal telangiectasia with intra- and subretinal exudation and retinal detachment (Fig. 12.2). Apparently bilateral Coats' disease is usually familial exudative vitreoretinopathy (p. 546) or another disorder. Coats' disease typically present in boys at a median age of 5 years, but there is a large range from neonate to adult, with severity inversely related to the age of presentation. There is no racial predisposition, and it is nonheritable in >95% of cases. Telangiectasia is temporal or inferior in the majority of cases, and anterior to the equator in half. B-scan ultrasound aids diagnosis. Fluorescein angiography may help identify the telangiectasia. Treatment is cryotherapy to telangiectatic vessels (or laser photocoagulation if less exudation). Vitrectomy has been considered in severe cases where laser and cryotherapy have failed. When there is macular involvement or extensive exudation, the visual prognosis is poor even after treatment.

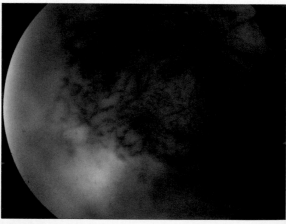

Fig. 12.2: Coats' disease. (Courtesy A. Alkaier)

Persistent Hyperplastic Primary Vitreous

Persistent hyaloid artery represents a remnant of the hyaloid vascular system. This occasionally runs from the disc to the lens; more commonly an anterior remnant gives a Mittendorf dot on the posterior lens surface or a posterior remnant gives a Bergmeister's papilla over the disc.

Persistent hyperplastic primary vitreous (PHPV) occurs when the primary vitreous fails to regress. It may be anterior or posterior. The commonest type is anterior with a microphthalmic eye and a vascularized retrolental mass. Cataract develops early. In the posterior form the lens is usually clear and there is a retinal fold or detachment. It is unilateral in >95% cases with no racial/sex predisposition and is nonheritable in >95%. Observe for angle closure glaucoma secondary to progressive anterior chamber shallowing or direct fibrovascular angle invasion. Exclude other causes of leucocoria (p. 561). Secondary tractional retinal detachment (usually tentlike or sickle-shaped) occurs in a minority of cases. Surgery is rarely required and would normally only be undertaken if the anterior chamber shallowing was causing glaucoma. The final vision is related to the extent of posterior involvement, development of glaucoma, or phthisis.

Toxocariasis

Ocular toxocariasis is caused by infection with the nematode *Toxocara cani* which is commonly found in dogs and is excreted in their faeces. If faecally contaminated matter is ingested, the ova develop into larvae in the gut and then travel to other organs. Ocular infection is always unilateral and presents in the age range 2–10 years as a severe endophthalmitis, or in a slightly older child with posterior or peripheral granuloma formation. Vitreous activity is very variable, and macular dragging or retinal detachment may occur. The eosinophil count may be raised on full blood count or aqueous examination. Immunodiagnostic tests are only about 50% sensitive. Treatment is with local or systemic corticosteroids and albendazole (10 mg/kg of body weight/day in two divided doses).

Retinopathy of Prematurity

Background Retinopathy of prematurity (ROP) is a proliferative retinopathy developing in immature retinal vessels. It is still an important cause of visual loss in premature babies (the major cause is cerebral visual impairment) especially in those of 23–26 weeks gestation. Despite a reducing incidence, >50% of babies <1000 g birth weight develop some ROP. Most ROP will regress, and in the UK only about 2% of screened babies require treatment.

Classification Categorized by the international classification of ROP (ICROP) on location, severity or stage, extent, and plus disease. Normal vascularization proceeds centrifugally from the optic disc to the ora serrata, reaching the nasal edge at about 36 weeks' gestation and the temporal edge at term; thus, any baby born prematurely will have immature retinal vascularization, increasing with decreasing gestation.

■ *Location*: described as 3 concentric zones centred on the disc (Fig. 12.3). Zone I extends 30 degrees from the optic disc, a radius of twice the distance from the disc to the fovea. To define the temporal edge of zone I clinically, view the posterior pole with a 28 D lens and align one edge of the lens with the nasal side of the disc: the temporal lens edge then aligns with the temporal zone edge. Zone II surrounds zone I, up to the nasal ora serrata. Zone III is the residual retina anterior to zone II.

■ *Stage*: Stage 1 is a thin white demarcation line at the junction of anterior avascular and posterior vascularized retina (Fig. 12.4). Stage 2 has a ridge at the avascular/vascular junction. Also included in this stage is 'popcorn' or small retinal tufts of new vessels posterior to the ridge. Stage 3 has neovascularization extending from the ridge into the vitreous. Stage 4, with partial retinal detachment, is subdivided into 4A which is extrafoveal and 4B which involves the fovea. Total retinal detachment is present in stage 5 disease. The most posterior disease present in an eye determines its staging.

■ *Extent*: recorded by the number of clock hours of retina involved.

■ *Plus disease*: is a marker of severity in active ROP and includes engorgement and tortuosity of the posterior pole vessels, iris vessel engorgement, poor pupil dilatation, and vitreous haze. The presence of plus disease is shown by the addition of a plus sign (+) to the staging. Plus disease involves

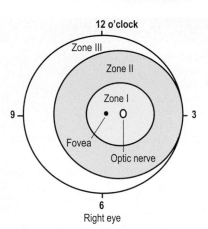

Fig. 12.3: Retinopathy of prematurity, zones I to III.

6 or more clock hours of vessel change. Pre-plus disease involves <6 clock hours and is an intermediate level between normal posterior pole vessels and frank plus disease (Fig. 12.5).

Extremely low birth weight babies may have a different morphology to typical ROP.

Aggressive posterior ROP (AP-ROP) is a deceptively featureless form of ROP which progress rapidly to stage 5 and does not progress through stages 1–3. It usually occurs in zone 1 but can occur in posterior zone 2. There is plus disease with flat brushlike neovascularization at a poorly defined vascular/avascular border.

Screening guidelines In the UK all babies ≤31 weeks gestation (including 31 weeks and 6 days) or ≤1500 g birth weight should be screened. For those <27 weeks gestational age (including 26 weeks and 6 days), start screening at 30–31 weeks post-menstrual age. For those born at or after 27 weeks, start at 4–5 weeks post-natal age. Note the different ways of expressing age. For example, a child born at 23 weeks would be screened 7–8 weeks after birth, and a child born at 28 weeks would be screened at 32–33 weeks gestational age. Examine every 1–2 weeks until vascularization progresses into zone 3. Severe ROP (stage 3 and above) develops between 33 and 43 weeks' gestation.

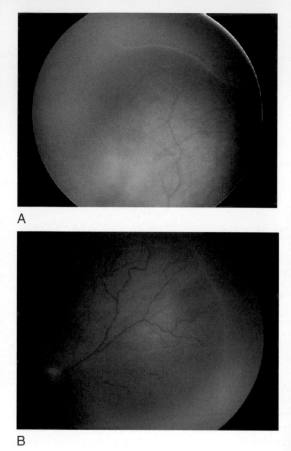

A

B

Fig. 12.4: **(A, B, C, D)** Stage 1 to 4 retinopathy of prematurity, respectively.

History A separate eye record sheet within the neonatal folder helps identify significant disease progression. Document gestational age, birth weight, postnatal age, and significant medical problems.

Examination Dilate with G. phenylephrine 2.5% and G. cyclopentolate 0.5% applied twice, starting 30 minutes before examination. Use an indirect ophthalmoscope and a wide-angle indirect lens (e.g. 28 D or 30 D). If a lid speculum or indentation is

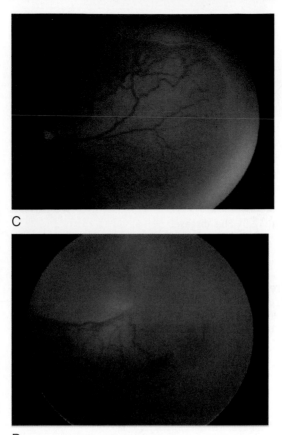

C

D

Fig. 12.4—cont'd.

required instil topical anaesthetic. Imaging using the RetCam can be undertaken, and requires a speculum and topical anaesthetic. Screening stresses the baby, so have a neonatal nurse assisting when examining any infant in an incubator or on oxygen.

Differential diagnosis The cicatricial form of ROP may appear similar to familial exudative vitreoretinopathy, Norrie's disease (abnormally vascularized retinal detachment ± hearing loss and developmental delay), and congenital retinal folds.

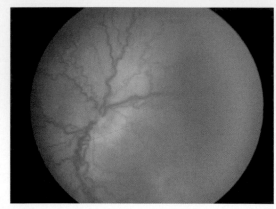

Fig. 12.5: Plus disease.

Treatment is advised for those defined as having type 1 pre-threshold disease (see below) or threshold disease. Review those with type 2 disease and if this progresses to type 1 disease or threshold, then treat.

■ Theshold.

Stage 3 ROP involving at least 5 contiguous or 8 cumulative clock hours in zone I or II, with plus disease.

■ Type 1 pre-threshold disease.

Zone I involvement of any stage with plus disease.

Zone I stage 3 with or without plus.

Zone II stage 2 or 3 with plus disease.

■ Type 2 disease.

Zone I stage 1 or 2 disease without plus.

Zone II stage 3 without plus.

Transpupillary diode laser is the usual treatment, but trans-scleral diode or cryotherapy can be used. Apply burns confluently to all avascular retina up to and just anterior to the ridge. Prescribe G. cyclopentolate 0.5% t.d.s. and prednisolone 0.5%/neomycin q.d.s. for 1 week post-treatment. Review in 1 week. Re-treatment may be required in up to 14% of babies and if required is usually at 2 weeks after the initial treatment. The majority have a favourable outcome (an essentially normal posterior pole).

Treatment for stages 4 and 5 ROP is currently not recommended in the UK.

Follow—up Long-term review is advised for all infants with stage 3 ROP or worse. Issues include subnormal vision, myopia, strabismus, and field loss.

Conjunctivitis of the Newborn (Ophthalmia Neonatorum)

Background Defined as conjunctivitis in neonates aged <4 weeks. The infection may be acquired during delivery (if the mother has vaginal infection or if born in an unhygienic environment) or from postnatal caregivers. Causes include *Chlamydia trachomatis*, *Staphylococcus aureus*, *Streptococcus viridans*, enterococci, *Neisseria gonorrhoeae*, and herpes simplex virus (HSV). Gram-positive cocci are the commonest pathogens.

Signs Look for injected conjunctiva, lid swelling, and discharge. Skin vesicles and keratitis occur with HSV. *N. gonorrhoeae* can cause corneal ulceration and perforation. The causative organism cannot be accurately diagnosed from the clinical presentation but gonococcal conjunctivitis tends to be more severe with earlier onset, usually 2–5 days after birth, whilst chlamydial infection has a creamy white discharge, a velvety conjunctival appearance, and presents at 5–12 days after delivery. Staphylococcal infection often produces a yellow discharge.

Differential diagnosis Conjunctivitis secondary to nasolacrimal duct obstruction. Test for mucopurulent reflux on lacrimal sac massage.

Investigations Arrange an urgent Gram stain to identify any Gram-negative diplococci (*N. gonorrhoea*) and take swabs for bacteria and *Chlamydia*. A special *Chlamydia* swab is required, with the specimen obtained from the everted lid – this must include conjunctival cells and not just exudate. Parents should be warned that the conjunctiva is friable and may bleed after taking the chlamydial swab. If the infant has chlamydial or gonococcal infection, both the mother and her partner require treatment and contact tracing.

Treatment If there is mild to moderate conjunctivitis without a history of maternal vaginal infection, treat empirically with lid hygiene and broad-spectrum topical antibiotic (e.g. ofloxacin 0.3% q.d.s. for 1 week.) until the microbiology results are available.

■ *N. gonorrhoea*: admit and treat with ceftriaxone 25–50 mg/kg i.m. or i.v. o.d. (max 125 mg) if only conjunctivitis. Some advocate a single i.v. injection, others advise 3 days of i.m. injections. Treat for up to a week if there is systemic infection. Coinfection with *Chlamydia* may occur.

- *C. trachomatis*: erythromycin syrup 50 mg/kg/day in four divided doses for 2 weeks. A second course may be required.

- Treat neonatal herpes infection with systemic aciclovir.

Follow–up In general, review outpatients once weekly until improving. If infection recurs, reconsider *Chlamydia* even if initial testing was negative. Observe for chlamydial pneumonitis (cough, nasal discharge, and tachypnoea).

Anterior Segment Dysgenesis

Background Anterior segment dysgenesis (ASD) describes a heterogeneous group of rare disorders characterized by variable maldevelopment of anterior segment structures including the cornea, iris, and drainage angle (Table 12.1). ASD is occasionally associated with systemic abnormalities. Glaucoma is a frequent complication and is often difficult to manage. Goniotomy or trabeculotomy may be required for infantile glaucoma; trabeculectomy with antimetabolites or drainage tubes may be required for juvenile glaucoma. A number of genes have been implicated in this group of disorders. At presentation, draw the family pedigree (p. 412), examine family members, and arrange review with an experienced clinician for genetic testing and counselling. Regularly review refraction, cornea, lens, IOP (use Tonopen if cornea involved), optic nerve, and field tests as required.

Aniridia A condition characterized by bilateral complete or partial iris hypoplasia with associated foveal hypoplasia, resulting in photophobia, reduced acuity (6/36–6/60), and nystagmus presenting in early infancy. Frequently associated ocular abnormalities, often of later onset, include cataract, glaucoma (up to 50%), and corneal opacification and vascularization (secondary to limbal stem cell deficiency). Aniridia may occur as an isolated abnormality without systemic involvement, or as part of the Wilms' tumour–aniridia–genital anomalies–retardation (WAGR) syndrome (PAX6 and adjacent Wilms' tumour, WT-1 locus). Aniridia may be familial or sporadic; both are caused by mutations or deletions of the PAX6 gene on 11p. Children with familial aniridia are not at significantly increased risk of Wilms' tumour and do not need ultrasound screening. Children with sporadic aniridia should be tested for deletion of the Wilms' tumour suppressor gene (WTS). Those with WTS deletion are at high risk of Wilms' tumour and need regular abdominal ultrasound. Usually corneal opacification occurs in adulthood but may occur in children, necessitating limbal stem cell transplant and corneal grafting. Correct any refractive errors with tinted spectacles.

Sclerocornea Describes opaque scleral tissue with fine vascular arcades extending into the peripheral cornea. There is a spectrum of severity from complete corneal opacification to a poorly defined limbus. Most (90%) are bilateral, but often asymmetrical. It is sporadic and nonprogressive and may be associated with: cornea plana (80%); microphthalmos; iridocorneal synechiae; persistent pupillary membrane; angle and iris dysgenesis; congenital glaucoma; coloboma; posterior embryotoxon; mental deficiency; deafness; craniofacial, digital,

Table 12.1: Anterior segment dysgenesis						
Signs	Posterior embryotoxon	Axenfeld's anomaly	Reiger's anomaly	Peter's anomaly type 1	Peter's anomaly type 2	Posterior keratoconus
Prominent Schwalbe's line	✓	✓	✓			
Iris strands to Schwalbe's line		✓	✓			
Hypoplasia of the anterior iris stroma			✓			
Strands from iris collarette to edge of posterior corneal depression				✓	✓	
Posterior corneal depression with variable overlying haze				✓	✓	✓
Central cornea				✓	✓	
Adherence between iris and cornea					✓	
Abnormal lens position/clarity					✓	
Glaucoma %	0	0*	60	50–70	0	

* Called Axenfeld's syndrome if glaucoma is present.

and skin abnormalities. The differential diagnosis includes interstitial keratitis (p. 167) and arcus juvenalis.

Posterior embryotoxon Anterior displacement and enlargement of Schwalbe's line is seen as an irregular circumferential ridge on the posterior corneal surface, just inside the limbus. Present in 10–15% of normal eyes. May be associated with primary congenital glaucoma, Alagille's syndrome, megalocornea, aniridia, corectopia, and Noonan's syndrome.

Axenfeld's anomaly Posterior embryotoxon with attached iris strands. Called Axenfeld's syndrome if glaucoma is present.

Reiger's anomaly Axenfeld's anomaly with hypoplasia and distortion of the iris stroma. May have corectopia or polycoria. Glaucoma occurs due to incomplete development of aqueous outflow pathways. Associated with oculodigital dysplasia, osteogenesis imperfecta and Down's, Ehlers Danlos, Noonan's, and Franceschetti's syndromes. Called Reiger's syndrome (or Axenfeld-Reiger syndrome) if there are skeletal abnormalities such as maxillary hypoplasia, abnormal dentition, micrognathia, hypertelorism, and other limb or spinal malformations.

Peter's anomaly Congenital central corneal opacity (Fig. 12.6) with iridocorneal ± lenticulocorneal adhesions. Bilateral in 80% with glaucoma in 50–70%. Usually sporadic, but when familial, autosomal recessive inheritance is the most common.

◼ *Type I*: usually has no other abnormality.

◼ *Type II*: may have abnormal lens position, cataract, microcornea, microphthalmos, cornea plana, sclerocornea, coloboma, aniridia and dysgenesis of the angle and iris. Corneal grafting is high risk, with many cases having a poor outcome.

Posterior keratoconus May represent a mild variant of Peter's anomaly.

Iridocorneal endothelial (ICE) syndrome Abnormal epithelioid endothelium migrates across the angle and iris, elaborating Descemet's membrane-like tissue. Membrane contraction then causes pupillary abnormalities (Fig. 12.7) and secondary glaucoma. Usually unilateral, progressive, and diagnosed in young to middle-aged patients, rather than in childhood. It is not inherited. Descemet's membrane has a beaten-metal appearance and there may be corneal oedema in relation to the IOP. The iris has stromal thinning, full-thickness holes, 'naevi', and broad tenting peripheral anterior synechiae, depending upon the subcategory. The IOP may be raised and the disc cupped. Perform gonioscopy at presentation, treat elevated IOP, and

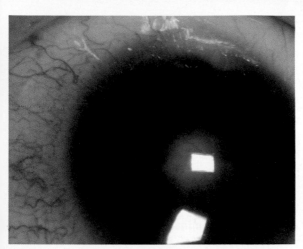

Fig. 12.6: Type II Peter's anomaly (Courtesy of DH Verity).

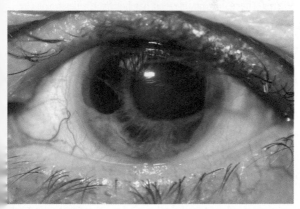

Fig. 12.7: Iridocorneal endothelial (ICE) syndrome (Courtesy PT Khaw).

epithelial oedema (G. sodium chloride 5% q.d.s. and reduce the IOP). May need corneal grafting eventually. Variations include:

- *Chandler's syndrome*: mild iris thinning and pupil distortion.

- *Cogan Reese syndrome*: pigmented iris nodules with variable iris atrophy.

- *Essential iris atrophy*: marked iris thinning, iris holes, and pupil distortion.

Nonaccidental Injury

Background Ophthalmological signs of nonaccidental injury (NAI) can be varied and include periorbital and conjunctival injuries, damage to the anterior segments and lens, and vitreoretinal injuries. One of the commonest ophthalmic manifestations is retinal haemorrhage. Retinal haemorrhages are usually reported in children below 1 year of age and there is about an 80% association between subdural haemorrhage and retinal bleeding in cases of inflicted injury. Retinal haemorrhages can be caused by trauma, both accidental and nonaccidental, and nontraumatically, including infection, raised intracranial pressure, blood disorders, and rare metabolic conditions. For this reason, never assume deliberate harm has, or has not, taken place.

History and examination As legal proceedings are likely to follow, make clear, timed and dated entries in the records, including when continuing onto a new record page. Clearly record the retinal haemorrhages with drawings and photographs.

Signs The morphology of retinal haemorrhage is determined by the anatomy of the layer in which it occurred, rather than by the cause, so the appearances of retinal haemorrhages cannot be used to determine the cause of the bleeding. Although perimacular folds and traumatic retinoschisis are usually only seen in cases of inflicted injury, they have rarely been described as occurring accidentally.

Timing The timing of retinal haemorrhages is only approximate. Superficial haemorrhage normally clears in under a week; deeper intraretinal haemorrhages usually clear in 4 weeks. Preretinal and vitreous haemorrhage take longer to resolve.

Management

- *Casualty*: refer immediately to a consultant ophthalmologist, and designated paediatrician or nurse. They will undertake further management and contact social services if necessary. Consultant examination should occur as soon as possible and within 48 hours.

- *Clinic*: arrange follow-up at 1 week to review any retinal haemorrhage and again clearly describe its morphology. Review until the retinal haemorrhages clear. Some children are left significantly visually impaired from associated damage to the visual pathways, and need long-term follow-up. Electrodiagnostic testing may be useful in these children. Surgery is rarely required but may have to be considered for nonclearing vitreous haemorrhage to prevent deprivational amblyopia.

Reduced Vision with an Otherwise Normal Examination

Background Reduced vision for age with an apparently normal examination may be due to ophthalmic or neurological disease. In the older child it may be functional. Some children will turn out to have subtle abnormalities on detailed examination which will identify the cause of reduced vision.

History Ask about prematurity, consanguinity, family history of ophthalmic disease, photophobia, night blindness, and evidence of field loss.

Examination Perform a full ophthalmic examination. In particular look for nystagmus, which when fine can easily be overlooked. Check for iris transillumination which will suggest albinism. Optic nerve abnormalities such as hypoplasia and atrophy can be subtle and difficult to identify; examine carefully with a direct ophthalmoscope. Check the pupil responses for an afferent defect or sluggish reactions. Small babies usually have small pupils, which may make pupil testing difficult. In older children, check colour vision. A careful examination should exclude albinism and optic nerve hypoplasia. Most retinal dystrophies have fundal abnormalities present by the time visual symptoms occur but in some cases, especially in infants, the early fundus appearance can be normal.

Investigation Perform electrodiagnostic tests if there is no obvious cause for visual loss. Consider paediatric neurological referral and neuroimaging.

Differential diagnosis Depends on the age at presentation.

■ Infants

1. *Cerebral visual impairment*: reduced vision due to damage to the cerebral visual pathways. Most patients have associated neurological deficits. The commonest cause is hypoxic/ischaemic damage, but it may be associated with intracranial infection, bleeding or hydrocephalus. Electrodiagnostic tests show post-retinal dysfunction.

2. *Delayed visual maturation (DVM)*: reduced visual function in a child <16 weeks old. Vision improves with time. Three categories are recognised: visual problem only (type 1), occurring as part of a generalized developmental delay or with fits (type 2), and in association with other ocular disease, particularly albinism (type 3). Electrodiagnostic

tests are normal for age. There is an increased incidence of reading problems in children who had DVM.

3. *Retinal dystrophies*: these may present in infancy or childhood. Most are progressive but some are stationary. They may involve either the rod or cone systems or inner retina. Nystagmus is common in early-onset forms. Electrophysiology is essential for diagnosis. There is an increased incidence of retinal dystrophies in children with high refractive errors.

4. Stationary dystrophies presenting in infancy include *congenial stationary night blindness (CSNB)*, and the *achromatopsias. Leber's congenital amaurosis* is an autosomal recessive, severe, early-onset rod–cone dystrophy. Affected infants have roving eye movements or nystagmus, high hyperopia, and poor pupillary light responses. Eye-poking is common. The initial fundus examination is usually normal but later in childhood a pigmentary retinopathy with optic disc pallor and retinal arteriolar narrowing develops. The electroretinogram (ERG) is severely abnormal or undetectable.

5. *Optic nerve hypoplasia*: may be unilateral or bilateral and of variable severity. The disc is very small and often appears grey. There may be a 'double-ring sign' with the true edge of the optic nerve being surrounded by the scleral opening which may be pigmented. There may be a history of maternal alcohol/drug ingestion. Bilateral cases may be associated with intracranial anomalies, for example septo-optic dysplasia (absence of septum pellucidum and agenesis of the corpus callosum) and pituitary stalk abnormalities. Endocrine abnormalities are common. Arrange neuroimaging and paediatric endocrinology referral.

■ Children.

1. *Neurological disease*: whilst rare, consider neurological diseases which in the early stages may have few ophthalmological signs, including Batten's disease and chiasmal tumours. Batten's disease (p. 497) has an electronegative response on the photoptic ERG; chiasmal disease shows postretinal dysfunction with hemisphere asymmetry.

2. *Retinal dystrophies*: these include CSNB, retinitis pigmentosa, and progressive cone dystrophy. ERGs are abnormal and can distinguish between the different dystrophies.

3. *Inherited macular dystrophies*: Stargardt's disease and X-linked retinoschisis have fundal abnormalities that may be subtle or absent in early disease.

4. *Inherited optic neuropathies*: dominant optic atrophy may be subtle and difficult to detect. Look for yellow/blue colour defect, and a central field defect. *Leber's hereditary optic neuropathy* typically presents in males aged 15–35 years and is caused by a mitochondrial DNA defect, with maternal inheritance. It presents with painless, central visual loss in the first eye, weeks to months prior to second eye involvement. VA worsens over weeks or months, often to 6/60, with colour vision affected early. The optic disc may be normal or hyperaemic with peripapillary telangiectasia in the early stages, but becomes atrophic later. See also page 666.

5. *Functional visual loss*: most commonly presents at age 10–12 years, with girls more frequently affected than boys. It is usually bilateral but can be unilateral. Check vision with neutralizing lenses and look for spiral visual fields. Examine pupils for an afferent pupillary defect. Do not diagnose this condition unless good vision can be demonstrated or appropriate electrodiagnostic testing and/or imaging have been undertaken. Encouragement and reassurance usually help. See also p. 677.

Management Establish the diagnosis and arrange genetic referral if appropriate. Involve paediatric and family support at an early stage. The provision of appropriate spectacle correction, low-vision aids, and educational support are very important. If photophobia is a prominent symptom, tinted spectacles or tinted contact lenses may help.

Optometry and General Practice Guidelines

If there is any doubt about the appropriate referral for a child with an eye problem, ask a pediatric ophthalmologist for advice or discuss with the local hospital eye service out of hours. The following guidelines for hospital referral urgency are not prescriptive, as clinical situations vary.

Same day

- Suspected nonaccidental injury (consult local guidelines first) — p. 578
- Papilloedema with neurological signs or systemically unwell (refer to neurology) — p. 644

Urgent (within 1 week)

- Disc swelling — p. 644
- Sudden onset of double vision — p. 585
- Sudden onset of squint with restricted eye movements — p. 585
- Absent red reflex, or suspected cataract at the 6–8 week postnatal check — p. 562
- Leucocoria — p. 561
- Abnormalities detected at the postnatal check, e.g. anophthalmos, microphthalmos, or colobomas — p. 558
- Neonatal conjunctivitis — p. 572
- Complete ptosis — p. 589

Soon (within 1 month)

- Juvenile arthritis
- Severe allergic eye disease — p. 124
- Staphylococcal keratoconjunctivitis — p. 117
- Children with significantly reduced vision bilaterally — p. 558

Routine

- Meibomian cysts (chalazion) — p. 28
- Squints — p. 583
- Allergic eye disease — p. 124
- Watery eyes — p. 65
- Recurrent conjunctivitis — p. 572

Chapter 13

STRABISMUS

Anatomy and Physiology

Extraocular muscles The actions of the extraocular muscles are summarized in Table 13.1.

The actions of the extraocular muscles are examined in the nine cardinal positions of gaze. This includes moving from the primary position (looking straight ahead) into the eight other cardinal positions, as illustrated in Table 13.2; this also shows the muscle pairs that move the eyes into these positions. Remember *SIN RAD*: *S*uperior muscles (superior rectus, superior oblique) *IN*tort; *R*ecti (superior rectus, inferior rectus) *AD*duct.

Binocular vision The ability to use both eyes simultaneously so that each eye contributes to a common vision perception. Classified as three grades:

- *Simultaneous perception*: the ability to simultaneously perceive two images, one formed on each retina.

- *Fusion*: sensory fusion is the ability to fuse these two images and perceive them as one. Bagolini glasses and the Worth four dot test can be used to confirm sensory fusion. Motor fusion is the ability to maintain sensory fusion through a range of eye movements. Motor fusion is essential to join diplopia because it allows similar retinal images to fall on corresponding retinal points in each eye. The prism fusion range is used to quantify motor fusion.

- *Stereopsis*: the perception of depth based on binocular image disparity.

Binocular single vision (BSV) The ability to use the foveae and other corresponding retinal points in both eyes to perceive a single image with stereopsis. Two types exist:

- *Normal retinal correspondence (NRC)*: the visual directions of both foveae are the same. The temporal retina of one eye corresponds with and has a common visual direction with the nasal retina of the other eye.

- *Abnormal retinal correspondence (ARC)*: a 'second-best' form of binocular vision in which, in the presence of a constant manifest strabismus, the fovea of the fixing eye corresponds

Table 13.1: The actions of the extraocular muscles

Muscle	Primary action	Secondary action	Tertiary action
Medial rectus	Adduction		
Lateral rectus	Abduction		
Superior rectus	Elevation	Intorsion	Adduction
Inferior rectus	Depression	Extorsion	Adduction
Superior oblique	Intorsion	Depression	Abduction
Inferior oblique	Extorsion	Elevation	Abduction

Table 13.2: The actions of the extraocular muscles examined in the nine cardinal positions of gaze

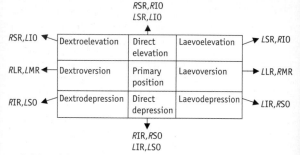

RSR,RIO
LSR,LIO

RSR,LIO ←

Dextroelevation	Direct elevation	Laevoelevation
Dextroversion	Primary position	Laevoversion
Dextrodepression	Direct depression	Laevodepression

→ LSR,RIO

RLR,LMR ← → LLR,RMR

RIR,LSO ← → LIR,RSO

RIR,RSO
LIR,LSO

R,right; L,left; S,superior; I,inferior; R,rectus; O,oblique.

with a nonfoveal area of the deviating eye, e.g. in a manifest left convergent strabismus the fovea of the right eye corresponds with an area of nasal retina in the left eye; all retinal areas (nasal and temporal) similarly adapt when both eyes are open. The angle of anomaly refers to the difference between the subjective and objective angles of deviation.

Suppression The cortical inhibition of the visual sensation from one eye, when both eyes are open. Suppression occurs to avoid diplopia or visual confusion. Suppression areas (scotomata) may vary in position, size, and density.

History and Examination

Background Eyes that are correctly aligned are described as orthophoric or 'straight'. A manifest deviation or heterotropia is when one or other visual axis is not directed towards the fixation point – esotropia if convergent, exotropia if divergent, hypertropia if up, and hypotropia if down. In heterophoria (latent deviation) both eyes are directed towards the fixation point but deviate on dissociation – esophoria (latent convergence), exophoria (latent divergence) or hyperphoria/hypophoria (latent vertical deviations). A constant deviation typically refers to a deviation that is present for near and distance, whereas an intermittent deviation is only present at one distance, e.g. near fixation, or certain conditions, e.g. without spectacles. A concomitant deviation occurs when the angle of deviation is the same in all directions of gaze, whichever eye is fixing, unlike an incomitant deviation where the angle between the two eyes is different in different gaze positions, or with asymmetrical accommodative effort.

History Ask about the presenting complaint and its duration. If diplopia (double vision) is a symptom, ask whether it is monocular or binocular, constant or intermittent, the position of gaze in which it occurs, or whether it produces vertical, horizontal or tilted images. Does it stop the patient from doing anything? Is the deviation socially embarrassing? Check medications and allergies. In children, take a birth history, ask about any family history of amblyopia, strabismus, or refractive error, and make brief developmental assessment if appropriate. Inquire about any previous ophthalmic treatment including spectacles, prisms, occlusion therapy, and surgery. Ask adults about their occupation and if they drive. If in doubt about a prior eye position or abnormal head posture, ask to see old photographs.

General examination and cover testing

- Measure VA and record refraction.

- Observe any abnormal head posture (AHP). The AHP may include head tilt, face turn, or chin elevation or depression. Deafness, torticollis, and cervical spine abnormalities may also cause an AHP.

    Observe ocular posture including an obvious manifest squint, wide epicanthic folds (pseudosquint), spectacles, and any spectacle prisms ('stick-on' Fresnel or incorporated prisms).

- Using a pen torch at 33 cm, observe the corneal reflections (CRs). Look for symmetry or asymmetry. Small manifest deviations may not be obvious by CRs. Note: CRs are central or slightly nasal in most people. Not all abnormal-appearing CRs are due to strabismus, e.g. high refractive errors can produce a pseudosquint – a pseudoesotropia in high myopia.

▣ Perform cover test (CT) at near (33 cm) to a light and then accommodative target (e.g. reduced Snellen letter at VA of worst eye, or pictures/toys for children). CT involves two manoeuvres.

   1. *Cover-uncover test*: to detect manifest strabismus. Cover one eye and look at the noncovered eye. Movement inward to take up fixation indicates an exotropia. Movement outward indicates an esotropia. If the eye is slow to fix the target, this may indicate poor VA or amblyopia. Note any manifest or manifest latent nystagmus (MLN) – horizontal jerky, often very fine nystagmus with fast phase towards the uncovered eye. Note any movement of the covered eye, particularly dissociated vertical deviation (DVD) associated with infantile esotropia.

   2. *Alternating cover test*: to detect latent strabismus. Alternately occlude left and right eye for 1–2 seconds each. Do not allow both eyes to view in between covering as fusion may then take place. A latent deviation sometimes becomes temporarily manifest after fusion is disrupted by testing. Note how fast the eyes resume binocular single vision (BSV) once testing is complete (rapid or slow recovery) indicating how well the deviation is compensated.

▣ Move the target occasionally to check fixation.

▣ Perform CT at distance to a suitably sized chart letter or picture/toy.

▣ Repeat CT with/without glasses, and then with/without AHP.

Eye movements (cranial nerves III, IV, VI)

▣ If suggested by the history, check for monocular diplopia by occluding each eye seperately. Note VA. If not already known, clarify if diplopia is horizontal, vertical, or tilted.

▣ Observe any head tilt, proptosis, ptosis, or lid retraction.

▣ Ask the patient to follow a light held at 50 cm and report if they see diplopia. Go from primary position and back again in the other 8 cardinal positions of gaze (p. 583). Ensure the CRs are always visible; the patient or examiner may need to lift the lids, particularly in downgaze. Check for lid-lag on downward smooth pursuit and any narrowing (Duane's syndrome) or widening (aberrant 3rd nerve regeneration or

Brown's syndrome) of the palpebral aperture on adduction; observe any pupillary changes, e.g. constriction of the pupil in adduction or other gaze position may occur with aberrant 3rd nerve regeneration.

◼ If diplopia occurs in any position, check which image disappears when an eye is covered; the more peripheral image comes from the eye with the paretic muscle(s).

◼ If CT shows a hypertropia/hyperphoria in the primary position (step 1) then do a CT in right and left gaze to see where the height is greatest (step 2). If greater in right gaze then repeat the CT up and down to the right. If the deviation is greater down to the right, a left 4th nerve palsy is suspected. Finally, compare CT (eyes in primary position, fixing at 3 metres) with the head tilted right and left, to see if the height differs (step 3). If the deviation is greater on head tilt left, a left 4th nerve palsy is likely. However, the head tilt test is not always reliable and other causes of hypertropia should not be ignored, e.g. thyroid eye disease. *Park's three-step test* refers to steps 1, 2, and 3 combined. Step 3 is also called the *Bielschowsky head-tilt test*. However, the diagnostic importance of testing in all 9 positions cannot be overemphasised. Vertical deviations can be associated with bilateral (often asymmetrical) muscle under- or overactions.

◼ Examine saccades in suspected supranuclear lesions to help differentiate newly acquired palsies from mechanical strabismus (normal in the latter). Position a target to the right and left of the patient's eyes, within the visual field; instruct the patient to look from one target to the other as quickly as possible, without moving the head. Repeat the test in the vertical plane. Compare the vertical and horizontal velocity of the excursion, as well as the velocity in each eye; e.g. a reduced excursion of the adducting eye on horizontal saccades may indicate an internuclear ophthalmoplegia (same side). Cerebellar disease and MS may produce hypermetric saccades (eyes overshoot the target). Myasthenia gravis and Parkinson's disease may produce hypometric saccades (eyes undershoot the target).

◼ Test convergence to a detailed target, and observe normal pupillary constriction.

◼ If required perform Doll's head manoeuvre to differentiate supranuclear from nonsupranuclear lesions (e.g. Steele Richardson Olszewski Syndrome). Ask the patient to fixate a target in the distance. Inform the patient that you are going to gently move the head right, left, up and down. Observe the extent of ocular rotations. Doll's head movements may be absent in supranuclear lesions.

■ Test optokinetic nystagmus with an OKN drum rotated slowly in front of the patient, both horizontally and vertically, and in both directions. Horizontal asymmetry may indicate a parietal lesion. Convergence retraction nystagmus with a downward moving drum (producing upward re-fixation saccades) suggests Parinaud's syndrome.

Amblyopia

Background Amblyopia is a condition of reduced visual function, in one or both eyes, which is not improved by the correction of any refractive error, or by removal of a pathological obstacle to vision.

Causes are form deprivation and abnormal binocular interaction producing degraded retinal images in the sensitive or critical period of visual system development, particularly in the first 2–3 years of life, decreasing with age, up to 7 years of age. During this sensitive period, amblyopia can develop as well as respond to treatment.

Classification

- *Strabismic amblyopia*: from a constant, unilateral, manifest strabismus.

- *Anisometropic amblyopia*: >1 dioptre interocular difference.

- *Ametropic amblyopia*: bilateral moderate to high refractive errors.

- *Meridional amblyopia*: astigmatism >1.5 dioptres.

- *Stimulus deprivation amblyopia*: lack of adequate visual stimulus in early life, e.g. cataract; ptosis.

History Take a full ophthalmic history noting any previous eye surgery, squint, refractive error, and relevant birth history such as premature delivery. Review previous VA data if available and note poor compliance with glasses or occlusion.

Examination Crowded or logMAR-based VA tests increase the sensitivity to detect amblyopia. If vision testing is unreliable or unachievable, compare fix and follow responses. Suspect amblyopia with constant unilateral strabismus; suspect equal vision (good or bad) with alternating strabismus. Refract and undertake a media and fundus examination. Assess eccentric fixation, which can occur in strabismic amblyopes – under monocular conditions the amblyopic eye does not fixate centrally, but instead with a nonfoveolar area of the retina. Classify as macular, paramacular, peripheral, steady, or unsteady.

In children >6 years old, the presence of motor fusion affects whether to treat or continue to treat, and the risk of causing potentially troublesome diplopia. If good motor fusion is present, certain cases can be occluded after the usual 7–8 year cut-off. If motor fusion is poor or absent, warn parents to stop occlusion if diplopia occurs. Also assess with the Sbisa bar. Place the Sbisa bar over the better eye and record the filter at which diplopia is appreciated. Readily appreciated diplopia indicates weak fusion or less dense suppression and occlusion should be avoided to reduce the risk of subsequent diplopia.

Treatment Prescribe the full spectacle correction to be worn full-time. If vision is 6/24 (0.7 logMAR) or worse, commence treatment (usually occlusion) at the same time; otherwise, reassess VA in spectacles at 6–8 weeks (some practitioners recommend waiting up to 12 weeks). Then commence therapy if:

- VA is stable at worse than 6/9.5 (0.2 logMAR).

- There is more than one logMAR (0.1) line interocular VA difference.

- VA cannot be reliably tested and there is fixation preference.

Occlusion normally starts with 2 hours per day part-time total (light and form deprivation) using an adhesive patch. Increase to 4 hours, and if necessary continue to double hours if VA fails to improve. If necessary, full-time total occlusion can be used for dense amblyopia, particularly if there is poor compliance with occlusion in the past, and/or a VA of 6/24 (0.7 logMAR) or worse.

Penalization is the optical reduction of form vision in the nonamblyopic eye, usually with G. atropine 1% once daily to the better eye. It compares well to occlusion, and is acceptable to carers, but there is a slower improvement.

In children <2.5 years use minimal occlusion because of the risk of occlusion amblyopia, e.g. 20–30 minutes/day, or fixing eye 3 days/nonfixing eye 1 day. If using optical penalization, reduce the frequency of installation of drops.

Stimulus deprivation amblyopia (e.g. cataract) requires a more intensive regimen.

The key to success is compliance. If this cannot be achieved, consider inpatient admission for treatment.

Follow–up Regular follow-up is required. Continue with the dose of occlusion that works for that patient, aiming to achieve 6/9.5 or better, or less than one line interocular difference. Once therapy has ceased, observe for visual regression until 8 years of age. If VA drops more than one line, re-commence occlusion.

Esotropia

Background Esotropia is a manifest convergent squint. The following relates to concomitant esotropia (angle of deviation the same in all positions of gaze and regardless of which eye is fixing). For incomitant strabismus see page 601.

Classification

■ *Primary esotropia*:

1. Constant.

   a. *Constant esotropia with an accommodative element*: esotropia at near and distance with hypermetropic correction. Increases without glasses. Formerly called partially accommodative esotropia.

   b. *Early-onset esotropia (infantile esotropia)*: esotropia at near and distance caused by failure of cortical motor fusion. Onset before 6 months of age. Associated with manifest latent nystagmus (MLN) and dissociated vertical divergence (DVD) where on cover test either eye elevates and extorts under cover.

   c. *Late-onset esotropia*: A sudden-onset esotropia for near and distance usually in a child >5 years, often with diplopia.

2. Intermittent.

   a. *Fully accommodative esotropia*: binocular single vision (BSV) with hypermetropic correction for near and distance. Becomes esotropic for near and distance on accommodation without correction.

   b. *Convergence excess esotropia*: BSV at distance and near when fixing a light; esotropia at near with an accommodative target. Usually associated with hypermetropia but patients can be emmetropic and rarely myopic. Associated with a high accommodative convergence/accommodation (AC/A) ratio.

   c. *Near esotropia*: BSV at distance; esotropia at near with both a light and accommodative target. Normal AC/A ratio.

   d. *Distance esotropia*: BSV at near; esotropia at distance. No limitation of abduction, unlike a lateral rectus palsy which can appear similar. Often associated with myopia; if not, consider neurological disease.

e. *Cyclic esotropia*: varies between straight and large-angle esotropia in rhythmic cycles, usually every 48 hours. Onset usually <5 years of age. Assess patients on alternate days to confirm the diagnosis. Rarely may occur in adults with a secondary squint. Can become a constant esotropia over time.

■ *Consecutive esotropia*: esotropia in a previously divergent eye. May be constant or intermittent. Usually follows surgical overcorrection.

■ *Secondary esotropia*: constant deviation secondary to visual loss or impairment occurring usually before 2 years of age.

History Ask about the nature of any double vision (rare in children), family history of strabismus, febrile illness (may precede accommodative esotropia), developmental delay, previous history of occlusion, spectacles, strabismus surgery, and birth history.

Examination Check VA, cover test with light and accommodative targets (near and distance, with and without spectacles), alternate cover test, and eye movements. 'V' patterns are common (p. 603). Obtain refraction (with cycloplegia in children).

Investigations Stereopsis, fusion, prism cover test, AC/A ratio, synoptophore, and postoperative diplopia test, as required.

Treatment More than one treatment option often applies.

■ *Optical correction*: fully correct any hypermetropia (minus working distance) and treat amblyopia if appropriate. If myopic, reducing the myopic correction may help maintain BSV but the patient must retain good VA to prevent amblyopia. Only in children <3 years might a low myopic correction be postponed. Executive bifocals (+3 D add) can help convergence excess esotropia, and the patient can then be weaned off as the condition stabilizes, e.g. postoperatively.

■ *Amblyopia therapy*: if <8 years (p. 589).

■ *Observe*: consecutive esotropia following exotropia surgery usually settles in a few months; correcting previously uncorrected low hypermetropia or prisms may help. Consecutive estropia should not be allowed to persist for more than 6 weeks without intervention. Consider botulinum toxin or further surgery if it persists. In children <8 years, monitor for amblyopia risk if suppression occurs.

- *Botulinum toxin*: useful in assessing the risk of postoperative diplopia in 'cosmetic' cases not expected to achieve BSV. Also diagnostically useful in cases with weak potential BSV to see if this can be restored, and where several previous squint procedures make surgery unpredictable.

- *Orthoptic exercises*: aim to improve the quality of BSV, and are based on physiological diplopia and using the relationship between accommodation and convergence (e.g. bar reading, stereograms) in carefully selected patients with fully accommodative or convergence excess esotropia, or as an adjunct to surgery.

- *Prisms*: may help small-angle deviations, especially in distance esotropia.

- *Surgery*: performed to improve the appearance of the eyes and, where possible, to restore binocular vision. In general, if surgery is aiming to restore binocular function, it is performed once hypermetropia is satisfactorily corrected and amblyopia treated. The timing of surgery to improve appearance is largely a matter of patient (or parent) preference.

  1. *Constant esotropia with an accommodative element*: operate if cosmetically unsatisfactory with glasses. Consider medial rectus recession (MR−) with lateral rectus resection (LR+) if the deviation is a similar size near and distance, or bilateral MR (bimedial) recessions if the deviation is larger at near. Undercorrect, as residual convergence tends to reduce over time: in the absence of BSV there is a high risk of consecutive exotropia.

  2. *Early-onset esotropia*: requires early surgery, preferably before age 1 year, for any chance of binocular vision, but most patients suppress and there is a risk of consecutive exotropia. Surgery may involve bimedial recession, or medial rectus recession/lateral rectus resection. Patients usually need more than one procedure; however, multiple procedures mean a higher risk of consecutive exotropia as many patients continue to suppress. For cosmetically poor DVD consider bilateral inferior oblique anterior positioning or bilateral superior recti recessions (with Faden procedure for worse eye, if asymmetrical).

  3. *Late-onset esotropia*: botulinum toxin or surgery if BSV not restored by glasses.

  4. *Convergence excess esotropia*: notoriously difficult to manage. Start with bimedial recessions, with further

Esotropia

surgery including Faden procedures or supramaximal medial rectus recessions.

5. *Near esotropia*: normally undertake bimedial recessions.

6. *Distance esotropia*: if not controlled with prisms, usually requires bilateral lateral rectus resections using adjustable sutures, although not all clinicians agree with this surgical approach.

7. *Cyclic esotropia*: consider medial rectus recession with lateral rectus resection as the deviation is usually a similar size near and distance.

Exotropia

Background Exotropia is a manifest divergent squint. The following relates to concomitant exotropia (angle of deviation the same in all positions of gaze and regardless of which eye is fixing). For incomitant strabismus, see page 601.

Classification

■ *Primary exotropia.*

1. Constant.

   a. *Early-onset exotropia*: typically associated with dissociated vertical deviation and manifest latent nystagmus. Much less common than early-onset esotropia and found particularly in Asian or African populations.

   b. *Constant primary exotropia*: rare. Exclude secondary exotropia or decompensating intermittent exotropia. Be suspicious of an associated neurological or developmental problem.

2. Intermittent.

   a. *Distance exotropia*: binocular single vision (BSV) at near; intermittent or constant exotropia at distance. Diplopia is very rare as suppression normally occurs on divergence. Subdivided into 2 types – true distance exotropia and simulated distance exotropia (see differential diagnosis below).

   b. *Near exotropia*: BSV for distance; exotropia for near. Commoner in adults than children, e.g. existing near exophoria decompensated by presbyopic correction.

   c. *Non-specific exotropia*: intermittent exotropia can present in any age group, and for either near or distance fixation.

■ *Consecutive exotropia*: usually follows surgery for esotropia after a variable period of time. Usually constant but can be intermittent.

■ *Secondary exotropia*: constant, secondary to visual impairment, usually >2 years of age.

Symptoms Ask about diplopia, although this is rare except in near and occasionally in consecutive exotropia. Intermittent exotropia commonly presents in toddlers or infants; ask about closure of one eye in bright sunlight. Ask about previous eye treatment or surgery.

Signs VA is reduced in secondary esotropia. Amblyopia is common in consecutive exotropia but rare in intermittent exotropia.

Examination Perform a cover test for near and distance with and without spectacles. Perform the alternate cover test; a slowly recovering latent deviation may decompensate (become manifest) later. Examine eye movements. Intermittent exotropia may have a 'V' exo or 'X' pattern and can have slight limitations of adduction. Consecutive exotropias may have limitation of adduction from previous squint surgery. Reduced convergence can be associated with near exotropia. If VA is reduced, carefully exclude intraocular disease. Obtain refraction.

Investigations The accomodative convergence/ accomodation (AC/A) ratio is often high (>5 : 1) in simulated distance exotropia, normal (3–4 : 1) in true distance exotropia, and low in near exotropia (<3 : 1). Consider postoperative diplopia testing if there is no BSV, e.g. consecutive or secondary exotropia.

Differential diagnosis Distinguish true from simulated distance exotropia. Simulated distance exotropia can be controlled for near by a high AC/A ratio and/or fusional convergence. Disrupt fusion by occluding one eye for >45 minutes then measure the maximum true near angle.

Treatment Treat amblyopia in children <8 years (p. 589). Give the full myopic correction (minus working distance). Use of minus lenses or reduced hyperopic correction can be considered in children to stimulate accommodative convergence to help control intermittent distance exotropia or to improve the cosmetic appearance in consecutive exotropia, but should avoid asthenopia and retain 6/6 VA. The effect of the full hypermetropic correction, which may increase the angle of squint, must be considered when planning surgery. Orthoptic exercises have a role in intermittent deviations <20 prism dioptres, and can be useful postoperatively, e.g. convergence exercises, stereograms. Treat any convergence insufficiency with exercises in near exotropia. Small to moderate-sized distance exotropia often remains stable without deterioration: consider surgery if control deteriorates or for cosmesis. Surgery is often the treatment choice to improve appearance in consecutive and secondary exotropia. Botulinum toxin is useful diagnostically where the quality of BSV is poor or where there is a risk of postoperative diplopia.

Warn the patient that surgery aims for an early postoperative esotropia, as the eyes drifts outward over a few months. Diplopia may occur during this period. Undertake lateral rectus recession (LR–) and medial rectus resection (MR+) in simulated distance exotropia and other exodeviations if the angle is of similar size for near and distance; or bilateral lateral rectus recessions in true distance exotropia or other exodeviations if the angle of deviation is much greater at distance. Consecutive exotropia usually requires exploration with medial rectus advancement and lateral rectus recession, using adjustable sutures in patients >10 years of age.

Microtropia

Background Optimal binocular single vision (BSV) exists with bifoveal fusion. A subnormal variation of BSV can exist with foveal (central) suppression. Microtropia is a small-angle squint (<10 prism dioptres) with foveal suppression in the deviating eye and subnormal stereopsis. Motor fusion is present but the range may be reduced. Microtropia is commonly associated with anisometropia and amblyopia in the deviating eye. Microtropia can also occur after surgical or optical treatment for a larger-angle squint and can be present with other strabismus, e.g. a fully accommodative right microtropia.

Classification

- *Microtropia with identity*: no manifest deviation on cover test because the eccentric point of fixation coincides with the angle of squint and is used for monocular and binocular fixation. There is abnormal retinal correspondence (ARC) with the angle of anomaly (angle of squint) equal to the angle of eccentricity (angle between abnormal point of retinal fixation and normal fovea (p. 583).

- *Microtropia without identity*: a minimal flick deviation is seen on cover testing. Usually but not always esotropic. Central or eccentric fixation and ARC are more common than normal retinal correspondence. The angle of anomaly is larger than the angle of eccentricity.

History and examination Take a full history, perform cover testing, examine eye movements, and refract. Anisometropia is common.

Investigations Assess fusion, stereopsis, and measure any deviation with a prism cover test. The simultaneous prism cover test, rarely used in practice, measures the manifest component of the deviation where there is an associated heterophoria. The 4-dioptre prism test (base out for suspected microesotropia) usually shows no movement when the prism is placed in front of the deviating eye due to central suppression.

Treatment Fully correct refractive error (minus working distance). Consider amblyopia therapy, but if motor fusion is absent or poor there is a risk of intractable diplopia in patients >6 years (p. 589). Treatment is unlikely to produce bifoveal fixation. Treat decompensated microtropias as for concomitant strabismus.

Accommodation and Convergence Disorders

Classification

- Isolated primary convergence insufficiency (CI).
- Primary CI with secondary accommodative insufficiency (AI).
- CI secondary to vertical deviation or decompensating near heterophoria (convergence weakness exophoria).
- Primary AI.
- Near reflex palsy (variably involving convergence, accommodation and pupil).
- Accommodative fatigue.
- Accommodative inertia.

History Patients can present at any age. Symptoms are associated with close work and include blurred vision, difficulty changing focus, horizontal diplopia, headaches, eyestrain, and nausea. Check medication, as this may contribute to reduced accommodative responses, particularly antidepressants, muscle relaxants, antihistamines, and some antihypertensives.

Examination Assess ocular motility, as decompensating vertical deviations may be unable to converge. Check the near pupil response. In patients with near reflex palsy or marked AI or CI the pupils may fail to constrict, or even dilate, on attempted near fixation. Consider neurological assessment in convergence and accommodation paralysis.

Investigations Test the near point of convergence (NPC). The patient follows a small detailed target as it is slowly moved to within 8–10 cm of the nose on an RAF rule. Test three times. CI is diagnosed if this is not achieved, or if only with effort. Check accommodation under emmetropic conditions using the RAF rule; bring the target progressively nearer until blurred. Alternatively, use increasing plus and then minus lenses to determine the accommodative facility. Reduced accommodation is commonly associated with CI. Examine the prism fusion range, as this is often reduced.

Treatment Leave asymptomatic adults without treatment. Consider treating asymptomatic children if they have any other binocular imbalance. Treat with orthoptic exercises (pen and jump convergence, dot cards, stereograms, and voluntary convergence).

Consider prisms if symptoms persist despite exercises. Convex lenses may be needed in those with AI. Botulinum toxin may provide some temporary relief in gross CI. Surgery is unhelpful, as CI recurs.

Incomitant Strabismus

Background Incomitant strabismus occurs when the angle of deviation differs depending upon the direction of gaze or according to which eye is fixing. It is associated mostly with defective eye movements, particularly neurogenic or mechanical lesions such as 3rd nerve palsy or thyroid eye disease, and less commonly with asymmetrical accommodative effort such as anisometropia.

History Establish when symptoms occurred (acute, chronic, congenital). Vague symptoms imply that the deviation is longstanding. Ask about diplopia (monocular or binocular; intermittent or constant; position of gaze when it occurs; vertical, horizontal, or tilted images), trauma, hypertension, diabetes, thyroid conditions, previous eye surgery or treatment. Neck ache may occur with recently acquired abnormal head posture (AHP). Longstanding AHP may be asymptomatic.

Examinations Note any AHP, nystagmus, lid malposition, and pupil reactions. Check spectacles for prisms. Perform cover test with and without any AHP. In paralytic strabismus the secondary deviation of the unaffected eye when fixing with the affected eye will be larger than the primary deviation when fixing with the normal eye, based on Hering's law of equal innervation. Examine ocular movements and perform cover tests in the nine cardinal positions to establish overactions, underactions, and where the deviation is greatest. Compare subjective diplopia with objective findings. Check for bilateral asymmetric underactions. Examine ductions (movements tested monocularly with fellow eye covered) to differentiate underactions versus (mechanical) limitations.

Investigations

- Note the angle of deviation in primary position, fixing right and left eyes, and relevant positions of gaze with the prism cover test (PCT). Look for binocular single vision (BSV), stereopsis, and sensory and motor fusion. Patients with severe head injuries may lose motor fusion with intractable diplopia.

- *Synoptophore*: useful if BSV is not present in free space and for measuring torsion.

- *Hess chart*: based on simultaneous perception. Compare the patient's results with the 'normal' grid on the chart. Different size fields show incomitance. Observe the deviation in the primary position. The smaller field indicates the primarily affected eye (primary deviation), the larger field shows the secondary deviation. The greatest inward displacement compared to the normal field shows the primarily affected muscle(s), or in mechanical limitations the greatest restriction of movement. In the larger field the greatest outward displacement from normal indicates the main overacting muscle(s) – the contralateral synergist according to Hering's law. Longstanding deviations may be more concomitant and identifying the primarily affected muscle can be difficult. In mechanical strabismus the outer field of the Hess chart tends to be compressed. A sloping field indicates an 'A' or 'V' pattern and not torsion.

■ *The field of BSV chart*: usually plotted on an arc perimeter – shows the size, position, and usefulness of the area of BSV.

■ *Imaging*: and other investigations may be required depending on the cause. See the appropriate sections for details (p. 612, 3rd nerve palsy; p. 615, 4th nerve palsy; p. 618 6th nerve palsy).

Treatment Initial management of acquired incomitance includes advice about the use of an AHP, stick-on prisms, or occlusion. The prism is usually placed on one eye: the paralytic eye or the eye with the worst VA. The prism can be tilted to join both vertical and horizontal diplopia. It can also be placed on the top segment (or bifocal segment) of spectacles as required. Aim to join diplopia in the primary position and depression at least. Diplopia on extremes of gaze may not be correctable with prisms as this may lead to overcorrection in another position of gaze. Monitor patients, reducing prism strength as they recover or stabilize. Occlusion. Occlusion, (graded frosting, foils, frosted tape, or lenses) is used for large deviations or large incomitance, unsatisfactorily controlled with prisms, or where there is a lack of fusion. Long-term prisms can be incorporated into glasses for small deviations. Orthoptic exercises have a limited role except for associated convergence insufficiency. Treat amblyopia if age <8 years (p. 589).

Surgery for acquired incomitance is indicated for symptomatic deviations such as unsatisfactory control with prism/large AHP, and when the deviation is stable for at least 6 months. The type and number of operations depends on clinical findings. For neurogenic strabismus, weaken the overacting muscle(s). For mechanical strabismus, weaken the tight muscle(s).

Alphabet Patterns

Background Alphabet pattern refers to a change in the angle of horizontal strabismus in up/downgaze.

Classification

- 'V': a 'V' pattern is a relative divergence of >15 prism dioptres on upgaze compared to downgaze. The normal physiological 'V' pattern measures <15 prism dioptres.

- 'A': a relative divergence of ≥10 prism dioptres or more on downgaze compared to upgaze.

- 'X': relative increase in elevation and depression, usually in an exodeviation.

- 'Y': relative exodeviation on upgaze. Downgaze and primary positions have similar deviations

- 'λ': relative exodeviation on depression. Upgaze and primary positions have similar deviations.

Aetiology The main causes are bilateral oblique and vertical rectus muscle dysfunction, e.g. inferior recti overactions producing adduction on depression ('V' pattern). Conversely, inferior recti underactions produces an 'A' pattern. Super oblique underaction can produce a 'V' pattern, and overaction can produce an 'A' pattern. High medial recti insertions can produce a 'V' Eso pattern and low lateral recti insertions a 'V' Exo pattern. There is a high incidence of 'A'/'V' patterns in children with craniofacial abnormalities.

Symptoms Possible diplopia where the deviation is greatest.

Signs Chin elevation or depression to achieve binocular single vision. May have vertical deviation in primary position if vertical recti/oblique actions are asymmetrical.

Examination Cover test for near, distance, depression, and elevation by moving the head up and down. Look for bilateral asymmetrical muscle dysfunctions during eye movement testing.

Investigations Hess chart: slanting sides indicate an 'A' or 'V' pattern.

Treatment Usually surgical. If there are oblique overactions these should be weakened. For a 'V' pattern, inferior obliques are recessed or disinserted. Superior oblique posterior tenotomies are used for 'A' patterns. Weakening the obliques may cause a relative esodeviation. Where no oblique overactions occur, transposing the horizontal recti by a half or full muscle width, as shown in Figure 13.1 below, can reduce 'A' or 'V' patterns. This can be combined with recession/resection of horizontal recti.

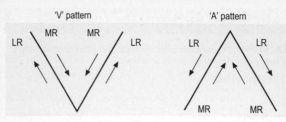

Fig. 13.1: Transposition of horizontal recti in 'A' and 'V' patterns. The arrows indicate the direction of muscle transposition.

Duane's Syndrome

Background Duane's syndrome is a spectrum of congenital motility disorders with anomalous innervation of the lateral rectus muscle, together with retraction of the globe, and narrowing of the palpebral fissure on adduction. There is hypoplasia of the 6th nerve nucleus and/or absence of the 6th nerve, with the lateral rectus being innervated by a branch of the 3rd nerve. Secondary myogenic factors are also involved.

The condition usually presents in childhood but mild cases are sometimes picked up incidentally in adults. It is more common for the left eye and females to be affected. The condition may also be bilateral, although very asymmetrical in some cases. Systemic abnormalities may coexist: hearing defects, ear malformations, Goldenhar's syndrome, Klippel-Feil syndrome, or spinal abnormalities.

Classification

- The essential underlying pathophysiology is similar in all types, but they differ in the degrees of abnormality of the lateral and medial rectus innervations (Table 13.3).

- Alternatively, Duane's syndrome is sometimes referred to as typical (mainly limited abduction), or atypical (mainly limited adduction).

History and examination Check for anisometropia and amblyopia. Observe any abnormal head posture (AHP): usually a face-turn to the affected side in types 1 and 3 and to the opposite side in type 2. Most patients have fusion and stereopsis, often maintained by the AHP. Diplopia is rare.

- *Cover test*:

  1. Types 1 and 3: orthophoria/esophoria/esotropia

  2. Types 2 and 3: exophoria/exotropia.

- *Ocular movements*: lids show narrowing of the palpebral fissure on adduction with retraction of the globe on attempted adduction (Fig. 13.2). The palpebral fissure often widens on abduction. Upshoot or downshoot of the eye may occur on

Table 13.3: Classification of Duane's syndrome		
	Abduction	**Adduction**
Type 1	Limited or absent	Normal or slight limitation
Type 2	Normal or slight limitation	Limitation or absent
Type 3	Marked limitation or absent	Marked limitation or absent

adduction. Retraction on adduction is often best observed from the side. Palpebral fissure changes can be subtle.

Treatment Treat associated refractive error and amblyopia if <8 years (p. 589). Prisms and botulinum toxin have a limited role.

Surgery: has a limited role and patients/carers must understand that normal eye movements cannot be restored. Indications include a large primary position deviation, noticeable AHP, marked globe retraction or up/downshoots, and large decompensating phorias.

- Type 1: ipsilateral/bilateral medial rectus recession(s).

  a. With large deviation and no abduction beyond midline: vertical muscle transposition (superior rectus and inferior rectus moved to lateral rectus).

- Type 2: ipsilateral/bilateral lateral rectus recessions.

  a. With globe retraction: ipsilateral medial and lateral rectus recessions.

  b. With up/downshoots: lateral rectus recession and splitting.

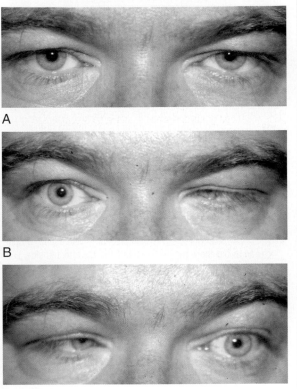

A

B

C

Fig. 13.2: Bilateral type 1 Duane's syndrome.

Brown's Syndrome

Background A condition with limited elevation in adduction due to mechanical restriction rather than inferior oblique paresis. Commonly congenial but can be acquired. May be constant or intermittent. Congenital cases were previously thought to be due to a short superior oblique tendon sheath, but are now considered to be caused by anomalies of the tendon–trochlear complex. Causes of acquired Brown's syndrome include trauma of the trochlear region, sinus surgery, inflammatory conditions, and following superior oblique surgery.

History and examination

- In congenital cases, parents may not notice reduced elevation but instead the overaction of the contralateral eye on elevation. Acquired cases usually complain of diplopia.

- *Abnormal head posture* (AHP): if present, this is usually a chin elevation but there may be a head tilt to the affected side ± face turn away from the affected side.

- *Cover test*: often straight in the primary position with binocular single vision (BSV) or less commonly, hypotropia in the affected eye/hypertropia in the unaffected eye.

- *Ocular movements*: features include limited elevation in adduction, usually good elevation in abduction (Fig. 13.3), overaction of the contralateral superior rectus, and no/minimal ipsilateral superior oblique overaction (Fig. 13.4). A 'V' pattern

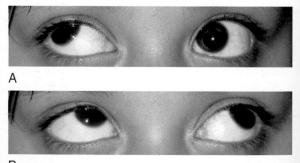

A

B

Fig. 13.3: Left Brown's syndrome.

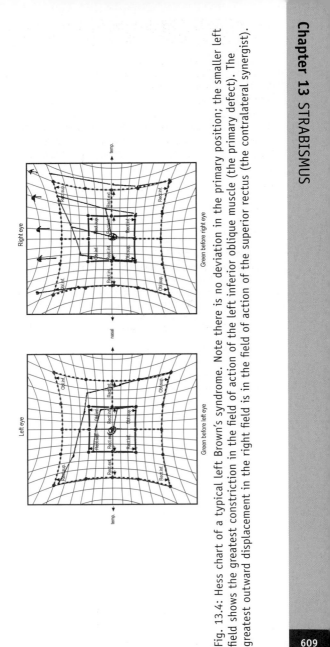

Fig. 13.4: Hess chart of a typical left Brown's syndrome. Note there is no deviation in the primary position; the smaller left field shows the greatest constriction in the field of action of the left inferior oblique muscle (the primary defect). The greatest outward displacement in the right field is in the field of action of the superior rectus (the contralateral synergist).

is often present. There may be down-drift in adduction and widening of the palpebral fissure in adduction. There is resistance to passive elevation of the eye in adduction (positive forced-duction test). Check for an audible/palpable click on elevation. Diplopia, if present, is usually on elevation.

Treatment

■ Treat any refractive error and amblyopia, if present (p. 589). Most patients do not require surgery as BSV is present in primary position and downgaze. Also, spontaneous improvement can occur in congenital cases, particularly in cases with a click/discomfort on elevation in adduction.

■ If associated with an acquired inflammatory condition local, peritrochlear steroid injections can be beneficial.

■ Surgery is indicated if there is significant hypotropia in the primary position or marked AHP. Surgical options include superior oblique tenotomy/tenectomy (be aware of the risk of palsy requiring further treatment), silicone band, or suture spacer on the tendon. Patients with Brown's syndrome secondary to trauma often have a poor surgical outcome.

Thyroid Eye Disease

Background Patients with thyroid eye disease (TED) may experience diplopia due to inflammatory change that is then followed by extraocular muscle fibrosis. For other aspects of TED, see page 81.

History Diplopia is commonly intermittent, vertical, and in either upgaze or primary position. It may be worse in the morning (fusion interrupted overnight) and evening (from decompensation).

Examination Note any abnormal head posture (commonly chin elevation to maintain binocular single vision because of limited elevation) perform cover test, and examine eye movements. A tight inferior rectus is most common (restricted elevation, maximum in abduction, hypodeviation, and possible excyclotorsion) followed by medial rectus (restricted abduction, esodeviation) and then superior rectus (limited depression maximum in abduction). Hypo- and esodeviations often coexist. Look for bilateral signs that may be asymmetric. An 'A' esodeviation is common, especially following orbital decompression.

Investigations Compare the Hess chart to ocular motility. Be aware that patients with moderately limited elevation may guess the upper points when plotting the Hess chart (using visual fields, or moving head). Consider testing field of binocular single vision and monocular eye movements (uniocular fixation).

Management Prisms are often helpful if diplopia is present in the primary position. Occlusion of one eye may be necessary for very large incomitant deviations. Await stability for at least 6 months before undertaking corrective surgery. Both horizontal and vertical surgery may be required. Use recession not resections, preferably with adjustable sutures. Recess the inferior rectus for hypotropia or restricted elevation. Recess the medial rectus for esotropia. Bilateral surgery is common, e.g. bilateral inferior recti recessions for bilateral limited elevation. Four muscles can be recessed at one operation (two in each eye); usually one eye has the medial and inferior recti on adjustable sutures.

3rd Nerve Palsy

Background Signs and symptoms vary depending on the site of the lesion. A painful, unilateral 3rd nerve palsy suggests a posterior communicating artery aneurysm, requiring an emergency neurological referral. Microvascular, pupil-sparing 3rd nerve palsies are commonly associated with diabetes and hypertension. Other causes of 3rd nerve palsy include trauma, neoplasm, infection, migraine, congenital cases, and giant cell arteritis (rare).

Signs A total 3rd nerve palsy affects all extraocular muscles except the superior oblique and lateral rectus, which act unopposed to give exotropia and hypotropia ('down and out') plus a dilated pupil with paralysis of accommodation. The extent to which the 3rd nerve is affected can depend on various factors, including aetiology, e.g. pupil-sparing 3rd nerve palsies are commonly ischaemic (microvascular). Superior division involvement produces ptosis and superior rectus underaction.

There may be aberrant regeneration as the affected nerve fibres are misdirected during recovery, producing retraction of the upper lid on attempted adduction ± depression, adduction on attempted elevation (+ rarely depression), pupil constriction on attempted adduction ± depression, retraction of the globe on attempted elevation ± depression. Aberrant regeneration is rare with microvascular causes.

History Ask about the duration of onset, diabetes, hypertension, headache, trauma, features of giant cell arteritis, myasthenia gravis, and MS.

Examination Check BP, other cranial nerves including visual fields, fundus for retinopathy and optic disc swelling. Examine the temporal arteries if aged >50 years. Exclude proptosis, lid fatigue with sustained upgaze, and Cogan's lid twitch (overshoot of lid when going from sustained downgaze to primary position). Check eye movements and cover test.

Investigation

- *Orthoptic testing*

- *Pupil sparing*: fasting glucose. ESR and CRP if age >50 years. Request CT or MRI if age <50 years and no diabetes or hypertension.

- *Pupil or other cranial nerves involved, or optic disc swelling*: urgent CT or MRI via a neurologist.

- *Myasthenia suspected*: consider Tensilon test via a neurologist, or 'ice-pack test' (an ice pack applied to lid for 10 minutes improves neuromuscular transmission and improves function).

■ *Congenital cases*: work-up for a possible neurological aetiology.

■ *Hess chart*: Figure 13.5.

Treatment

■ Treat amblyopia in children <8 years old (p. 589). Prisms may help in isolated muscle cases.

■ Surgery only achieves a limited area of binocular single vision at best. The main aim is to improve the appearance. Residual diplopia can be treated with an occlusive contact lens.

1. *Exotropia with hypotropia*: large lateral rectus recession, and resection of medial rectus with supraplacement of the insertions. Consider recessions of contralateral synergists.

2. *Mainly exotropia*: large lateral rectus recession and resection of medial rectus with temporary traction sutures. Nasal transposition of the vertical rectus muscles.

3. *Superior division*: Knapp procedure for hypotropia.

4. *Inferior division*: inverse Knapp for hypertropia on depression.

Follow–up Review isolated pupil-sparing cases at 1 week, then monthly. Expect improvement in presumed microvascular cases and arrange CT or MRI if not evident in 6–12 weeks, or if any aberrant regeneration occurs.

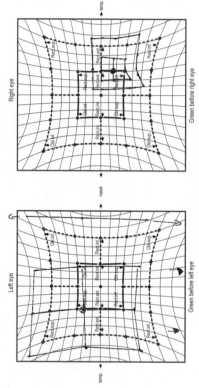

Fig. 13.5: Hess chart of a total right third nerve palsy. This shows the primary deviation with the right eye exotropic and hypotropic (right lateral rectus and superior oblique functioning). The right affected eye has the smaller field and is markedly constricted in the fields of action of the affected muscles (right superior, medial and inferior recti and inferior oblique). The large left field shows the secondary deviation and overactions of the contralateral synergists (Sherrington's law).

4th Nerve Palsy

Background May be uni- or bilateral, congenital (abnormal superior oblique tendon/trochlea) or acquired (head trauma; trochlear/orbital injury; ENT surgery; sinus infections, or vascular). May also be idiopathic or associated with hypertension and diabetes, or more rarely demyelination, giant cell arteritis, tumours, and aneurysms.

Symptoms Vertical diplopia ± torsional and horizontal components.

Signs A left superior oblique palsy may have a head tilt ± slight face turn to right, with chin depression. Cover testing shows left hyperdeviation, greater for near, with slight esodeviation. Excyclotorsion may be present. Hyperdeviation and diplopia increase in dextrodepression but this is less common in congenital cases. Torsional diplopia is maximum on laevodepression. The Bielschowsky head tilt test (p. 587) may show a positive result – an increased hyperdeviation on head tilt left – but not all practitioners feel it is reliable.

History and examination Diplopia is a presenting sign in acquired cases – usually vertical, on depression and to one side; diplopia may also have horizontal and tilted components. In congenital cases diplopia is less common as a presenting symptom. Such cases may present at any age because of signs of decompensating or abnormal head posture (AHP) noticed by others.

Investigations

- *Full orthoptic testing* including vertical fusion range.
- *Synoptophore*.
- *Hess chart*: Figure 13.6.
- *Blood tests*: fasting glucose. ESR and CRP if age > 50 years.
- *CT or MRI*: request if age <50 years and no diabetes or hypertension, or if failure to improve after 6 weeks. Image urgently via neurologists if there are other signs, including cranial nerve palsies.

Differential diagnosis

- *Congenital versus acquired*: acquired cases are more likely to experience diplopia, especially with subjective torsion, have binocular single vision, and normal (6 dioptres) vertical fusion range. Congenital cases may have contralateral facial

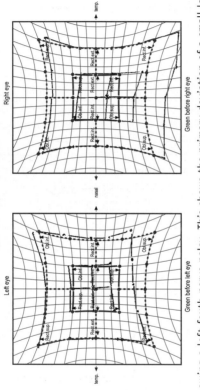

Fig. 13.6: Hess chart showing a left fouth nerve palsy. This shows the primary deviation of a small left hypertropia. The smaller left field shows greatest constriction in the field of action of the superior oblique. The left fields also shows a small overaction of the unopposed ipsilateral antagonist – left inferior oblique. The right field shows the larger secondary deviation – right hypotropia (Hering's law) and the greatest enlargement is in the field of action of the right inferior rectus (contralateral synergist – Sherrington's law), and a slight underaction of the right superior rectus (secondary inhibitional palsy of contralateral antagonist).

hypoplasia, a large vertical fusion range (but not always), and often have a longstanding AHP which can be seen in old photographs.

■ *Unilateral versus bilateral*: assume bilateral until proved otherwise. Bilaterality is suggested by a 'V' esodeviation, a right over left in laevodepression and left over right in dextrodepression (may be very asymmetrical), and ≥10 degrees of excyclotorsion on the synoptophore in depression.

■ *Other diseases*: consider myasthenia gravis, skew deviation, and orbital disease.

Treatment

■ *Medical*: prisms (and/or AHP) may control small deviations. Joining the vertical diplopia often allows patients to then fuse a remaining slight horizontal deviation, if present. Prisms cannot join torsional diplopia. Treat any amblyopia in children <8 years (p. 589).

■ *Surgery*: options for hyperdeviation include:

1. Ipsilateral inferior oblique weakening if <15 prism dioptres in primary position.

2. Superior oblique tendon tuck if superior oblique underaction exceeds inferior oblique overaction, particularly in congenital cases.

3. Ipsilateral superior rectus recession.

4. Contralateral inferior rectus recession.

For bilateral acquired cases perform bilateral Harado-Ito procedure to correct torsion first.

Follow-up

■ All patients are seen every 1–2 months whilst being monitored for stability/recovery.

■ Unilateral cases of vascular origin usually recover within 6 months. Congenital cases, as the deviations tend to be larger, often require surgery as do large unrecovered vascular or more frequently bilateral traumatic superior oblique palsies. Small unrecovered deviations with vertical/horizontal diplopia can be managed long-term by incorporating prisms into spectacles.

6th Nerve Palsy

Background Several possible causes include:

- *Adults*: microvascular (particularly if aged >50 years, hypertensive, or diabetic), MS, neoplasm, head trauma, infection (bacterial or viral), raised intracranial pressure, and idiopathic.

- *Children*: similar to adults except microvascular causes are unlikely. Transient 6th nerve palsies may occur in neonates. 'Benign 6th nerve palsy of childhood' may occur 1–3 weeks after a febrile viral illness.

Symptoms Horizontal diplopia greater looking to the affected side and in the distance. Diplopia may be constant in total 6th nerve palsy.

Signs Patients may have a head turn to the same side, limited abduction, and esodeviation most easily detected with cover test and a distant target, comparing findings in extreme left and right gaze. Nuclear lesions are accompanied by a gaze palsy to the same side because of involvement of the conjugate gaze mechanism. Pontine lesions may be accompanied by a 7th nerve palsy, and cavernous sinus disease is often accompanied by 3rd , 4th and trigeminal division of 5th nerve palsies. Look for bilaterality.

History and examination See page 612.

Investigations

- *Orthoptic testing*: a prism cover test (PCT) in right and left gaze at distance quantifies incomitance and is useful diagnostically and preoperatively. There is usually motor fusion and stereopsis at near.

- *Hess chart*: Figure 13.7.

- *Blood tests*: fasting glucose. ESR and CRP if >50 years old.

- *MRI and CT*: request if age <50 years and no diabetes or hypertension, or if failure to improve after 6 weeks. Image urgently via a neurologists if there are other signs, including other cranial nerve palsies.

Management Most microvascular palsies and childhood postviral palsies resolve spontaneously, so offer prisms or, for large very incomitant deviations, occlusion. If stable and symptomatic after more than 6 months, consider surgery. The selected operation depends on the abduction status (check with

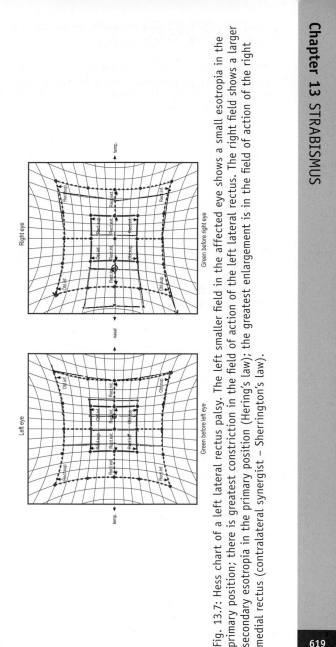

Fig. 13.7: Hess chart of a left lateral rectus palsy. The left smaller field in the affected eye shows a small esotropia in the primary position; there is greatest constriction in the field of action of the left lateral rectus. The right field shows a larger secondary esotropia in the primary position (Hering's law); the greatest enlargement is in the field of action of the right medial rectus (contralateral synergist – Sherrington's law).

diagnostic botulinum toxin to medial rectus). If there is abduction beyond the midline, the palsy is incomplete, so perform medial rectus recession and lateral rectus resection. If not, the palsy is complete, so undertake transposition of the vertical recti to the lateral rectus border and botulinum toxin to the ispilateral medial rectus. Treat bilateral palsies like unilateral ones, but these often need second-stage surgery.

Follow–up Monitor for stability or recovery. Review every 1–2 months. Unilateral cases of vascular origin usually recover within 6 months. If recovery does not take place, smaller unrecovered deviations can be managed long-term by incorporating prisms into spectacles. Larger/very incomitant deviations may require surgery.

Optometry and General Practice Guidelines

General comments

All children under the age of 5 years with suspected strabismus and amblyopia should be assessed by an orthoptist. However, those who are older than 5 years may be seen initially by a community optometrist. The risk of amblyopia and strabismus is increased in children with a family history of squint, amblyopia or a high refractive error (particularly hypermetropia), and children born prematurely or with developmental delay.

Optometrists

Preschool children who are found to have abnormal amounts of hypermetropia (>+3.5 dioptres), or anisometropia (>1.0 dioptre), or astigmatism (>1.5 dioptres) are at risk of developing strabismus and amblyopia. To prevent this, a spectacle correction is required. If in doubt about management, discuss with a Hospital Eye Service.

General practice

Never delay referral for suspected squint as it is very rare for a child to 'grow out of it'. Squint or limited eye movements due to trauma, even when the eye does not appear inflamed, should be seen the same day. Childhood refractive errors (without squint) are usually treated by an optometrist experienced in refracting children.

The following guide to referral urgency is not prescriptive, as clinical situations vary.

Same day

■ 3rd nerve palsy with pupil involvement p. 612

■ Orbital blow-out fractures p. 101

■ 6th nerve palsy with papilloedema (refer to neurology) p. 618

Urgent (within 1 week)

■ Sudden onset of squint with diplopia in a child >5 years p. 585

■ Sudden onset of double vision p. 585

■ Squint with other neurological symptoms or signs p. 585

Routine

Chapter 14

NEURO-OPHTHALMOLOGY

History and Examination

History Ask about past medical history, drug history, family history, and occupation. Smoking, alcohol use and diet may be particularly important. The history is guided by the presenting complaint. The following symptoms and signs are relatively common and are dealt with elsewhere:

- *Transient visual loss*: page 634.

- *Headache*: page 649.

- *Anisocoria*: page 632.

- *Diplopia*: page 585.

- *Ptosis*: page 26.

Examination Basic neuro-ophthalmic examination includes: near and distance VA, colour vision, confrontation field tests, pupil tests, cover tests, eye movements, cranial nerves, fundoscopy including optic nerve examination, and other tests as indicated. Full neurological examination may be required.

- *Cover test and eye movements:* see page 585.

- *Pupils:*

    1. Observe: look for anisocoria, ptosis, and iris abnormality (heterochromia, rubeosis, posterior synechiae, coloboma).

    2. Check the near response using an accommodative target (some patients find it easier to converge on their own finger).

    3. Test pupillary constriction to light: dim the lights and ask the patient to look at a distance target. Check the direct response (pupil constriction in the same eye) and consensual response (fellow eye constriction). Use a very bright light such as an indirect ophthalmoscope.

4. Look for a relative afferent pupillary defect (RAPD) using the swinging light test. Ask the patient to fix on a distant object. Shine light in one eye for 3 seconds, then move to the other for the same interval. Repeat as required but do not spend longer on one eye than the other as this may bleach the retina and create an artificial RAPD. If the left optic nerve is damaged, shining the light in the right eye will produce a normal efferent response in the right and left pupil. Moving the light to the left eye then causes a paradoxical dilatation of both pupils as the stimulus intensity is effectively diminished (left RAPD). Retinal disease, if extensive enough, will also impair the pupil light reflex. Only one functioning pupil is required to test for an RAPD; for example, in a patient with a 3rd nerve palsy with a fixed dilated pupil the test can be carried out as above but only the active pupil is observed. Remember that in bilateral symmetrical optic nerve disease the pupil deficit will be balanced and no RAPD will be elicited.

■ *Confrontation visual field testing:*

1. Establish the VA and explain that you are testing peripheral vision.

2. Ask the patient to cover one eye with the palm of their hand: 'Look at my nose: are any parts of my face missing or blurred? Can you see both my eyes?'

3. Hold up both your palms, one in each hemifield and ask, 'Is each hand equally clear, are there any differences or does each hand look the same?'

4. Now ask the patient to fix on your eye. Always begin by testing for a defect to hand movements. Advance your hand, with fingers moving, from the periphery towards fixation, asking the patient to report when they see movement. A patient will not be able to count fingers in a visual field region in which he or she cannot detect hand movements.

5. Ask the patient to fixate on your eye and hold up a finger in one quadrant; ask how many fingers can be seen. Repeat in each quadrant, presenting 1, 2, or 5 fingers (3 or 4 is too difficult). This will identify areas where vision is better than hand movements.

6. In visual field areas where finger-counting vision has been established look for red desaturation using a red target such as a 4 mm hat pin (a red bottle top may also be used but it is too large for the blind spot or small

scotomas). Compare subjective colour intensity in four quadrants whilst fixating your eye. Simultaneously holding two red pins either side of the vertical midline (in each eye separately) may help detect bitemporal red desaturation from pituitary tumours or a relative homonymous hemianopia.

7. Test the midperipheral and central field with the red target. 'Tell me when you first see the red colour, rather than the pin, and tell me if it then disappears or the colour changes at any point.' Move obliquely in each quadrant from periphery to fixation, equidistant between you and patient. Compare to your own monocular visual field. Look for scotomas.

8. Consider comparing the blind spot size with your own using the red target.

9. It is possible to ascertain the isopter to a small white target such as a 4 mm white hat pin. Failure to detect the white target indicates greater severity of loss than is revealed by the 'red desaturation' technique. Similarly, the white target can also be used to plot scotomas and the blind spot.

10. Test the fellow eye.

11. If any defect is detected, draw fields and arrange formal testing. Document the left eye visual field on the left side of the page; the right visual field on the right side of the page (opposite convention to VA).

12. For the interpretation of common field defects, see page 639.

■ *Colour vision.*

Optic nerve damage can result in loss of colour saturation and poor colour discrimination before significant acuity loss is present. This is very helpful in determining the likely cause of visual loss (i.e. refractive, lenticular, retinal, optic nerve, postchiasmal) and is usually tested with Ishihara plates. The procedure is as follows:

1. Patients should wear reading correction if required.

2. Cover one eye and ask patient to read through the book. Allow 2 or 3 seconds per plate only.

3. Patients with VA better than 6/60 can usually complete the test, but do not proceed if they cannot see the first test plate. Test patients before examining them with bright lights (e.g. fundal examination or RAPD check) or allow them

several minutes to recover after such examination. Patients who have had dilating drops can still perform the test but may need to use a +1.00 or +2.00 lens. Consider testing red desaturation instead if VA is very poor (see below).

4. Score the number of plates read out of 13, 17, or 21 depending on which book is used (1/17 or 'control only' if only the test plate was read). Record the reading distance and any refractive correction.

5. There are some plates which only some patients with congenital anomalous colour vision (Daltonism) will be able to read. Do not include these when testing for acquired visual loss unless the patient has Daltonsim.

6. Patients who cannot identify numerals (e.g. small children) can be asked to trace the outline of the numbers with their finger or trace the wiggly line across the page in the colour plates at the end of the book.

7. The Ishihara book comes with instructions on how to interpret performance on the missed plates in cases of Daltonism. The missed and misread numbers should be the same using each eye.

■ *Red desaturation.*

Ask the patient to report any difference in the appearance of a red target viewed with each eye in turn.

■ *Cranial nerves.*

    I. Rarely formally tested; ask about sense of smell and if food tastes different.

    II. Test VA, pupil reactions, visual field and colour vision.

III, IV, VI. See eye movements examination (p. 585).

    V. Warn the patient then test corneal sensation by lightly touching a wisp of cotton-wool on the peripheral cornea. Sensation may be decreased in contact lens wearers, recurrent herpetic keratitis, or if anaesthetic drops have been instilled to check IOP. Check skin sensation to light touch and pin prick on the face. Ask the patent to clench the teeth together and feel for contraction of the masseter muscles. Ask the patient to open the mouth against the resistance of your hand and look for jaw deviation towards the weaker side.

    VII. Ask the patient to show their teeth (smile), purse lips, blow out cheeks against the resistance of your fingers, raise eyebrows (forehead wrinkling is spared in central/upper motor neurone lesions) and screw up eyes (assess Bell's phenomenon). Look for loss or asymmetry of nasolabial folds. Assess for lagophthalmos and corneal exposure by asking the patient to close the eyes lightly.

VIII. Ask about hearing loss and vertigo. Cover one ear and whisper a number in the other for the patient to repeat. To test more formally, check that a 256 Hz or 512 Hz tuning fork held on the midline forehead (Weber's test) is heard equally in both ears, and that air conduction persists after audible bone conduction (with the tuning fork held on mastoid) ceases (Rinné's test).

IX, X. Ask the patient to open their mouth and say 'Ahhh!'. Look for symmetrical elevation of the uvula, or deviation away from the affected side. Ask about any choking or problems swallowing. Test the gag reflex with an orange dressed stick if concerned.

XI. Ask the patient to lift both shoulders and press down to check power. Ask the patient to turn the chin towards one shoulder and press against this action with your palm. With the other hand, feel the muscle bulk of sternocleidomastoid.

XII. Observe the patient's tongue when it is in their mouth for fasciculations or wasting. Ask the patient to stick out their tongue (deviates to the weaker side).

■ *Cerebellar tests.*

1. Listen to the patient's speech, which may be slurred or interrupted and staccato. Ask them to say 'British constitution' or 'Baby hippopotamus.'

2. Dysdiadochokinesis: Ask the patient to place one hand palm down and then rapidly turn it palm up and palm down again, repeating this about 10 times. Compare with the other side. This is often a little asymmetrical in people who are strongly right or left handed.

3. Ask the patient to touch their nose and then touch your finger held about 50 cm in front of them, then to touch their nose again. Repeat this, moving your own finger further away to make the patient stretch to reach it. In cerebellar disease past-pointing occurs and an intention tremor appears or increases as the target is approached.

4. Examine gait, which in cerebellar disease will be broad-based. If uncertain, ask the patient to walk 'heel-toe' (as if on a tight rope), which will exaggerate minor degrees of gait ataxia.

5. If gait is unsteady, perform Romberg's test of dorsal column function (proprioception). Ask the patient to stand still with feet together and eyes open. If the patient cannot do this, abandon the test. See how steady the patient is for 15 seconds then ask the patient to close their eyes. In cerebellar disease there should be little difference in balance whether the eyes are closed or open, whilst in dorsal column disease the patient will become more unsteady when the eyes are shut. Do not let the patient fall!

6. If the patient has binocular double vision, consider patching one eye for steps 3 to 5.

Investigations

Computed tomography (CT)

See page 75.

Magnetic Resonance Imaging (MRI)

Useful for imaging the anterior and posterior visual pathways (including optic nerve, chiasm, optic tracts, optic radiation and visual cortex), brain, soft tissue or vascular masses, and nonorganic, nonmetallic foreign bodies (FB). Does not show bone or calcium well. More expensive and less readily available than CT, and less useful for some orbital disease. Contraindications include a pacemaker and possible metal FB. Patients with clipped intracranial aneurysms need documentation to show that their clip is not ferromagnetic.

■ Commonly used sequences:

a. T_1 *image*: best for structural definition of anatomy. Water (vitreous and CSF) appears black (hypointense), fat is hyperintense, which degrades orbital images (Fig. 14.1).

b. T_2 *image*: best for identifying diseased tissue. Water appears white, so pathological oedema shows as a high signal; fat is also hyperintense (Fig. 14.2).

c. *Fat suppression*: Suppression of high signal from orbital fat allows clear definition of the optic nerve and extraocular muscles (Fig. 14.3).

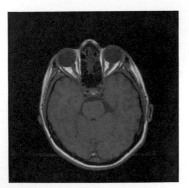

Fig. 14.1: Normal T_1 axial MRI.

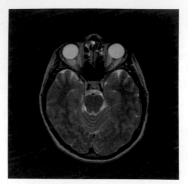

Fig. 14.2: Normal T$_2$ axial MRI.

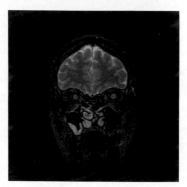

Fig. 14.3: Normal T$_2$ coronal MRI with fat suppression (see also Fig. 14.17).

d. *Fluid-attenuated inversion recovery sequence* (FLAIR): CSF appears dark, making it easier to detect small T$_2$-hyperintense lesions (e.g. MS plaques) adjacent to the lateral ventricles.

e. *Short tau inversion recovery sequence* (STIR): ideal for imaging the intraorbital optic nerve as orbital fat is supressed but water (inflammatory oedema) can still be seen as high signal.

f. *Gadolinium contrast*: useful when looking for lesions with disrupted vessel permeability. Consider if suspected meningioma, acoustic neuroma, lymphoma, metastatic disease, optic neuropathy (e.g. sarcoid), or active MS plaques. Contrast enhancement can be seen on T_1 weighted images but not on T_2 weighted images.

■ Common examples:

a. *Optic nerve disease*: judge size on coronal sections. Acute optic neuritis shows high signal on T_2 imaging and gadolinium enhancement. The acute phase, anterior ischaemic optic neuropathy shows no abnormality. Both will show high signal chronically due to Wallerian degeneration.

b. *Vascular imaging*: blood flow produces a 'flow void' on MRI, appearing as low signal in most of the above sequences. Lack of flow void implies complete or partial occlusion. Consider axial T_2 cuts to look for dural sinus thrombosis or carotid artery dissection. MR angiography (MRA): can confirm blood flow without contrast injection, but may fail to detect very slow flow. MRA excludes clinically significant intracranial arterial aneurysms of >3 mm but has not yet completely replaced intra-arterial angiography, e.g. in acute, painful 3rd nerve palsy with pupillary involvement. CT angiography and MR venography are also available.

c. *Stroke*: early (within 1–8 days) CT excludes clinically significant haemorrhage and allows early aspirin use. CT may be normal for the first 24 hours after a nonhaemorrhagic cerebral infarct. MRI may not detect acute intracerebral haemorrhage but is more sensitive for diagnosing small infarcts such as brainstem lesions. Diffusion weighted images (DWI) on MRI and FLAIR imaging are the most sensitive way of detecting early ischaemic CVAs.

Anisocoria

History Ask who first noticed the anisocoria (difference in pupil size) and attempt to establish the duration. Review of old photos such as a bus pass may help. Magnification may be required to assess pupil size. Exclude a history of neck or chest surgery/injury, limb weakness, difficulty focusing, diplopia, and ptosis.

Examination Identify which pupil is abnormal by examining first in the dark then in the light. Greater anisocoria in the dark indicates impaired dilatation (sympathetic dysfunction): greater anisocoria in the light indicates impaired constriction (parasympathetic dysfunction). Physiological anisocoria is usually ≤2mm and the difference is the same at all light levels. Examine the pupils (p. 623) and the iris on the slit lamp.

Differential diagnosis of an abnormally large pupil Consider Adie's pupil (below), 3rd nerve palsy, dilating drops, traumatic mydriasis, iris rubeosis, Urrets-Zavalia syndrome (iris atrophy following corneal graft), and physiological anisocoria.

■ *Adie's tonic pupil (Holmes-Adie pupil)*: Presumed postviral denervation of the sphincter pupillae and ciliary muscle produces anisocoria and difficulty focusing. Owing to reinervation, accommodation recovers in a few weeks but the sphincter pupillae becomes partially innervated by lens fibres. Signs thereafter include light-near dissociation (slow or absent constriction to light but prompt constriction on attempted near vision), segmental sphincter palsy on slit lamp examination which gives rise to so-called vermiform movements of the iris, and absent limb reflexes. Slow dilation following accommodation (tonic constriction) differentiates it from Argyll Robertson pupils. Exclude ptosis and diplopia (3rd nerve palsy). Whereas normal pupils do not usually constrict to G. pilocarpine 0.125%, Adie's pupil does (denervation hypersensitivity), but this test has only moderate specificity, as preganglionic lesions do likewise. Further investigations are not normally required. Arrange routine referral to a neuro-ophthalmologist. Long-term follow-up is not required. It is often bilateral but asymmetric. The affected pupils eventually become small.

Differential diagnosis of an abnormally small pupil Consider Horner's syndrome (below), pilocarpine drops, uveitis/posterior synechiae, chronic unilateral aphakia, and physiological anisocoria.

- *Horner's syndrome*: Sympathetic denervation produces miosis and mild ptosis. It may be preganglionic or postganglionic. Preganglionic (central) causes include lung and breast malignancy, sympathetic chain schwannoma, and cervical spine damage (e.g. C8 or T1 disc prolapse). Postganglionic causes include internal carotid dissection, neck tumours, cavernous sinus disease (especially if 6th nerve palsy coexists), and cluster headache. The diagnosis of Horner's syndrome is *C*onfirmed by *C*ontinued pupil *C*onstriction despite G. *C*ocaine 4% (delay further pharmacological testing for 2 days after cocaine testing). Preganglionic causes produce ipsilateral anhydrosis of the face (ptosis, miosis, anhydrosis) and the pupil dilates with G. hydroxyamphetamine 1% (no effect if postganglionic). Investigations depend on the likely cause, but if painful request urgent T_2 weighted MRI axial scans to exclude carotid dissection. This is associated with a high risk of embolic stroke within 10 days and anticoagulation is indicated. Congenital preganglionic Horner's syndrome typically has iris heterochromia and is seen on old photographs. Acquired childhood cases require investigation to exclude neoplasia, particularlarly cervicothoracic neuroblastoma, though most are benign.

Transient Visual Loss

Background Transient visual loss has numerous causes. A careful history is crucial.

History Ask about: duration; whether one or both eyes are affected; total blackness (arterial occlusion) or just blurred; patchy grey blobs (spasm of choroidal vessels); cardiovascular risk factors; TIAs or strokes; known carotid disease; headache; migrainous aura; dizziness, hearing, or speech problems; loss of balance; haloes; eye pain; abnormal clotting (DVTs); scalp tenderness; jaw claudication (over 50 years). Specific precipitants may suggest the diagnosis:

■ *Bright light*: chronic retinal ischaemia due to carotid insufficiency.

■ *Eye movements*: space occupying orbital lesions or optic nerve tumour.

■ *Prolonged reading or evening onset*: intermittent angle closure glaucoma.

■ *Exercise*: pigment dispersion syndrome.

■ *Standing up*: usually indicates reduced perfusion pressure including postural hypotension, carotid insufficiency, and giant cell arteritis (precedes nerve infarction). Papilloedema may produce brief monocular or bilateral obscurations with either standing up or stooping down.

Examination Check BP in both arms (sitting and standing if appropriate); radial pulse; cardiac and carotid auscultation; temporal artery palpation (in patients over 50 years); VA; confrontation visual fields; colour vision; RAPD; corneal clarity (oedema or endothelial pigment); iris rubeosis; gonioscopy (is angle closeable?); IOP; dilated fundoscopy (especially retinal vessels for emboli, venous dilation, retinal haemorrhages and optic disc for swelling); assess central retinal artery perfusion pressure (p. 483); other tests as indicated.

Differential diagnosis See Table 14.1.

■ The following are the more common or serious causes:

1. Carotid or cardiac emboli: see below.

2. Carotid dissection: may have neck pain and Horner's syndrome.

3. Migraine: usually hemianopic, positive features, with zig-zags typical (p. 652).

Table 14.1: Causes of transient visual loss

Visual loss lasting less than 1 minute		Visual loss lasting 5–30 minutes	
Monocular	Binocular	Monocular	Binocular
Carotid insufficiency	Bilateral carotid insufficiency	Retinal arterial embolus	Migraine
Giant cell arteritis	Bilateral papilloedema	Retinal vasospasm	Occipital embolus
Papilloedema	Vertebrobasilar insufficiency	Choroidal vasospasm	
	Cardiac dysrhythmia	Retinal migraine (controversial)	
	Postural hypotension	Angle closure glaucoma	
	Occipital epilepsy	Pigment dispersion syndrome	

Patients often incorrectly describe hemianopic visual loss as being loss from one eye only.

4. Giant cell arteritis: see page 655.

5. Vertebrobasilar ischaemia: page 673.

6. Intermittent angle closure glaucoma: page 325.

■ Also consider:

7. Occipital embolus: may cause hemianopic loss or transient blindness.

8. Retinal arterial embolus: typically, a curtain descent to a blackout.

9. Retinal vasospasm: more likely a whiteout.

10. Choroidal vasospasm: vision disappears in patches.

11. Cardiac dysrhythmia: blindness may precede loss of consciousness or occur in isolation.

12. Occipital epilepsy: usually hemianopic with positive symptoms such as coloured circles.

Management Investigation and treatment depends on the likely cause. In the case of transient monocular blindness, emboli usually arise from the aorta, carotids, or heart valves. Most commonly, they are cholesterol, platelet-fibrin, or calcific, but septic, amniotic fluid, air, fat or talc (i.v. drug users) may rarely occur in specific situations. If likely, start oral aspirin 75 mg o.d.

and check BP, FBC, ESR, glucose, and lipids as a minimum. Arrange carotid Doppler and echocardiogram and refer to a stroke physician. Warn patients that intervention may be indicated if investigations reveal internal carotid artery stenosis or valvular heart disease. A statin is likely to be indicated. In the case of posterior circulation transient blindness, or transient hemianopia, a cardiac source is more likely and atrial fibrillation or a paroxysmal dysrhythmia must be considered.

Nystagmus

Background Nystagmus is a rhythmic, often rapid, involuntary eye movement. If a patient is unaware of oscillopsia (visual field appearing to move) then nystagmus is probably congenital. This includes most causes of pendular nystagmus due to low vision (e.g. albinism, Leber's congenital amaurosis) and congenital motor nystagmus. The latter is usually horizontal in all directions of gaze, uniplanar, and often accompanied by an abnormal head posture to achieve best vision, usually with a head turn to match gaze direction to the null position of the nystagmus (the eye position that minimizes the nystagmus).

Examination Observe and document whether the nystagmus is pendular or jerk. Document whether vertical or horizontal and the direction of the fast phase. Is it present in primary position? The magnification provided by the direct ophthalmoscope can be used to observe low-amplitude nystagmus in the primary position. Is it always horizontal and uniplanar with a null point (e.g. congenital motor nystagmus)? Is the direction of the fast phase always in the direction of gaze (gaze evoked) or not (vestibular, congenital). Is there a torsional component? Examine the eyes in primary position for several minutes. Does the nystagmus change direction in a regular cycle (periodic alternating nystagmus)? Look for the following patterns.

Gaze evoked nystagmus Jerk nystagmus occurs in the same direction as the patient's gaze, but is absent in the primary position. Seen in cerebellar and brainstem disease and with some drugs (anticonvulsants, sedatives). A few beats of nystagmus at the extremes of gaze may be normal.

Acquired pendular nystagmus May occur with severe visual loss, brainstem strokes, and MS. Consider gabapentin (100 mg t.d.s. increasing slowly to 300 mg t.d.s.) or baclofen (5 mg daily increasing to a maximum of 10 mg t.d.s.).

Downbeat nystagmus Often most obvious on downward and lateral gaze, the direction of the fast phase is downwards. Seen with Arnold-Chiari malformations and cerebellar degenerations.

Upbeat nystagmus Seen with intrinsic brainstem disease. Up- and downbeat nystagmus will be present in primary position and this distinguishes it from vertical gaze evoked nystagmus.

Convergence retraction nystagmus Test with an optokinetic (OKN) drum rotating the stripes downwards to induce attempted up saccades. This results in convergence and retraction rather than up saccades and is typically seen in *Parinaud's syndrome*, also called dorsal midbrain syndrome: causes include pinealoma, head trauma, arteriovenous malformation, MS, and basilar artery CVA. Parinaud's syndrome may have light-near dissociation of pupils, lid retraction, and spasm/paresis of convergence/accommodation. It is not a true nystagmus.

See–saw nystagmus One eye elevates and intorts whilst the other depresses and extorts then vice versa. Occurs with suprasellar lesions. May have a fast phase or be a variant of pendular nystagmus.

Periodic alternating nystagmus Horizontal jerk nystagmus that changes direction every few minutes. May be congenital or occur in a variety of vestibulocerebellar diseases and occasionally following severe bilateral visual loss. Consider gabapentin (100 mg t.d.s. increasing slowly to 300 mg t.d.s.) or baclofen (5 mg daily increasing to a maximum of 10 mg t.d.s.). Try baclofen first.

Peripheral vestibular nystagmus Unidirectional, uniplanar with a torsional element, and greatest amplitude with gaze in the direction of the fast component. Associated with paroxysmal vertigo, tinnitus, and hearing loss. Occurs in acute labyrinthitis, Menière's disease, and benign positional vertigo.

Central vestibular nystagmus Chronic jerk nystagmus, uni- or bidirectional, that varies with the direction of gaze. Often but not always torsional. Pure torsional nystagmus is of central vestibular origin. Vertigo, deafness, and tinnitus are less of a feature than in peripheral vestibular nystagmus. Caused by a variety of brain stem diseases, e.g. MS, CVA, tumour.

Visual Field Defects

Background The accurate delineation of visual field defects is critical to the diagnosis of visual pathway lesions. Visual field defects are frequently asymptomatic and may be detected on routine screening (usually by an optometrist) or when field tests are preformed for some other reason. An awareness of the various artefactually produced field defects is important.

Symptoms Patients are less likely to notice field defects from optic nerve or visual pathway lesions if these spare the central field. Retinal lesions often produce positive scotomas with patients aware of photopsia within the visual field defect.

History Ask when and how the field defect was first noticed. Sudden onset or gradual? Any recovery? Ask about cardiovascular risk factors, photopsia, pain, headache and other neurological symptoms, and symptoms of pituitary disease (amenorrhoea, hypothyroidism, loss of libido, headache, and acromegaly).

Examination Check BP, cranial nerves, VA, colour vision, RAPD, formal fields, eye movements, IOP, assess angle, and dilated fundoscopy. Exclude ptosis, and disc cupping, pallor, or swelling. Many field defects are relative, and not absolute.

Differential diagnosis Abnormal visual fields may be caused by retinal pathology (e.g. retinal detachment or vein occlusion). Cataract may cause a globally decreased field but not focal defects. A homonymous hemianopia should not cause a decreased VA. Glaucoma can cause a range of field defects but confirm that the field defect corresponds to the sectoral neuroretinal rim thinning; colour vision is relatively well preserved until late in the disease, unlike optic nerve disease.

- *Left homonymous hemianopia* (Fig. 14.4): consider a right postchiasmal lesion such as occipital lobe CVA or tumour. The more congruous the field defect, the nearer to the occipital lobe, but a large lesion affecting both temporal and parietal lobes (the entire optic radiation) could also cause this.

- *Left superior homonymous quadrantanopia* (Fig. 14.5): probably right inferior occipital cortex but consider right temporal lobe lesion. Inferior homonymous quadrantanopia may be caused by a parietal lobe lesion. The defect may be relative or absolute. The vertical meridian will be absolutely respected but usually not the horizontal meridian.

- *Bitemporal superior quadrantanopia* (Fig. 14.6): typically caused by pituitary tumours but will be relative; the defect will

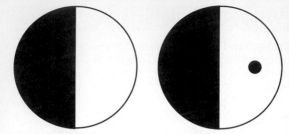

Fig. 14.4: Left homonymous hemianopia.

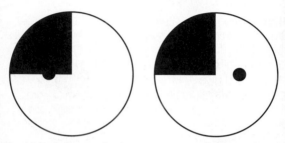

Fig. 14.5: Left superior homonymous quadrantanopia.

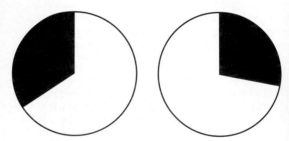

Fig. 14.6: Bitemporal superior quadrantanopia.

respect the vertical meridian but not the horizontal meridian. As the defect progresses, the bitemporal hemianopia will become more complete but usually asymmetric and eventually with evidence of optic neuropathy on one or other side. A craniopharyngioma may cause a bilateral inferotemporal quadrantanopia but is more likely to give rise to a combination of optic nerve, chiasm and tract deficits.

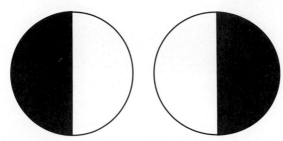

Fig. 14.7: Complete bitemporal hemianopia.

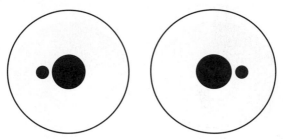

Fig. 14.8: Central scotoma.

- *Complete bitemporal hemianopia* (Fig. 14.7): may occur with compressive lesions of the chiasm but such a clear-cut deficit is typically only seen in cases of traumatic chiasmal transection.

- *Central scotoma* (Fig. 14.8): the commonest cause is age-related macular degeneration. In the case of optic nerve disease, such a symmetrical picture is more likely to be toxic, nutritional, or an inherited condition. Cone dystrophy can produce a similar picture.

- *Superior altitudinal hemianopia in the left eye* (Fig. 14.9): typically seen with nonarteritic anterior ischaemic optic neuropathy but also normal pressure glaucoma (usually bilateral and with arcuate defects in the lower field also), hemicentral vein occlusion, branch retinal artery occlusion, ptosis (less severe), sector panretinal photocoagulation (PRP) laser, and inferior retinal detachment.

- *Concentric peripheral field loss* (Fig. 14.10): may be seen in retinitis pigmentosa, chronic atrophic papilloedema (e.g. idiopathic intracranial hypertension), end-stage glaucoma,

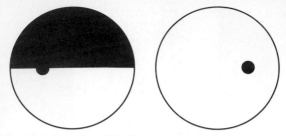

Fig. 14.9: Superior altitudinal heminaopia in the left eye.

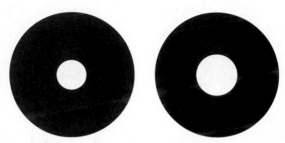

Fig. 14.10: Concentric peripheral field loss.

PRP, central retinal artery occlusion with cilioretinal artery sparing (usually unilateral), optic neuropathies, and in vigabatrin toxicity.

Investigations Most afferent visual system deficits affect the central 10° of the visual field. A Humphrey 24–2 threshold field is therefore suitable for most indications, including subtle chiasmal lesions. Review the reliability indices (p. 284). Goldmann kinetic perimetry (Fig. 14.11) may be preferable for medically unexplained visual loss (p. 677), patients who cannot adequately perform a Humphrey test, and conditions such as idiopathic intracranial hypertension and vigabatrin-associated visual field loss where peripheral loss may be outside the area tested by a Humphrey. Goldmann field tests are also useful for patients with very large central scotomas (e.g. severe optic neuritis) who may see nothing on a Humphrey. The remaining peripheral field can still be used to assess progression or improvement of the condition in such patients.

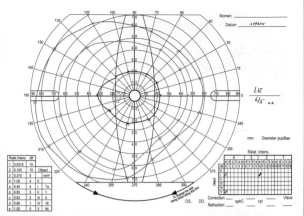

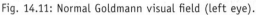

Fig. 14.11: Normal Goldmann visual field (left eye).

Management This depends on the cause of the field loss. Consider eligibility to drive (p. 688) and test binocular Estermann field if in doubt.

Optic Disc Swelling

Background Papilloedema refers exclusively to optic disc swelling caused by raised intracranial pressure (ICP). There are many other causes of disc swelling.

History Take a full systemic, neurologic, and ophthalmic history. Headache from raised ICP may be stereotypic (p. 650).

Examination Check BP, cranial nerves (raised ICP may cause a 6th nerve palsy), VA, colour vision, pupils, refraction, dilated fundoscopy, and general examination as indicated by the history. Pulsating retinal veins exclude raised ICP (but only at the time the observation is made) but the converse is not true as absent spontaneous venous pulsations may be normal. Severe papilloedema causes blurring of the disc margin and nerve fibre layer thickening that obscures disc vessels. The normal optic disc cup is absent. Flame haemorrhages at the optic disc may occur, particularly in acute anterior ischaemic optic neuropathy (AION) and also acutely in raised intracranial pressure (Fig. 14.12). In central retinal vein occlusion (CRVO) there will be haemorrhages on the disc but also throughout the affected retina.

Differential diagnosis Consider: raised ICP; meningitis; posterior uveitis (panuveitis); infiltration or inflammation, e.g. leukaemia, sarcoid; demyelinating optic neuritis; posterior scleritis; compressive optic neuropathy, e.g. thyroid eye disease or sheath meningioma; malignant hypertension; diabetic papillopathy; Irvine-

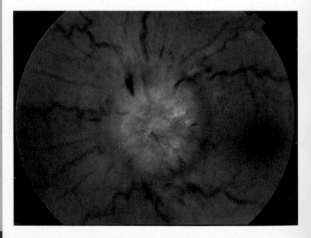

Fig. 14.12: Papilloedema.

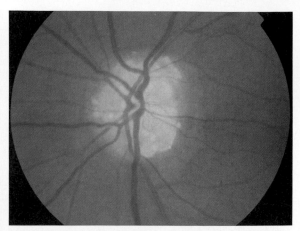

Fig. 14.13: Optic disc drusen.

Gass syndrome; AION; CRVO; Leber's hereditary optic neuropathy; carbon dioxide retention; hypoparathyroidism; uraemia.

Optic disc swelling may be simulated (pseudopapilloedema) by small hypermetropic discs, tilted discs, and disc drusen.

Optic disc drusen (Fig. 14.13) are calcified deposits in the optic nerve head which may be clearly visible but if buried may simulate disc swelling. They are sometimes associated with arcuate field loss. Drusen involute in later life. No treatment is available.

Investigations Arrange formal perimetry. If papilloedema is suspected, request neuroimaging and liaise urgently with neurology. If imaging shows no cause for raised ICP, lumbar puncture may be required to measure ICP. Photograph the optic discs. Consider fundus photos using angiography filters to show drusen autofluorescence (Fig. 14.14), or alternatively disc drusen are visible using ultrasound examination (calcium also shows on CT).

Management Treat the underlying cause. If pseudopapilloedema is suspected, repeat disc photography, fields, VA, and colour vision after several months to check there has been no change, as this would suggest another diagnosis.

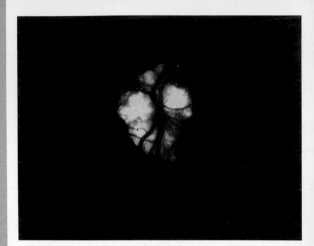

Fig. 14.14: Optic disc drusen autofluorescence.

Idiopathic Intracranial Hypertension

Background A condition with raised intracranial pressure (ICP) but no mass lesion or hydrocephalus. Previously referred to as pseudotumour cerebri and benign intracranial hypertension. The syndrome known as idiopathic intracranial hypertension (IIH) occurs in women of childbearing age with a history of recent substantial weight gain. However, the same clinical picture may be associated with prolonged therapy with tetracyclines (most commonly minocycline for acne), anabolic steroids, danazol, exogenous growth hormone, hypervitaminosis A, isotretinoin, tretinoin, nalidixic acid, lithium, ciclosporin, pregnancy (probably related to weight gain), several endocrine disorders, chronic meningitis (especially in sarcoidosis), and vasculitis rarely. Dural sinus thrombosis is another cause of the pseudotumour syndrome, especially in association with prothrombotic disorders such as Behçet's disease, pregnancy, antiphospholipid syndrome, protein S deficiency, protein C deficiency, oral contraceptive pill use, and Factor V Leiden mutation. In cases of dural sinus thrombosis the onset is more likely to be subacute. Also consider sleep apnoea syndrome, especially in obese males.

Symptoms Include headache (94%), unilateral or bilateral transient visual obscurations lasting seconds (68%), pulsatile tinnitus (58%), photopsia (54%), retrobulbar pain (44%), diplopia (38%), and loss of vision (26%). Headache may be throbbing, wake the patient from sleep, and be exacerbated by recumbent posture and Valsalva. It may improve on rising in the morning but get worse during the day.

Signs The patient is often very obese. There is bilateral papilloedema and there may be a unilateral or bilateral 6th nerve palsy. Visual fields may be severely constricted.

History and examination Take a full medical history and record medications, particularly those for acne. Check for neck stiffness, temperature, BP, VA, colour vision, confrontation visual fields, and IOP. Exclude vitritis and scleritis. Perform a full neurological examination and measure weight.

Differential diagnosis Consider any cause of papilloedema or disc swelling (p. 644). Exclude intracranial space occupying lesions (SOL), subarachnoid haemorrhage, meningitis, malignant hypertension, and dural sinus thrombosis.

Investigations Any patient presenting with headache and bilateral disc swelling needs urgent neuroimaging to exclude imminent coning. In the pseudotumour syndrome MRI will not show hydrocephalus or a mass lesion, but there is usually evidence of chronic raised ICP (dilated optic nerve sheaths and so called 'empty sella'). Dural sinus occlusion (by thrombosis or small SOL) is usually visible on brain MRI but MR venography may clarify. Once normal imaging has been obtained, arrange neuro-ophthalmological referral for lumbar puncture and perimetry. CSF constituents are normal and lumbar CSF pressure is raised ($>20\,cmH_2O$, but usually $>25\,cmH_2O$). Request FBC, ESR, autoantibody screen, syphilis serology, U&E, calcium, phosphate, and glucose (should all be normal).

Treatment

- Lumbar puncture is a useful holding move.

- Weight loss: refer to a dietician and/or obesity specialist.

- Cease any drug thought to have precipitated the condition.

- Acetazolamide 250 mg b.d. p.o. if not contraindicated (warn about possible side effects). Higher doses may be required. The use of other diuretics is controversial but bendroflumethiazide (which has carbonic anhydrase activity) 2.5–5 mg o.d. is effective.

- If vision deteriorates or headaches persist despite medical management consider a CSF diversion procedure (lumboperitoneal or ventriculoperitoneal shunt). Optic nerve sheath fenestration is indicated for visual failure without headache.

- The use of corticosteroids is contraversial.

Follow–up Once the diagnosis is confirmed, see at 2–4 weeks with repeat field test, then less often if responding. The condition usually resolves spontaneously following cessation of the drug which initiated it, or after weight loss.

Headache and Facial Pain

Background Headache is one of the commonest of all symptoms. Patients seen in eye clinics usually have headaches localized to one or both eyes, associated visual symptoms, or concern that eye-strain is causing the headaches. Headache may be a manifestation of eye disease, or systemic disease may manifest with headache and altered vision.

History Ask about the mode of onset and duration of the headache, how often it occurs, the site, and relieving or exacerbating factors. The pain itself may have a throbbing quality, be constant or paroxysmal. Associated features may include: blurred vision; field defect; scintillating scotoma; nausea; photophobia; phonophobia; autonomic symptoms such as lacrimation, nasal congestion or Horner's syndrome; scalp tenderness; jaw claudication; anisocoria, or tinnitus.

Examination Check BP (ensure the cuff pressure is high enough to occlude the radial pulse to ensure correct systolic measurement in patients with possible malignant hypertension), cranial nerves, VA, colour vision, pupils, confrontation fields, IOP, drainage angles, and fundoscopy (exclude disc swelling and retinal haemorrhage). Palpate the temporal arteries in those over 50 years. Consider refraction and orthoptic review.

Differential diagnosis

- *Tension headache*: a common, benign, headache that feels like a tight band across the forehead, around the head, or sometimes at the back of the head and involving the muscles in the back of the neck.

- *Chronic daily headache*: symptoms vary but pain is constant (24 hours a day) and not relieved by analgesics. Analgesic overuse is common. Insomnia usually coexists.

- *Atypical facial pain*: this condition has similar characteristics to chronic daily headache in that pain is unremitting but it is unilateral and usually localized to the cheek and periorbital region. Exclude local causes and treat as for chronic daily headache.

- *Herpes zoster associated pain*: Characteristic pain precedes the appearance of a V_1 rash. Postherpetic neuralgia occurs in 10% of cases. For managements, see page 182.

- *Trigeminal neuralgia*: must be lancinating (flashes of pain) most commonly in V_3 territory but can affect the brow or cheek. Patients are aware of triggers such as touch, cold, or chewing.

Responds to carbamazepine or gabapentin. Refer to a neurologist.

■ *Other neuralgic facial pain*: damage to the sensory nerves emerging from the orbit may result in neuralgic pain, particularly with a history of trauma or surgery, with sensory disturbance in the distribution of the affected nerve. Tapping the nerve produces pain: local anaesthetic relieves it. Refer to a pain specialist.

■ *Ocular causes*: significantly raised IOP (almost always >35 mmHg) produces ache around the eye. Uncorrected refractive error usually produces ache between the eyebrows. Scleritis causes a deep boring pain which may wake the patient from sleep.

■ *Giant cell arteritis*: must be considered. See page 655.

■ *Raised intracranial pressure*: produces headache with nausea and vomiting, often worse on waking, coughing, and bending over. A whooshing tinnitus is often present. Look for absent spontaneous venous pulsations. Check eye movements, pupil size, and reaction. Sixth nerve palsy may be a false localizing sign. Full neurological examination is essential. See page 647. Drowsiness and/or unilateral dilated pupil are serious signs suggesting coning and the need for urgent neurological intervention to prevent death. Contact a neurologist immediately if these signs are present.

■ *Low pressure headache*: most commonly seen following lumbar puncture but chronic CSF leak may occur for a variety of reasons. The essential feature is that the headache is totally relieved by lying flat.

■ *Sinus infection*: the patient typically has pyrexia, tenderness over the affected sinus (usually ethmoid), and pain worse on bending forward. Optic neuropathy can occur with severe infection or an expanding mucocele. Imaging (plain films are useful) shows opacification of the affected sinus; however, incidental sinus disease is common.

■ *Malignant hypertension*: headache ± blurred vision. Look for retinopathy. Can cause confusion and fits.

■ *Subarachnoid haemorrhage*: sudden onset of severe headache 'like being hit over the head with a hammer'. Neck stiffness, decreased consciousness, or other neurological signs may be present. A diagnostic finding is subhyaloid haemorrhage. Lay the patient flat and do not allow the patient to sit up even to go to the toilet if this diagnosis is likely. Needs immediate admission and investigation. Painful 3rd nerve palsy with pupil involvement may indicate an expanding posterior communicating artery aneurysm and imminent rupture. Anterior communicating artery aneurysm may affect the optic nerve in a similar fashion.

■ *Meningitis*: features include photophobia, neck stiffness, possible decreased consciousness or neurological signs, and pyrexia. Purpuric or petechial rash suggests meningococcal meningitis. Test passive neck flexion looking for stiffness ± pain (but may be normal in children). If passive straight leg raise causes pain, suspect meningism (or nerve root entrapment). Meningococcal meningitis can kill within hours; if suspected, give intravenous benzylpenicillin immediately (300 mg in infants, 600 mg child 1–9 years, 1200 mg >10 years or adult).

■ *Migraine*: see page 652.

■ *Cluster headache*: paroxysmal attacks of severe pain, red watering eye, transient or permanent postganglionic Horner's syndrome, and nasal stuffiness/rhinorrhoea. Patients pace around rather than lie still as with migraine. Usually lasts around 30 minutes, occasionally longer. Characteristically, a daily headache for several weeks, usually occurring at the same time of day, that then disappears for months or years. Usually affects middle-aged men, and may be precipitated by alcohol. Refer to a neurologist.

■ *SUNCT syndrome*: Short-lasting Unilateral Neuralgiform headache attacks with Conjunctival injection and Tearing. Severe orbital, periorbital, forehead, or temple pain lasts from 5 seconds to a few minutes. Occurs from once daily to more than 60 times per hour. As with cluster headache, the dysautonomic features are an essential element.

Migraine

Background Migraine affects 15% of people, women more than men, with peak prevalence age 35–45 years.

Symptoms Visual aura may be hemianopic or affect the entire visual field. A slowly enlarging scotoma with a shimmering border evolves over a period of minutes, but usually resolves completely within 30 minutes. Zig-zag lines (fortification spectra/teichopsia) are pathognomonic. Vision recovers fully within 1 hour. Headache may occur about 30 minutes after the visual aura has resolved. Headache is typically unilateral, throbbing, and associated with nausea, photophobia, and phonophobia. It is usually exacerbated by movement and therefore relieved by lying down in a dark, quiet room. Nonvisual aura (vertigo, paraesthesia), migraine without aura (common migraine) and aura without headache (acephalgic migraine) can all occur.

History Ask patients about the nature of the attack, or past history of typical migraine headache in their early twenties. This may not be present in elderly patients presenting with aura without headache. If the visual aura is always restricted to the same hemifield this may very rarely be due to an occipital lobe lesion (such as an arteriovenous malformation, AVM).

Examination Ocular examination is normal. Field tests may be abnormal during an attack. Occasionally, persistent defects are seen, usually homonymous hemianopic scotomas. A 3rd, 4th or 6th nerve palsy (ophthalmoplegic migraine) occurs in children more frequently than adults, usually lasting for days or weeks. Perform dilated fundoscopy to exclude a retinal tear, embolus, or haemorrhage. Check BP, VA, colour vision, confrontation fields, and optic disc appearance. The occurrence of retinal migraine is controversial but nonembolic transient visual loss is sometimes referred to as retinal migraine. Similarly, ophthalmoplegic migraine is nosologically unclear.

Differential diagnosis Consider any cause of transient visual loss (p. 634) including amaurosis fugax, ocular ischaemia, narrow angle glaucoma, occipital epilepsy, retinal hole, tear or detachment, and occipital lobe AVM, or tumour (rare).

Investigations Not required unless atypical. Acephalgic migraine in older patients is *not* equivalent to a TIA.

Treatment Reassure the patient. Advise to pull over the car if they develop an attack whilst driving. Paracetamol or aspirin and an antiemetic relieve headache and nausea if taken early.

Avoid precipitating factors such as red wine or cheese if any can be identified.

Follow–up Refer to the GP or a neurologist, particularly if the headache is disabling and frequent (more than twice per month), needing prophylactic treatment to prevent headache (e.g. propranolol, pizotifen, or amitryptiline), or atypical features are present requiring investigation. Specific antimigraine agents are available for acute attacks but are best prescribed in neurology or general practice.

Ischaemic Optic Neuropathy

Anterior ischaemic optic neuropathy (AION) is caused by infarction of the optic nerve head. It may be nonarteritic, or arteritic (giant cell arteritis, GCA).

Nonarteritic anterior ischaemic optic neuropathy

Background Increased risk if male, systemic arteriopathy, aged 40–60 years, or disc vessel crowding (small hypermetropic discs, disc drusen). Occasionally precipitated by severe hypovolaemia or anaemia, e.g. cardiac surgery. Excluding an arteritic cause is key but GCA is rare under 65 years; other types of vasculitis may occur in younger age groups but this and thrombophilia are rare causes of AION.

Symptoms Typically sudden, painless, nonprogressive partial monocular vision loss. Sometimes asymptomatic.

Signs Optic disc swelling that may be sectoral, with flame haemorrhages and occasionally a macular star. Longstanding cases show sectoral disc atrophy corresponding to the field defect.

History and examination Ask about the speed of visual loss and any recovery. Importantly, exclude symptoms of GCA (see below). Record: refractive error; VA (typically 6/12–6/60); Ishihara plates (reduced); RAPD (expected); confrontation fields (typically, unilateral altitudinal hemianopia); dilated peripheral fundoscopy (exclude peripheral haemorrhage, vitritis, periphlebitis). Draw or photograph the optic disc. Confirm pulsatile, nontender, temporal arteries, full eye movements, and no lid-lag or proptosis.

Differential diagnosis The differential is similar to GCA (see below).

Consider posterior ischaemic optic neuropathy following face-down spinal surgery, radiotherapy, and hypotension/hypovolaemia/haemodialysis. This produces no disc swelling, is often bilateral, with worse VA, and a poor prognosis. There is no proven treatment.

Investigations Check ESR and CRP (mandatory) ± temporal artery biopsy; FBC; fasting blood glucose; lipids; BP; and Goldmann or 24–2 Humphrey field test. If disc drusen are suspected, consider USS or disc photos for autofluorescence.

Treatment

■ *Casualty*: start aspirin 75 mg o.d. if there are no contraindications. Review all vascular risk factors. Exclude GCA and if in doubt discuss with a senior colleague. Request review at 6 weeks.

■ *Clinic*: recheck clinical findings, particularly fields. Early stepwise progression occurs but is unusual. Neuroimaging is not required unless findings are atypical. Expect three lines of VA improvement in 30%. AION is unlikely (5%) to recur in the same eye after nerve fibre atrophy relieves disc vessel congestion. Studies suggest a 15–50% risk of fellow eye involvement. Review in 6 months then discharge if stable.

Giant cell arteritis (temporal arteritis)

Background Occlusive arterial inflammation causes optic disc ischaemia and sudden, usually total, unilateral visual loss. It is an ophthalmic emergency, as the second eye may develop irreversible visual loss within hours. Patients are usually elderly and never <50 years. Associated with polymyalgia rheumatica.

Symptoms These include new headache, scalp tenderness, loss of appetite, weight loss, limb girdle pain (worse in the morning, relieved by movement), and ischaemic jaw pain on chewing. Prodromal episodic transient visual loss, often on standing due to poor perfusion, occurs in 10%. Ophthalmoplegia may occur.

Signs Common features include thickened temporal arteries which may be nonpulsatile and tender, RAPD, and pale disc swelling ± flame haemorrhages. VA is usually ≤ count fingers. Central retinal artery occlusion and retinal cotton-wool spots may occur. Optic nerve ischaemia may be retrobulbar.

History and examination Ask about polymyalgia rheumatica and steroid contraindications or recent withdrawal. Record: temporal artery findings, VA, Ishihara plates, confrontation fields, eye movements, proptosis, RAPD, dilated fundoscopy, disc appearance, and any vitritis. Measure BP and BM before starting steroids.

Differential diagnosis Disc infarction is sectoral in nonarteritic AION but total in GCA. Disc infarction makes the diagnosis of GCA relatively easy, but it can be more difficult in those presenting with headache only, or ophthalmoplegia, postural transient monocular visual loss, or posterior nerve ischaemia (and no disc swelling).

Investigations ESR >47 and CRP >25=97% probability of GCA if the clinical features fit. Normal ESR is ≤ age/2 in men;

(age +10)/2 in women. Thrombocythaemia is common. Numerous other causes of raised ESR include infections that may worsen with steroids. Temporal artery biopsy (see Box 14.1) should be arranged but should not delay treatment. Choroidal hypoperfusion on fluorescein angiography suggests GCA.

Treatment Give *stat* methylprednisolone 1 g in 500 mL normal saline over 30 minutes and oral ranitidine 150 mg b.d. Substitute oral prednisolone 100 mg if arranging i.v. treatment will cause delay. Admit if elderly or cardiac disease. Expect a dramatic improvement in systemic symptoms in 24 hours. Continue i.v. steroids for 3 days then switch to oral prednisolone 100 mg daily. Osteoporosis prophylaxis is mandatory as treatment will be required for many months. For this and other aspects of long term steroid use, see p. 342.

Follow–up Review at 1 week then monthly with repeat ESR. Taper steroids only when the patient is asymptomatic and the ESR has fallen substantially.

Box 14.1: Temporal artery biopsy (Fig. 14.15)

May be positive after months of steroids, but aim to do within a week. If negative it does not exclude GCA, as skip lesions occur.

1. Consent

   Benefit: confirm diagnosis (in approximately 35%).

   Risk: bleeding, infection, scar. Scalp necrosis is very rare. Repeat biopsy is sometimes required. Damage to the facial nerve is theoretically possible but very rare in practice. Stroke has been reported but is extremely rare.

2. Mark tender areas of artery to biopsy with a surgical pen. If not obvious, mark the frontal branch.

3. Infiltrate with lidocaine 2% with adrenaline (≤10 mL).

4. Open skin with a No. 15 blade directly over the artery. Control bleeding with cautery.

5. Blunt dissect with blunt-nosed scissors, down to temporal fascia.

6. Identify and bluntly dissect around the artery. Before removing, tie two pairs of 4/0 Vicryl suture around either end, at least 3 cm apart. Avoiding crush artefact. Ensure haemostasis.

7. Close with Vicryl (4/0 subcutaneous tissues; 7/0 skin). Let skin sutures dissolve or remove at 1 week.

8. Apply a compression bandage for 24 hours. Avoid excessive compression over the auricular cartilage (risk of ischaemia).

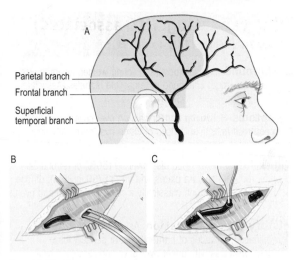

Parietal branch

Frontal branch

Superficial
temporal branch

Fig. 14.15: Temporal artery anatomy and biopsy.

Demyelinating (MS-associated) Optic Neuritis

Background Typically occurs in young women (average age 31) who have spent childhood in temperate latitudes. Associated with multiple sclerosis (MSAON).

Symptoms Headache and/or pain on eye movements (92%) then progressive, uniocular loss of vision over days. Photopsia may occur.

Signs These include optic disc swelling (50%) or retrobulbar neuritis, reduced Ishihara plates and VA (≤6/60 in 35%), diffuse field loss in 48% (though classically a central scotoma) and uveitis in 3%.

History and examination Ask about symptoms of demyelination: episodes of paraesthesia or sensory loss; transient weakness with onset over days and resolution over weeks; bladder dysfunction; vertigo; diplopia; Lhermitte's symptom (electric sensation down the spine and into the limbs on neck flexion). Ask about Uhthoff's symptom (see below). Record: BP, cranial nerves, saccades, cerebellar signs, proptosis, ocular inflammation, VA, Ishihara plates, confrontation fields and dilated fundoscopy.

Differential diagnosis Question the diagnosis if any of the following are present: age >60 years or born and raised in tropical latitudes; severe pain interrupting sleep; very rapid and severe visual loss (<48 hours, <CF vision); simultaneous bilateral involvement; pain for >2 weeks; optic disc haemorrhage; family history of Leber's hereditary optic neuropathy (LHON); known sarcoidosis, collagen vascular disease or cancer. Consider the following alternative diagnoses:

- *Orbital*: thyroid eye disease (not usually painful) and myositis (painful but causes ophthalmoplegia; visual loss is rare).

- *Ocular*: posterior uveitis, neuroretinitis, central serous retinopathy, and scleritis.

- *Optic neuropathy*: compressive (optic nerve, orbital, or intracranial tumours are rarely painful), paranasal mucocele (usually painful and subacute onset; mucocele may closely mimic MSAON), inflammatory (sarcoid, autoimmune disease), ischaemic (arteritic or nonarteritic: do not usually produce retro-orbital pain), nutritional (B_{12}, folate, alcohol), hereditary (LHON), and syphilis.

■ *Systemic disease*: severe hypertension, raised intracranial pressure (occasionally causes unilateral disc swelling), acute disseminated encephalomyelitis, and Devic's disease (bilateral optic neuritis is the rule).

Investigations If the clinical picture is typical of MSAON and if spontaneous recovery has occurred, no investigations are mandatory. Refer the patient to a neurologist for discussion. *In atypical cases investigation is mandatory*: In the acute-phase MRI, STIR orbital sequences show high signal/swelling of the optic nerve. T_1 orbital scan with fat suppression shows gadolinium enhancement of the optic nerve. In the chronic phase there is no enhancement but T_2 high signal is seen. Also in the chronic phase, with good recovery of acuity, the typical VEP finding is a substantial delay with preserved amplitude; this is unusual in any other cause of optic neuropathy. Consider: FBC, syphilis serology, sACE, ANA, ESR, ANCA, B_{12}, folate, CXR, lumbar puncture.

Key study *Optic Neuritis Treatment Trial*[1] Intravenous steroids hastened visual recovery and reduced the risk of MS at 2, but not 5 years. Neither oral nor intravenous treatment offered any long-term visual benefit. Note that some inflammatory optic neuropathies (e.g. sarcoid and autoimmune disorders) may require steroids to prevent severe visual loss.

Treatment

■ *Casualty*: refer to clinic within 1 week. Offer analgesia but if pain is severe (e.g. through the night) reconsider the diagnosis.

■ *Clinic*: expect 93% to improve by 5 weeks; 70% recover near-normal vision, but this may take 1 year. May recur (19% at 5 years), or affect the other eye within months (17%).

Mention the association with MS but emphasise that it tends to be a relatively benign form. If the patient wants to know the risk, refer to a neurologist who may order an MRI scan. If there are no white-matter lesions, the incidence of a second episode is 22% within 10 years. One lesion gives a 51% risk that rises with more lesions.

No treatment is required after a single episode. In relapsing remitting MS, beta-interferon reduces the number of relapses by one-third. A beneficial effect on long-term disability has not been proven.

In children, bilateral optic neuritis may follow viral infection or immunizations. The risk of MS is low. Treat with i.v. methylprednisolone 15 mg/kg for 3 days if there is significant visual loss.

Follow-up Review every few months initially. Discharge if stable at 1 year. Refer to a neurologist if symptoms of MS occur.

Other ocular features of MS

- *Uhthoff's phenomenon*: transiently decreased vision with exertion or in hot conditions.

- *Intermediate uveitis*: sheathing of retinal venules may be seen.

- *Cranial nerve palsy*: commonly 6th, but any may be affected.

- *Internuclear ophthalmoplegia*: the ipsilateral eye fails to adduct or adducts slowly, whilst the contralateral eye has horizontal nystagmus on abduction.

- *Wall-eyed bilateral internuclear ophthalmoplegia* (WEBINO): both eyes have no adduction. Prisms may reduce diplopia.

- *One-and-a-half syndrome*: one eye has no voluntary horizontal movements and the other can only abduct. If supranuclear, the palsy is overcome by dolls-head movements. Other supranuclear gaze palsies may occur.

- *Cerebellar disease*: dysmetric saccades and gaze-evoked nystagmus.

- *Acquired pendular nystagmus*: associated with reduced acuity; the amplitude may differ greatly in the two eyes.

Traumatic Optic Neuropathy

Background Caused by direct head, face, or orbital trauma. Rarely surgically induced. May be unilateral or bilateral. So-called 'indirect' injury to the optic nerve occurs following a blow to the brow which can be relatively minor with no other injuries, no fractures, and no loss of consciousness.

Symptoms Sudden loss of vision at the time of injury. May progress initially as soft tissue swelling compresses the nerve or if there is a haematoma.

Signs RAPD, VA decreased (6/6 to NPL), variable field loss, and decreased colour vision. The optic nerve may initially appear swollen or avulsed but is usually normal, with later atrophy.

History and examination Record Glasgow coma scale and ensure extraocular injuries are treated. Exclude orbital, anterior, and posterior segment injuries (pp. 101, 205, and 551, respectively). Check VA, RAPD, Ishihara colour vision, confrontation fields, eye movements, IOP, and dilated fundoscopy, noting disc, or retinal abnormalities. Avoid dilating if the patient requires neuro-observations for other injuries.

Differential diagnosis Visual loss is usually maximal at the instant of injury; any delay in loss may indicate a haematoma in the orbit or in the optic nerve sheath. Consider occipital infarct, vitreous haemorrhage, retinal detachment, retinal commotio, globe rupture, traumatic cataract, and lens dislocation.

Investigations Arrange an urgent CT scan of the brain and orbits looking for displaced orbital fracture, and orbital or intracranial haemorrhage, particularly if the patient has a decreased Glasgow coma scale. Liaise with other specialties as required. Arrange field testing if general health permits.

Treatment About 30% improve spontaneously. High-dose steroids have been advocated but there is no evidence that treatment will influence the outcome. Consider immediate lateral cantholysis if the orbit is tense and retrobulbar haemorrhage is suspected. Surgical decompression is rarely indicated unless there is evidence of optic nerve compression by a haematoma or bone fragment.

Follow–up Review with regular field tests for the first year. Check eligibility to drive.

Compressive, Infiltrative, and Inflammatory Optic Neuropathy

Background A wide range of orbital and systemic conditions may rarely involve the optic nerve.

Symptoms Visual loss over hours to weeks, severe periocular pain, pain on eye movements, or headache may occur. May be unilateral or bilateral. Compressive lesions usually cause gradual, painless, monocular loss of visual field or VA that may go unnoticed for months.

Signs Findings include reduced VA and colour vision, RAPD (if unilateral or asymmetric), visual field loss, optic nerve swelling, or atrophy. Examination may be normal.

History and examination Record the duration of symptoms and speed of visual loss. Ask about any obscurations on sustained eccentric gaze. Take a complete history and systems review. Look for typical features of demyelinating optic neuropathy (p. 658). Record VA, colour vision, RAPD, IOP, eye movements, and dilated fundus exam. Exclude vitritis and thyroid eye disease. Check orbital signs (p. 72), cranial nerves, and confrontation visual fields. Look for optic disc venous collaterals suggesting optic nerve sheath meningioma. Physician review is advisable.

Differential diagnosis Consider: neoplasm (leukaemia, lymphoma, secondaries); syphilis; sarcoid; TB; autoimmune disease; collagen vascular disease; vasculitides; sinus disease/ mucocele; HIV; thyroid eye disease; pituitary tumour; craniopharyngioma; fibrous dysplasia; Paget's disease; sphenoid wing meningioma; frontal lobe tumour; optic nerve glioma or meningioma; nasopharyngeal carcinoma; ophthalmic or carotid artery aneurysm; other optic neuropathies (demyelinating, traumatic, nutritional, toxic, radiation).

Investigations Initially, send for FBC and film, ESR, CRP, U&E, LFT, glucose, ANA, sACE, TPHA, ANCA, protein electrophoresis, and CXR. Request MRI of brain and orbits and formal perimetry (Goldmann or Humphrey). Consider Mantoux and HIV testing if the history is suggestive, and Lyme serology in endemic areas. Consider lumbar puncture.

Treatment Treatment should not usually be started until a diagnosis is established but if an inflammatory cause is suspected treatment should not be delayed beyond a few days. Consider admission for investigation. Discuss systemic steroids with a neuro-ophthalmologist in severe or rapidly progressive cases, but beware of TB.

- *Casualty*: if visual loss is progressing rapidly arrange admission for investigations; otherwise, arrange an early clinic appointment.

- *Clinic*: review results of imaging. Treatment depends on the diagnosis. If a suprasellar tumour is present, involve an endocrinologist.

Follow–up Long-term management of the underlying aetiology by a neuro-ophthalmologist and appropriate multidisciplinary team is usually required.

Nutritional and Toxic Optic Neuropathy

Background In developed nations this condition typically affects male alcoholic smokers but also those with poor diet, B_{12} deficiency, or on certain drugs, e.g. ethambutol, isoniazid.

Symptoms Painless, bilateral, central scotoma or reduced vision occurring over days to weeks.

Signs Sluggish pupil reactions (but usually no RAPD because eyes are affected equally), decreased colour vision and VA, and field defects. Optic discs usually appear normal but are occasionally mildly swollen and may appear atrophic later.

History and examination Ask about alcohol intake, smoking, abuse of methanol, dietary intake (vegan?), medications, any overdoses (quinine), pernicious anaemia, stomach resection or other causes of malabsorption. Record VA, colour vision, confrontation visual fields, and dilated fundal appearance. Exclude proptosis and dysmotility.

Differential diagnosis Consider other optic neuropathies (compressive, demyelinating, traumatic, infiltrative, inflammatory, radiation) and quinine overdose.

Investigations Arrange an MRI scan to exclude a compressive lesion. Check serum B_{12}, folate, syphilis serology, FBC and film, and LFTs to detect undeclared alcohol abuse. Investigate for infiltrative, inflammatory, or inherited optic neuropathy if indicated (p. 662 and p. 666). Request Humphrey 24–2 visual field test (colour perimetry may reveal larger central scotomas).

Treatment

- *Casualty*: advise to stop smoking and drinking alcohol and improve diet, if appropriate, and offer referral to alcohol or smokers' support services. Prescribe multivitamins. Refer to neuro-ophthalmology clinic within 1 month.

- *Clinic*: confirm the diagnosis, check results, and repeat VA, colour vision, visual fields, and dilated fundoscopy. In tobacco amblyopia or if B_{12} deficient use intramuscular hydroxocobalamin 1 mg daily for 2 weeks, then 1 mg twice weekly until no further improvement then 1 mg every 2 months for 6 months. Do not use cyanocobalamin.

Follow–up Review initially in a few weeks to confirm the diagnosis then 3–6 monthly. A slow recovery is expected if smoking stops. The role of vitamins is uncertain but advisable.

Hereditary Optic Neuropathy

Background Hereditary optic neuropathies may be autosomal dominant (Kjer or dominant optic atrophy), mitochondrially inherited (Leber's hereditary optic neuropathy, LHON), or associated with other syndromes (Behr, Wolfram, Friedrich's Ataxia, Charcot-Marie-Tooth) or neurological problems (deafness, peripheral neuropathy, ataxia).

Clinical features

■ *Dominant optic atrophy*: affects children but usually presents in adult life with reduced vision (>6/18 in 40%; only 17% are <6/60) that tends to be very slowly progressive over years. Optic atrophy may be an incidental finding. Rarely, patients may have nystagmus. Family history is usually positive.

■ *Leber's hereditary optic neuropathy*: affects any age but typically those 15–35 years. About 60% of males and 10% of females with a mutation will develop subacute sequential optic neuropathy with visual loss to 6/60 or worse. The second eye is affected within 15 months. Telangiectatic disc vessels sometimes occur, causing disc swelling that does not leak significantly on fluorescein angiography. Only 4% of those with 11778 mitochondrial DNA mutation improve, compared to 40% of those with the less common 14484 mutation. Only 50% of cases will have a positive family history; ask about affected male cousins on the maternal side of the family.

Differential diagnosis Consider other causes of bilateral symmetrical optic neuropathy (mostly nutritional or toxic). It is very unlikely for bilateral central scotomas to be compressive in aetiology. MS and normal tension glaucoma may cause progressive bilateral optic atrophy. ERG excludes cone dystrophy.

Investigations Request an MRI of the brain and orbits. Consider investigating other causes of optic neuropathy if in any doubt about the diagnosis. If LHON is suspected, arrange ECG because of the association with cardiac conduction defects, and genetic screen after counselling. For dominant optic atrophy genetic testing will soon be available but if not use VEP/ERG to confirm optic neuropathy.

Treatment

■ *Casualty*: suggest patients stop smoking and avoid alcohol. Refer to clinic soon if LHON is suspected or routinely if dominant optic neuropathy with clear family history and longstanding visual loss.

■ *Clinic*: draw the family pedigree (p. 412) and establish the inheritance pattern. Arrange genetic counselling, sight-impaired registration, and low-vision aids as appropriate. Refer to a neurologist if other neurological features are present.

Follow-up Annual review once the diagnosis is established.

Radiation Optic Neuropathy

Background Radiation to the anterior visual pathways can cause an optic neuropathy months or years after the treatment, but usually within 1–3 years. It is bilateral in 75% of patients. The cumulative radiation dose is usually >2400 cGy with 75% receiving >5000 cGy. Chemotherapy and diabetes increase the risk. The mechanism is likely to be microvascular.

Clinical features Rapid, progressive, painless, visual loss that stabilizes after a few months (<6/60 in 85%, 45% become NPL). There is decreased colour vision, field loss, and an RAPD. The disc is initially normal, then becomes atrophic. Cataracts, and radiation retinopathy that mimics diabetic retinopathy are typical and disc swelling may occur if the eye has been irradiated.

Differential diagnosis Consider recurrence of the primary disease, radiation-induced malignancy, raised intracranial pressure, venous sinus thrombosis, postchiasmal radiation damage, and other optic neuropathies (compressive, demyelinating, traumatic, infiltrative, inflammatory, and nutritional).

Investigations T_1 and T_2 weighted MRI is normal but optic nerves enhance with contrast for the first few weeks. Arrange a Humphrey 24–2 field test.

Treatment

- *Casualty*: refer to clinic within 1 month.

- *Clinic*: arrange imaging and exclude other diagnoses. Arrange low-vision aids, partially sighted/blind registration as appropriate. There is no proven treatment although hyperbaric oxygen is sometimes tried.

Follow–up Review every 2–3 months until the vision stabilizes, then annually.

Optic Nerve Tumours

Background Optic nerve glioma typically develops early in life and 90% are diagnosed by age 20 years. Optic nerve sheath meningioma is unilateral in 95% with a peak incidence in the third to sixth decades and a 4:1 female preponderance. Rarely, malignant glioma causes visual loss over several weeks in adults.

Symptoms Gradual painless loss of vision often described as fogging or dimming. Gaze-evoked amaurosis occurs with optic nerve sheath meningiomas. Sudden visual loss occurs rarely when the tumour bleeds into itself. Children may present with strabismus.

Signs Features include loss of colour vision and VA, any type of visual field loss, disc swelling, optic atrophy or optic disc collateral vessels, particularly with meningiomas. Proptosis and limitation of eye movements may occur from a splinting effect of a large tumour. Tumours may compress the eye and induce hyperopia. Signs are usually unilateral, rarely bilateral, but glioma of the chiasm causes bilateral signs

History and examination Record the duration and progression of symptoms, VA, colour vision, confrontation visual fields, RAPD, eye movements, measure proptosis, dilate and examine optic discs and fundi. Exclude vitritis.

Differential diagnosis Consider optic neuropathy (traumatic, compressive, demyelinating, infiltrative, inflammatory, radiation, nutritional, and toxic) and normal pressure glaucoma.

Investigations Arrange Humphrey 24–2 field test and imaging:

■ *Glioma*: CT or MRI shows enlargement (classically fusiform) of the nerve with minimal contrast enhancement (Fig. 14.16).

■ *Meningioma*: fat suppression (STIR) MRI characteristically shows bright enhancement with gadolinium (Fig. 14.17). Calcified psammoma bodies may show up on CT. Diffuse optic nerve thickening is typical with a tram-track sign of enlarged nerve sheath.

Treatment

■ *Casualty*: if available, order an MRI scan and arrange early (4–6 weeks) neuro-ophthalmic follow-up.

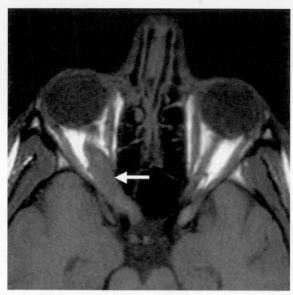

Fig. 14.16: Right optic nerve glioma (T₁ weighted MRI).

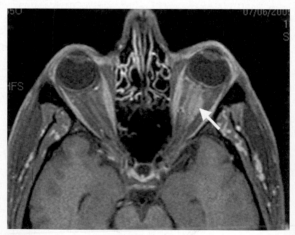

Fig. 14.17: Left optic nerve meningioma (Gadolinium-enhanced, fat-suppression MRI).

■ *Clinic*:

1. Glioma:

   a. *Children* generally follow a benign course so observe, but exclude neurofibromatosis type 1 (29% have NF-1). Tumours are usually only treated if there is hypothalamic involvement or progressive visual loss. Avoid radiotherapy as chemotherapy is much safer. Surgical excision is usually reserved for blind eyes with unacceptable proptosis.

   b. *Adult* gliomas may be highly aggressive, often presenting with bilateral simultaneous visual loss from chiasmal involvement; there may be pain, and most die within 12 months despite treatment.

2. Meningioma: treat with stereotactic fractionated conformal radiotherapy in selected cases, which should stabilize or improve vision. Surgery may be required if intracranial extension threatens vision from the other eye.

Follow—up Lifelong annual review is required in case of progression and need for treatment.

Cerebrovascular Disease

Background Disease of the carotid artery can cause monocular visual symptoms. Vertebrobasilar insufficiency can result in recurrent episodes of bilateral, simultaneous, transient visual loss. Occlusion may be due to cardiac emboli and typically affects elderly arteriopaths.

History Record the duration of visual loss and speed of onset. Ask about scintillations, coloured circles, hemianopia, halos, postural hypotension, and symptoms of vertebrobasilar ischaemia (especially loss of balance and dizziness). Assess cardiovascular risk factors including smoking and diabetes.

Examination Record VA, colour vision, confrontation visual fields, RAPD, dilate and check fundus for emboli, disc swelling, and hypertensive changes. Listen for a heart murmur, carotid bruit, and examine the peripheral pulse rate and rhythm, BP lying and standing and in both arms, cranial nerves, and cerebellar function.

Clinical features Consider the following manifestations of cerebrovascular disease and whether urgent onward referral is required.

▮ Carotid territory:

1. *Transient monocular visual loss*: see page 634.

2. *Ocular ischaemic syndrome*: see page 483.

3. *Carotid dissection*: there may be a history of trauma which may be minor. Features include pain in the neck, jaw or throbbing headache, ipsilateral Horner's syndrome (32%), transient visual loss, TIAs (30%), or embolic CVAs (46%). Arrange axial MRI of the neck ± MRA. Anticoagulate for 3 months. Associated with Ehlers-Danlos and Marfan's syndromes, pseudoxanthoma elasticum, and cystoid medial necrosis.

4. *Takayasu's disease*: a rare vasculitis which affects large vessels such as the aorta and carotids. Ocular ischaemic syndrome may result and cases may present to eye clinics.

5. *Moya Moya*: if carotid occlusion occurs early in life (radiotherapy, idiopathic) collateral vessels develop and ischaemic complications of the abnormal vasculature develop in later life.

6. *Giant carotid aneurysm in cavernous sinus*: may cause retro-orbital pain and compressive optic neuropathy. The 3rd, 4th, 5th (V_1 and V_2) and 6th nerves may be affected.

Lesions are extradural so rupture is less likely to be fatal than an intradural berry aneurysm. Endovascular embolization may be required if visual loss progresses.

7. *Carotid cavernous fistula*: see page 675.

8. *Vasculitis*: see page 655.

- Vertebrobasilar territory:

    1. *Occipital stroke*: produces a congruous homonymous hemianopia of sudden onset, often with macular sparing. Usually ischaemic rather than haemorrhagic. Bilateral cortical blindness may result from 'top of the basilar' artery occlusion.

    2. *Anton's syndrome*: patients with bilateral cortical blindness and damage to the visual association areas may deny blindness and claim to see normally. Extrastriate strokes may produce selective disorders of submodalities of vision such as colour (cerebral achromatopsia), spatial vision (Balint's syndrome), or face recognition (prosopagnosia).

    3. *Vertebrobasilar dissection*: features include bilateral transient visual obscurations lasting 1–5 minutes, transient vertigo, hearing abnormalities, dysarthria, diplopia, unilateral limb numbness or weakness, perioral numbness or tingling, reduced coordination and gait instability, and sudden loss of consciousness. Eye examination is usually normal. There may be abnormal eye movements, nystagmus, and other cerebellar or brainstem signs if seen during an episode. Patients with marked stenosis of the vertebrobasilar circulation may precipitate symptoms by neck movements or postural changes. Imaging confirmation may be problematic. Anticoagulation is advised.

    4. *Basilar thrombosis*: may begin with focal brainstem signs and may progress to a fatal outcome. Urgent referral is essential.

    5. *Transient homonymous hemianopia*: may be considered a type of TIA caused by emboli, usually lasting a few minutes but may last several hours. Consider migraine as an alternative explanation (p. 652).

    6. *Transient binocular visual loss*: consider basilar artery emboli and postural hypotension.

- Dural sinus thrombosis:

    1. Produces headache, papilloedema, and visual obscurations (p. 647).

Differential diagnosis Consider hypotension, bilateral carotid disease (symptoms may occur on exposure to bright light), giant cell arteritis, narrow angle glaucoma, occipital epilepsy, migraine (lasts longer with scintillations), and raised intracranial pressure (lasts seconds not minutes).

Investigations Request Humphrey 24–2 field test and other tests as detailed below.

Management

- *Casualty*: for presumed atherosclerotic disease start aspirin 75 mg o.d. if not contraindicated. Advise smokers to stop. Check FBC, ESR, CRP lipids, fasting glucose, and refer to clinic soon or to a neurologist.

- *Clinic*: confirm the diagnosis, check results, and refer to stroke assessment clinic for further management, e.g. MR angiography, transoesophageal echocardiogram, ECG, 24-hour ECG, and anticoagulation.

Follow–up Check visual fields and VA remain stable and exclude disc swelling. Follow for about 1 year then discharge if there are no new symptoms.

Carotid Cavernous Fistula

Background Occurs when the arterial circulation connects directly to the venous circulation in the cavernous sinus. May follow blunt head trauma (80%) or occur spontaneously, especially in hypertensive patients. May be high-flow (direct) or low-flow (indirect, dural arteriovenous malformations).

Symptoms Direct lesions produce a sudden onset of a whooshing noise in the head. Vision may be blurred with minor ocular discomfort. The indirect type is less severe, slower onset, and tinnitus may be absent.

Signs Patients are apyrexic, usually with unilateral proptosis. Eye movements are limited by a combination of nerve palsy and swelling. There is conjunctival chemosis (Fig. 14.18) with engorged vessels that become arterialized, with a spiral appearance near the limbus. Other features include exposure keratopathy, raised IOP with increased pulse pressure, poorly reactive mid-dilated pupil, and congested retinal veins. Central retinal vein occlusion and optic disc swelling may occur.

History and examination Document any history of head trauma, hypertension, previous thyroid problems, or diplopia. Lid

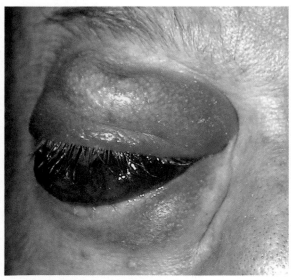

Fig. 14.18: Carotid cavernous fistula.

retraction is not seen. Record temperature, proptosis, eye movements, VA, confrontation fields, corneal exposure, IOP, and RAPD. Listen for an orbital bruit with the bell of the stethoscope over the globe, forehead, and temple.

Differential diagnosis Consider severe scleritis, cavernous sinus thrombosis, and orbital disease including thyroid, cellulitis, abscess, neoplasia, and inflammatory lesions (idiopathic, myositis, Wegner's).

Investigations Arrange urgent ultrasound to look for dilation and reversed flow in the superior ophthalmic vein. Request vascular sequence CT/MRI, or digital subtraction angiography (DSA) that commonly reveals an enlarged superior ophthalmic vein and cavernous sinus ± proptosis, enlarged extraocular muscles, and increased fat vascular markings. Request FBC, ESR, glucose, and TFTs.

Treatment Admit patients. Prescribe topical lubricants and treat elevated IOP with drops ± oral acetazolamide. Record daily VA, Ishihara plates, fields, and IOP. Life-threatening nose bleeds may occur, occasionally requiring emergency carotid ligation. Some fistulas also drain into the cerebral venous system and predispose to cerebral vascular accidents.

Direct carotid cavernous fistulas usually require embolization to close them, with 85% success. Indirect fistulas often close spontaneously and may be observed if the vision is not deteriorating; if progressive visual loss occurs then consider endovascular fistula embolization. Some fistulas close following angiography alone without any attempt at embolization. Thrombosis of the superior ophthalmic vein may cause a paradoxical worsening of proptosis for a few weeks before symptoms improve. Stereotactic radiosurgery has been used occasionally. Avoid glaucoma filtration surgery as suprachoroidal haemorrhage may result.

Follow−up Until resolution occurs.

Medically Unexplained Visual Loss

Background There are four types of medically unexplained visual loss:

- Undiagnosed organic disease.

- Malingerers with a secondary gain.

- Psychosomatic visual loss, often due to serious emotional stress. Patients genuinely believe they have lost vision. Also called hysterical, functional, or nonorganic loss.

- Munchausen's syndrome and Munchausen's by proxy.

For children with reduced vision but an otherwise normal examination, see also page 579.

Clinical features Malingerers typically have unilateral blurred vision. Functional loss is bilateral in 70%. VA is typically 6/12 to NPL. Examination is normal, although note any evidence of self-harm or eye rubbing.

History and examination A full history is essential. Ask if there is any ongoing litigation or compensation claim or any stressful event, e.g. divorce, bereavement. Observe behaviour. Is navigation consistent with VA? Test VA at 6 and 2 metres to see if the Snellen fraction is similar. Test near VA and Ishihara plates: are these consistent with the VA.

Place a +1 dioptre lens in one side of a trial frame, and cover fellow eye. Explain that you are adding a stronger (−1 dioptre) lens to see if a spherical equivalent of zero improves vision. Use an OKN drum to elicit nystagmus or move a mirror in front of the patient who will track their reflection unless genuinely NPL. Check for an RAPD.

Differential diagnosis Exclude the following by thorough history and examination: tear film abnormality; keratoconus; refractive error; presbyopia; intermediate uveitis; central serous retinopathy; macular dystrophy; central retinal artery occlusion; drug toxicity (e.g. quinine); amblyopia; optic nerve/chiasm disease, especially retrobulbar neuritis; traumatic optic neuropathy; and cortical blindness.

Investigations A Goldmann field may show spiralling (Fig 14.19) but tired patients may also show this. Hospital refraction is advisable. Electrodiagnostic testing is very useful to confirm the integrity of the visual pathways and MRI of brain and orbits are sometimes required. Fluorescein angiography is occasionally helpful.

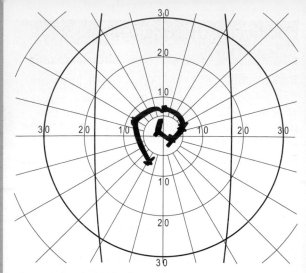

Fig. 14.19: Spiral field on a Goldmann field test.

Treatment

■ *Casualty*: for malingerers explain that the eye findings are not typical of the proposed injury mechanism, that there is no objective evidence of irreversible visual loss, and that a follow-up appointment by a senior colleague is appropriate to check that everything has resolved. Those with functional loss should be reassured that there is nothing seriously wrong and that stress is a likely explanation. Tell them their vision should improve and this will be confirmed in clinic. Routine clinic appointments are adequate unless the diagnosis is uncertain.

■ *Clinic*: confirm the diagnosis. Functional loss does not exclude eye disease.

Follow—up Review until the vision has recovered fully. Most children and adolescents recover with reassurance. Adults tend not to improve as quickly if the secondary gain or psychological illness persists. Liaise with the patient's general practitioner about psychological assessment if appropriate.

Systemic Disease Associations

Chronic progressive external ophthalmoplegia (CPEO) A feature of many different mitochondrial myopathies. Presents with bilateral ptosis with ophthalmoplegia later. May have generalized muscle weakness. Usually symmetrical so no diplopia, except for reading. Consider prisms on reading glasses, ptosis props, or cautious lid-raising surgery. For Kearn-Sayre syndrome (CPEO with pigmentary retinopathy) see page 497.

Progressive supranuclear palsy Also known as Steele-Richardson-Olszewski syndrome. Loss of downward saccades occurs first, then up saccades, and eventually complete ophthalmoplegia. There is progressive dementia, and stiff neck and trunk leading to falls. MRI shows midbrain atrophy with dilated ventricles. The differential includes parkinsonism, diffuse Lewy body disease, and multisystem atrophy. Avoid bifocals.

Myotonic dystrophy Autosomal dominant with genetic anticipation. This means that trinucleotide repeat sequences become ever longer with each generation and this typically results in progressively more serious disease with each generation.

- *Systemic features*: frontal balding, sunken temples, long face, peripheral weakness and wasting of muscles with myotonia, testicular atrophy, cardiac conduction defects, nocturnal hypoventilation, ± mild intellectual impairment.

- *Ocular features*: bilateral ptosis ± orbicularlis weakness, slow saccades, varying degrees of ophthalmoparesis, cataracts in almost all patients (coloured crystals), retinal pattern dystrophy.

Sturge–Weber syndrome Sporadic condition.

- *Systemic features*: port wine stain, ± epilepsy, hemiplegia, and intracranial calcification on skull X-ray.

- *Ocular features*: homonymous field defect, glaucoma, and diffuse choroidal haemangioma. Consider in cases of unilateral glaucoma as patients may have covered the naevus with make-up.

Tuberose sclerosis Autosomal dominant disease with multiple hamartomas affecting many systems.

- *Systemic features*: ash leaf spot, shagreen patch, adenoma sebaceum over nasolabial folds, subungal fibromas, epilepsy, periventricular astrocytic hamartomas, and mental retardation may occur.

■ *Ocular features*: retinal hamartomas (50%) may be flat, translucent lesions or multinodular 'mulberry' lesions (astrocytic hamartomas) – these are benign and rarely enlarge; optic nerve hamartoma; hypopigmented patches on iris.

Neurofibromatosis type I Dominantly inherited.

■ *Systemic features*: 6+ café au lait spots; neurofibromas; axillary freckling; phaeochromocytomas; meningioma; multiple tumours of the brain, spinal cord, and nerves.

■ *Ocular features*: optic nerve glioma (15%, only 1% progress and need treatment); >1 Lisch nodules (iris hamartomas present in 90% of those aged >6 year); congenital glaucoma; upper eyelid plexifrom neurofibroma (± ipsilateral glaucoma); retinal hamartomas; choroidal hamartomas; thickened corneal nerves; pulsatile proptosis (absent greater wing of sphenoid).

Neurofibromatosis type II Dominantly inherited.

■ *Systemic features*: bilateral vestibular schwannomas; meningioma (4%); other CNS tumours; café au lait spots (60%).

■ *Ocular features*: early-onset cortical or posterior subcapsular cataracts (81%); retinal hamartomas (combined hamartomas of retina and RPE, 22%); optic nerve sheath tumours; Lisch nodules are rare.

Von Hippel–Lindau syndrome Dominantly inherited.

■ *Systemic features*: cerebellar, brainstem or spinal haemangioblastomas (25%); phaeochromocytomas; renal cell carcinoma. Regular imaging is required to look for tumour development.

■ *Ocular features*: Retinal capillary angiomas characterized by a large feeder artery and dilated draining vein. Leakage may cause decreased vision, exudate deposition or serous retinal detachment. Treatment is with extensive laser photocoagulation or cryotherapy.

Wyburn–Mason syndrome Retinal racemous angioma associated with intracranial arteriovenous malformation. Request brain MRI.

Ataxia telangiectasia (Louis–Bar syndrome) Autosomal recessive. The most common progressive ataxia of childhood. Thymic hypoplasia and defective immune system results in recurrent infections. Conjunctival telangiectasia is common.

Optometry and General Practice Guidelines

General comments

Many neuro-ophthalmic symptoms are non-specific and it is not always clear if they should be managed by a general practitioner, neurologist, ophthalmologist, or other specialist. Thus, transient loss of vision might reflect systemic disturbance such as hypoglycaemia or hypotension, carotid emboli, or raised intraocular pressure (IOP).

Headache can be caused by several eye conditions and the following questions may help:

- Is the headache precipitated by visual attention? This may suggest refractive error or ocular muscle imbalance.

- Is headache associated with a red eye? This may suggest uveitis, scleritis, or acute angle closure glaucoma. Mild or moderately raised IOP does not usually cause headache or a red eye.

- Is headache associated with blurred vision? Consider high IOP, uveitis, raised intracranial pressure, optic neuritis, and migraine. A careful history can usually distinguish migrainous photopsia from those associated with retinal detachment (p. 556).

General practice

Although rare in general practice, always consider giant cell arteritis in those aged over 50 years with jaw claudication and temporal tenderness, especially those with polymyalgia rheumatica; an ESR and or CRP is helpful in this setting. Assessment of refraction, anterior chamber depth, IOP, dilated fundoscopy, optic discs, ocular muscle balance, and screening field tests can usually be undertaken via an optometrist and will help exclude many eye conditions associated with headache. Note that patients with good visual acuity but hemianopia are usually suitable for partial-sight registration by an ophthalmologist and this may confer some benefits.

Optometrists

An asymptomatic visual field defect picked up on routine screening should usually be repeated. Many defects will disappear as the patient learns how to perform the test. If a superior field defect is present, exclude ptosis. Tape the drooping lid up whilst the test is repeated. Exclude obvious optic disc and retinal disease with dilated fundal examination. Homonymous visual field defects (p. 639) suggest postchiasmal lesions and require relatively urgent medical assessment. For glaucomatous field defects, see page 329.

The following guide to referral urgency is not prescriptive, as clinical situations vary.

Immediate

<table>
<tr><td>■ Giant cell arteritis</td><td>p. 655</td></tr>
</table>

Same day

<table>
<tr><td>■ Acute 3rd nerve palsy (consider referral to a neurologist or neurosurgeon)</td><td>p. 631</td></tr>
<tr><td>■ Transient visual loss without features of migraine</td><td>p. 634</td></tr>
<tr><td>■ Optic disc swelling with headache or transient visual loss</td><td>p. 644</td></tr>
<tr><td>■ Anisocoria or Horner's syndrome with head or neck pain. Consider carotid artery dissection</td><td>p. 632</td></tr>
<tr><td>■ Sudden-onset visual field defect. Consider:</td><td></td></tr>
<tr><td> 1. Retinal detachment</td><td>p. 529</td></tr>
<tr><td> 2. Retinal artery occlusion</td><td>p. 478</td></tr>
<tr><td> 3. Retinal vein occlusion</td><td>p. 474</td></tr>
<tr><td> 4. Ischaemic optic neuropathy</td><td>p. 654</td></tr>
<tr><td> 5. Stroke (refer to neurology)</td><td>p. 672</td></tr>
</table>

Urgent (within 1 week)

<table>
<tr><td>■ Sudden onset of symptomatic (oscillopsia) nystagmus. Consider ENT referral if deafness, vertigo or tinnitus are prominent features. Also consider neurology referral</td><td>p. 637</td></tr>
</table>

Soon (within 1 month)

<table>
<tr><td>■ Optic disc swelling with no headache, no eye pain and normal vision</td><td>p. 644</td></tr>
</table>

References

1. *Optic Neuritis Treatment* Trial. Am J Ophthalmol 2004;
   137:77–83.

Appendix 1

Cardiorespiratory Arrest

Act quickly – 'time is (cardiac) muscle'.

Confirm diagnosis Unconscious patient, apnoeic, with absent carotid pulse.

Treatment Administer a precordial thump only if the arrest was witnessed or monitored and a defibrillator is not immediately available. Recheck the carotid/femoral pulse. If absent, perform *Adult Basic Life Support* (Fig. A1.1) while waiting for a defibrillator.

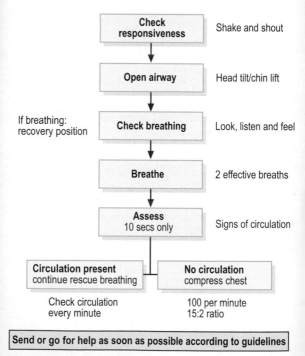

Fig. A1.1: Adult basic life support (Courtesy of Resuscitation Council, UK).

Ventilate to produce visible chest lifting. Compress 4–5 cm. Enlist help. Once cardiac arrest confirmed, follow *Advanced Life Support* algorithm (Fig. A1.2).

■ First set of shocks is 200 J, 200 J, then 360 J. Thereafter, all shocks 360 J. If three shocks are required, administer within 1 minute. After each set, only check the carotid pulse if the waveform is compatible with a cardiac output.

■ Epinephrine (adrenaline) dose is 1 mg i.v. every 3 minutes. If i.v. access fails, give 2–3 mg down the endotracheal tube (diluted to 10 mL with sterile water).

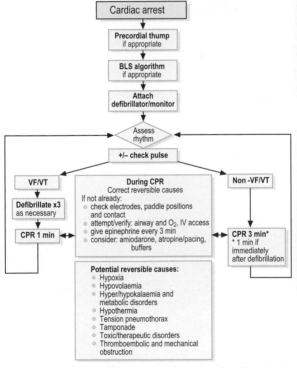

Fig. A1.2: Advanced life support algorithm for the management of cardiac arrest in adults (Courtesy of Resuscitation Council, UK).

■ Allow no more than 2 minutes between shocks three and four. Do not interrupt CPR for more than 10 seconds, except to defibrillate.

■ Asystole must be confirmed: exclude incorrectly attached leads, check the gain, and ensure the rhythm is being checked through leads I and II to exclude fine ventricular fibrillation (VF).

Appendix 2

Anaphylaxis

Signs Suspect anaphylaxis if, after exposure to a potential allergen, the patient develops: wheeze, breathlessness and cyanosis, tachycardia, hypotension, urticaria and erythema, angioedema or other soft tissue swelling (eyelids, lips).

Treatment

1. If possible, remove the cause.

2. Give epinephrine (adrenaline) 0.5 mg i.m. (equivalent to 0.5 mL of 1 : 1000 solution). If required, repeat every 10 minutes, until there are signs of clinical improvement.

3. Establish i.v. access. Give chlorpheniramine 10 mg i.v. over 1 minute.

4. Give hydrocortisone 100 mg i.v.

5. Administer 100% oxygen. Upper airway obstruction from laryngoedema may cause respiratory distress. Consult an anaesthetist, as patient may require endotracheal intubation or emergency tracheotomy.

6. If systolic BP <90 mmHg, administer 500 mL of i.v. colloid, over 15–30 minutes.

7. Attach an ECG monitor.

8. Nebulized salbutamol can also be given if there is bronchospasm.

9. Admit to ward for 24 hours, as relapses can occur.

10. Discuss with the duty physicians regarding further management, especially if the patient remains hypotensive or wheezy (admission to intensive care unit may become necessary).

If the anaphylactic reaction was caused by drug administration, this must be reported to the Committee on the Safety of Medicines (complete yellow cards at the back of the British National Formulary).

Appendix 3

Visual Standards for Driving

Table A3.1: Guide to fitness to drive (United Kingdom)	
Visual function	**Group 1 entitlement (includes motor cars and motor cycles)**
Acuity	Read in good light (with the aid of glasses or contact lenses if worn) a registration mark fixed to a motor vehicle and containing letters and figures 79 mm high and 57 mm wide (i.e. pre 1.9.2001 font) at a distance of 20.5 m, or at a distance of 20 m where the characters are 50 mm wide (i.e. post 1.9.2001 font). If unable to meet this standard, the driver must not drive and the licence must be refused or revoked.
Cataract	Must meet acuity standards above. In the presence of cataract, glare may prevent the ability to meet the number plate requirement, even with apparently appropriate acuities.
Monocular vision	Complete loss of vision in one eye. Must notify DVLA but may drive when clinically advised that driver has adapted to disability AND the prescribed eyesight standard in the remaining eye can be satisfied AND there is normal monocular visual field in the remaining eye.
Visual field defects	Driving must cease unless confirmed able to meet following standard: visual field of at least 120° on the horizontal measured using a target equivalent to the white Goldman III4e settings. In addition, there should be no significant defect in the binocular field which encroaches within 20° of fixation above or below the horizontal meridian.

Group 2 entitlement (includes large lorries and buses)

New applicants are barred in law if the visual acuity, using
  corrective lenses if necessary, is worse than 6/9 in the better eye
  or 6/12 in the other eye. Also, the uncorrected acuity in each eye
  MUST be at least 3/60.
'Grandfather Rights' allowing reduced standards may apply if licence
  issued prior to 1.1.1997. Contact DVLA.

Must be able to meet the above prescribed acuity requirement. In
  the presence of cataract, glare may prevent the ability to meet
  the number plate requirement, even with appropriate acuities.

Complete loss of vision in one eye or uncorrected acuity of less
  than 3/60 in one eye. Applicants are barred in law from holding
  a Group 2 licence.
'Grandfather Rights' allowing reduced standards may apply if
  licence issued prior to 1.1.1997. Contact DVLA.

Normal binocular field of vision is required.

(Continued on next page)

Table A3.1: Guide to fitness to drive (United Kingdom)—cont'd

Visual function	Group 1 entitlement (includes motor cars and motor cycles)
Diplopia	Cease driving on diagnosis. Can resume driving once confirmed to the Licensing Authority that the diplopia is controlled by glasses or by a patch which the licence holder undertakes to wear while driving. A stable uncorrected diplopia of 6 months' duration or more may be compatible with driving if there is consultant support indicating satisfactory functional adaptation.
Night blindness	Cases will be considered on an individual basis.
Colour blindness	Need not notify DVLA.
Blepharospasm	Consultant opinion required. If mild, driving can be allowed subject to satisfactory medical reports. Control of mild blepharospasm with botulinum toxin may be acceptable provided that treatment does not produce debarring side effects such as uncontrollable diplopia. DVLA should be informed of any change or deterioration in condition. Driving is not permitted if condition severe, and affecting vision, even if treated.

Source: DVLA, Swansea, 'At a Glance Guide to the Current Medical Standards of Fitness to Drive – A Guide for Medical Practitioners.' Readers are advised to check all details are correct before issuing advice, as they may be subject to change. Visit: www.dvla.gov.uk/at_a_glance/ch6_visual.htm

Group 2 entitlement (includes large lorries and buses)

Recommended permanent refusal or revocation if insurmountable diplopia. Patching is not acceptable

Group 2 acuity and field standards must be met and cases will then be considered on an individual basis.

Need not notify DVLA.

Consultant opinion required. If mild, driving can be allowed subject to satisfactory medical reports. Control of mild blepharospasm with botulinum toxin may be acceptable provided that treatment does not produce debarring side effects such as uncontrollable diplopia. DVLA should be informed of any change or deterioration in condition. Driving is not permitted if condition severe, and affecting vision, even if treated.

Appendix 4

Suture Material

Sutures

- Sutures can be divided into absorbable/nonabsorbable, and monofilament/multifilament (braided) (Table A4.1).

- Absorbable sutures are absorbed by proteolysis of natural material or hydrolysis of synthetic materials; hydrolysis causes less tissue reaction. Nonabsorbable sutures become encapsulated by fibrosis.

- Compared to multifilament sutures, monofilament sutures are more resistant to infection, have a lower coefficient of friction (easier to pass through tissue), lower tensile strength, lower flexibility, and are harder to tie.

- Sutures may be coated to reduce their coefficient of friction and dyed to increase their visibility.

Needle types

- The needle is divided into three parts: the point, the body, and the swage.

- The point extends from the tip to the maximum cross-section of the body. There are five types: spatulate, round bodied/taper point, cutting point, reverse cutting point, and tapered spatulate (Fig. A4.1). The body incorporates the needle length, and is the grasping area that transmits the penetrating force to the point. The body can be oval, round, triangular, side-flattened rectangular, or trapezoidal. The longitudinal shape of the body can be straight, half-curved, curved, or compound curved. The suture attaches to the swage, creating a continuous unit.

- A needle has five measurements:

  1. *Chord length*: linear distance from the point of a curved needle to the swage. This determines the width of the bite.

  2. *Needle length*: distance measured along the needle from the point to the swage; detailed on the packaging.

Table A4.1: Summary of types of suture materials

Suture	Type	Tensile strength	Tissue reaction
Absorbable			
Polyglactin 910 (Vicryl)	Mono- or multifilament	24–30 days	Mild
Polyglycolic acid (Dexon)	Multifilament	24–30 days	Mild
Plain gut*	Monofilament	5–7 days	Marked
Chromic gut*	Monofilament	10–21 days	Moderate
Nonabsorbable			
Polyamide (Nylon)	Monofilament	High; approximately 10% of strength lost per year	Mild
Silk	Multifilament	Moderate; lost by 1 year	Marked
Polypropylene (Prolene)	Mono- or multifilament	High; maintains strength over 2 years	Minimal
Polyester (Mersilene)	Monofilament	High; maintains tensile strength indefinitely	Minimal

Have been phased out as of 2002 in the UK, France, Germany, Spain, Austria and Japan.

Points of configuration

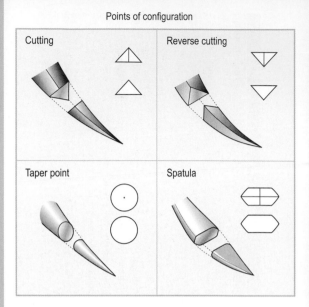

Fig A4.1: Examples of types of needles.

3. *Radius*: distance from the body to the centre of the circle along which the needle curves; this determines bite depth.

4. *Diameter*: thickness of the needle; a smaller-diameter needle requires less force and causes less trauma.

5. *Bicurve*: two radii on a needle; the radius near the point is usually shorter than that near the swage.

Needles may be coated with silicone to permit easier passage through tissues. Needles are made of stainless steel; the tip should not be touched with the needle holders to avoid blunting.

Table A4.2 summarizes the types of needle and suture materials recommended for use on named tissues.

Table 4.2: The type of needle and suture materials recommended for use on named tissues

Site	Suture types	Remove (days)	Needle type
Periocular skin	6/0 Nylon for most facial trauma.	Day 5	Reverse cutting point
	6/0 Silk: more comfortable than Nylon but may produce more scarring. Used for some oculoplastic procedures.	Day 5	
	6/0 Vicryl: may be appropriate for young children if avoids general anaesthesia to remove sutures	Absorbable	
Lid margin	6/0 Silk	Day 5–7	Reverse cutting point
Conjunctiva	8/0 Vicryl	Absorbable	Spatulate, round body
Sclera	7/0 Nylon behind the insertion of the muscles, 7/0 Nylon or 7/0 Vicryl between muscle insertions and the limbus. Avoid Vicryl if ruptured globe repair.	Permanent (Nylon) Absorbable (Vicryl)	Tapered spatulate
Cornea	10/0 Nylon	Usually weeks/month, depending on use	Tapered spatulate
Iris	10/0 Prolene	Permanent	Round bodied

Appendix 5

Ophthalmic Surgical Instruments

Forceps Ophthalmic forceps have three parts: tip, shaft, and handle. The term 'platform' refers to the last 5–7 mm of the shaft and includes the tip. There are three main types:

- *Toothed*: for holding tissues.

- *Notched*: also used for holding tissues but causes less trauma.

- *Tying*: for holding and tying sutures. Most are designed to close incrementally with increasing pressure.

Colibri forceps incorporate two types by adding a tying platform to the toothed forceps. The shaft can be straight, angled or curved. Commonly used ophthalmic forceps include (Fig. A5.1):

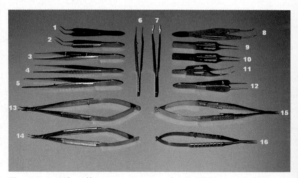

Fig. A5.1: Miscellaneous commonly used instruments.

Forceps		Notes
1.	Kelman-McPherson	Long angled shaft used for intraocular work, especially lens positioning.
2.	Rhexus forceps	Long angled shaft with further angle at tip. Used to grasp the lens capsule during capsulorrhexis. Commonly used version is Utrata forceps.
3.	Jayles	Plain handle and small interdigitating teeth.

4.	Toothed Castroviejo	The interdigitating teeth are forward angled.
5.	Moorfields	Flat handled with grooves on the handle and at the tip to allow firm grasping of the conjunctiva.
6&7.	Folding and insertion forceps	Designed to fold then insert intraocular lenses during cataract surgery.
8.	Max-fines	Plain curved platform commonly used for removing corneal sutures
9.	Suture tying	Fine plain forceps used for suture tying. Often blue in colour.
10.	Notched	Plain platform with curved notch at end. Various uses especially holding corneal or scleral wounds whilst suturing. Also called 'blue grooved'.
11.	Colibri	Ideal for holding the cornea or sclera whilst suturing.
12.	St. Martins	Short wide flat handle, interdigitating teeth commonly used during strabismus surgery. Can damage conjunctiva.

Needle holders Should be held like a pen, grasping at the junction of the upper one-third and lower two-thirds of the needle. Six main types are used during suturing. The type selected depends on the size of the needle used. Most needle holders now have the option of being locking or nonlocking. The platform that holds the needle can also be straight or curved. The handle can be flat or round.

Needle Holder		**Notes**
13.	Barraquer	Used for suturing skin and sclera. Round handled.
14.	Troutman	Finer than Barraquer. Also round handled. Useful for suturing conjunctiva.
15.	Castroviejo	Has a locking system that allows for a firm grasp; used for closing the sclera in vitreoretinal surgery and tying sutures tight over scleral explants. Flat handled.
16.	Titanium micro needle holder	For use with fine sutures (e.g. 10/0 Nylon) during corneal surgery; usually blue in colour.

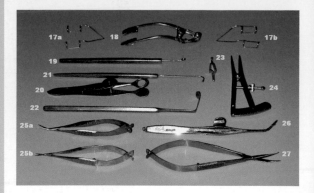

Fig. A5.1—cont'd.

Instrument		Notes
17.	Kratz Barraquer lid speculum	Wire speculum that produces a fixed opening of the palpebral fissure. The Kratz Barraquer (17a) has open wires and Barraquer (17b) has closed wires; the former is the commonly used 'phako speculum'. Pierce speculum is similar but allows adjustment of interpalebral distance.
18.	Langs lid speculum	Allows the width of the palpebral fissure to be adjusted; has guards to keep the eyelashes out of the operating field. Clark speculum is similar but has open wire loops to hold lids apart.
19 & 20.	Currette and chalazion clamp	Clamp controls bleeding and provides a rigid surface for incision and then currettage of cyst contents.
21.	Squint hook	Used for isolating extraocular muscles in squint and conventional retinal detachment surgery
22.	Fison retractor	Commonly used to retract conjunctiva and Tenon's capsule,
23.	Bulldog clamp	Used to clip sutures to avoid entanglement.
24.	Calipers	The pointed tips of the caliper can be used to mark the sclera, measure corneal diameter, and extraocular muscle position. Should usually be checked against a ruler.

25.	Vannas scissors	Fine scissors suitable for intraocular use. Can be angled (25a) or straight (25b).
26.	Dewecker scissors	Designed for cutting iris (iridectomy) but also suitable for prolapsed vitreous.
27.	Westcott scissors	Curved tips allow easy dissection of Tenon's capsule down to sclera during strabismus and vitreoretinal surgery. Tips of blades can be rounded or pointed. Use the former for blind procedures such as subtenons anaesthesia. Similar to Castroveijo scissors and often called 'spring scissors'.

Appendix 6

Use of the Operating Microscope

Modern operating microscopes have several important attributes including coaxial illumination, stereo-optics, fully adjustable eyepieces, and foot-controlled zoom and focusing.

The important steps in using the microscope are:

- Before surgery

  1. Set the eyepiece interpupillary distance and move the observer's viewing system to the correct side (left or right).

  2. If wearing spectacles during surgery, ensure the eyepiece focus is set to zero and that the 'spacers' (adjustable pads that separate your eye from the eyepiece) are out.

  3. If not wearing spectacles, set the eyepiece focus to your refraction and put in the spacers so you can rest your eyebrow on them during surgery.

  4. Reset the microscope focus and XY to the centre of their travel (look for a Reset or Centre button).

  5. Ensure the patient is comfortably positioned under the microscope.

  6. Adjust the surgeon's chair as required.

  7. Scrub, prep, and drape.

- At the start of surgery

  1. Adjust the position of the table, foot controls, microscope height, and importantly the eyepiece tilt so that your lower spine is straight or slightly extended, but never flexed.

  2. When comfortable, set any wheel locks on the surgeon's chair or mobile microscopes.

- During surgery

  1. Most microscopes are parfocal; that is, the focus and zoom are independent.

  2. However, increasing magnification reduces the depth of focus and may blur the image if the focal plane is far from the surgical plane.

3. To prevent this, focus the microscope under low magnification then zoom in on a defined object such as a blood vessel, adjusting the focus to maintain a clear image.

4. Zoom back out to the minimum magnification required to perform each task: this increases the depth of field (to avoid focusing too often) and field of view (to see the effects of manipulations on neighbouring structures).

5. This also helps overcome involuntary accommodation that is a common problem for inexperienced surgeons. If things start to blur transiently, zoom in, refocus, and zoom out. Alternatively, focus the microscope so that it moves from above down

6. Some hand tremor is normal under the microscope; concentrate on breathing normally to help reduce excessive sympathetic activity. Avoid breath-holding during difficult manoeuvres.

7. Using arm rests and resting your hands on the patient's forehead may help avoid excessive arm and upper body tension.

8. Avoid gripping the instruments too tightly as this reduces fine motor control and causes fatigue.

Appendix 7

Ophthalmic Drug Use in Pregnancy

Systemic absorption of topical eye medication may occur through conjunctival vessels or nasal mucosa. The latter is more common with drops than ointment. Systemic absorption may be reduced by nasolacrimal occlusion or eyelid closure for a few minutes after instillation, by avoiding the instillation of different drops in succession (since this increases the percentage of drops entering the nose and hence systemic absorption), and by blowing the nose after drop instillation into the eye. However, the amount of systemic absorption remains highly variable. In all categories of drug risk, any medication is advised to be used only when *the benefit to the mother outweighs the risk to the fetus*. Drugs should be prescribed using the lowest concentration at the minimum effective dose for the shortest duration of time to have their desired effect. For some drugs, there is conflicting data for their use and in many instances the toxicity advice refers to systemic and not topical use. Absence of a drug from Table A7.1 does not imply safety. Do not rely solely on the table, as the potential fetotoxic effects of topical ocular drugs are often uncertain, and the recommendations for systemic administration may not apply. If possible, avoid drugs in the first trimester. In each therapeutic group in the table, the drugs listed are those that are customarily used in ophthalmology in the UK.

Drug classification

- *Category 1* Animal studies imply a low risk in pregnancy *or* the constituents of the medication are individually known to be of low risk. Also included in this category are drugs where the dose administered is so low that the systemic concentration is negligible.

- *Category 2* Animal studies have shown adverse effects on the fetus, but there is some data for safety of use in human pregnancy. This group is further subdivided into *A* (lower-risk) and *B* (higher-risk) drugs. Lower-risk drugs include those drugs where there has been established experience with their systemic use in human pregnancy and therefore it can be extrapolated that their topical use is associated with lower risk. The higher-risk group includes drugs in which data relating to use in pregnancy is more limited and therefore the effects of the drugs is less predictive in pregnancy. Use of these drugs in pregnancy stems from anecdotal experience.

■ *Category 3* Drugs with positive evidence of human fetal risk. This does not automatically mean they cannot be used in pregnancy.

Table A7.1 should only be used in conjunction with up-to-date guides such as the British National Formulary, the National Teratology Information Service (Tel: +44(0)191 232 1525, *www.nyrdtc.nhs.uk/Services/teratology/teratology.html*), and the Medicines Information Department at Moorfields Eye Hospital (Tel: +44(0)20 7566 2369).

Sources: National Teratology Information Service guidelines, British National Formulary, Medicines Information Department (Moorfields Eye Hospital).

We are most grateful to Miss Jill Bloom, Senior Pharmacist in the Medicines Information Department at Moorfields Eye Hospital, and to Dr Patricia McElhatton, Consultant Teratologist and head of the National Teratology Information Service.

Ophthalmic drug use in pregnancy

Table A7.1: Drug use in pregnancy

Medication group		Category 1	Category 2A	Category 2B	Category 3
	Lubricants	Hypromellose Carbomers Polyvinyl alcohol Povidone Simple eye ointment/paraffins Carmellose Sodium chloride 0.9% Hydroxyethylcellulose			
Antiinfectious	Antibacterial	Fusidic acid Vancomycin (s & t) Penicillins (s & t) Cephalosporins (s & t) Metronidazole (s) Erythromycin (s & t) Clindamycin (s) Azithromycin (s) Polymyxin B Tetracycline (s, 1st trimester)	Chloramphenicol	Quinolones Aminoglycosides (gentamicin, neomycin, framycetin, tobramycin) Sulphonamides (s) Trimethoprim (s & t) Clarithromycin (s)	Tetracycline group (s, 2nd & 3rd trimester)

Medication group		Category 1	Category 2A	Category 2B	Category 3
Antiinfectious	Antifungal	Clotrimazole Amphotericin	Miconazole Econazole Natamycin	Fluconazole (s)	
	Antiviral	Aciclovir (s & t) Famciclovir (s) Valaciclovir (s)		Ganciclovir (ins & t) Trifluorothymidine (trifluridine)	
	Antiamoebic	Polyhexanide/PHMB Chlorhexidine	Propamidine		
Pressure lowering medications		Beta blockers	Pilocarpine α_2 agonists α agonists Carbonic anhydrase inhibitors (s & t)	Prostaglandin $F_{2\alpha}$ analogues Glycerin (s) Mannitol (inj)	
Antiinflammatories		NSAIDs (s & t; in 1st & 2nd trimester only except for ketorolac)	Corticosteroids (s & t, except rimexolone) Aspirin (s; low dose) Ketorolac (s & t; in 1st & 2nd trimester)	Rimexolone (very limited data)	NSAIDS (s & t; in 3rd trimester)
Antiallergic		Mast cell stabilizers (s & t)	Antihistamines (s & t, less data available)		

(Continued on next page)

Ophthalmic drug use in pregnancy

Table A7.1: Drug use in pregnancy—cont'd				
Medication group	Category 1	Category 2A	Category 2B	Category 3
Diagnostic	Fluorescein Tropicamide (but see Misc.) Cyclopentolate (but see Misc.) Rose Bengal	Phenylephrine Fluorescein (inj)		
Miscellaneous	Lidocaine (inj & t) Paracetamol (s) Sodium citrate Ascorbate (s & t) Acetylcysteine Sodium chloride 5%	Tropicamide (multidosage) Cyclopentolate (multidosage) Atropine Homatropine Hyoscine Ciclosporin (s & t) Mycophenolate (s) Local anaesthetics (except lidocaine) Botulinum toxin (inj) Povidone iodine	Verteporfin (inj) Indocyanine green (inj)	Cyclophosphamide (s) Azathioprine (s)

Where no abbreviation is used, this refers to the topical medication only.
Otherwise: s, systemic; t, topical; ins, intraocular insert; inj, injection; iv, intravenous.

Appendix 8

Reading Test Types

Held at 15 inches=38 cm

N4.5

As we walked along the edge of the river, the mild breeze rustling the trees whose boughs were bent over the water by the weight of their leaves, I could not help but recall those happy memories of childhood.

N5

with the actual experience of it all being quite overwhelming. I could not help but wonder who had been here before me, what feet had tread the same marble tiles that I stood on now.

N6

What a difference a day makes. One day, you find yourself hard up, wandering where you are going to get your next meal; the next day, just like a fairy-tale ending, a rich uncle claims you to be his long-lost nephew.

N8

but it was the music lessons I looked forward to the most. That one hour spent in the music room was my escape from all the troubles around me. It just took a few bars on the piano for my spirits to lift.

N9

There is nowhere that can compare to Paris in the springtime. It is known as the most romantic city in the world and no wonder! The blossoms on the trees, the cafes by the riverside

N10

yet the face in the photograph was strangely familiar – the same arched brows, the same deep-set grey eyes, even the same twist to the mouth in that familiar

N12

The little girl was playing on the swings with her mother tenderly watching over her. Her elder brother was amusing himself on the seesaw, all the while trying to gain

N14

as the columns became broader, the room became narrower, so that by the time we reached the end of the walk

N18

The sand was a pearly white, much whiter than I had imagined it to be.

N24

great flocks of birds were heading south for

N36

over the rooftops

N48

elephant trunks

Appendix 9

Amsler Chart

Chart to be held at a comfortable reading distance (Fig. A9.1).

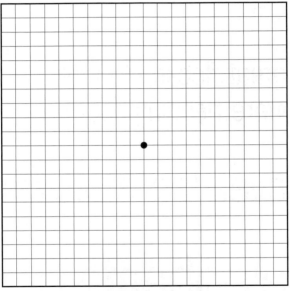

Fig. A9.1: Amsler chart. (Chart reproduced with kind permission of Keeler Ltd, Windsor, UK.)

Appendix 10

Contact Details

British Retinitis Pigmentosa Society Head Office P.O.Box 350 Buckingham MK18 1GZ Tel: 01280 821334 www.brps.org.uk	Medical Defence Union 230 Blackfriars Road London SE1 8PJ Tel: 020 7202 1500 www.the-mdu.com
Drivers Medical Group, DVLA Swansea SA99 1TU Tel: 0870 600 0301 (8.15am to 4.30pm Monday to Friday) www.dvla.gov.uk	Medical Protection Society 33 Cavendish Square London W1G 0PS Tel: 0845 605 4000 www.medicalprotection.org
The Dystonia Society 46/47 Britton St. London EC1M 5UJ Tel: 020 7490 5671 www.dystonia.org.uk	Moorfields Eye Hospital City Road London EC1V 2PD Tel: 020 7253 3411 www.moorfields.nhs.uk
British Medical Association BMA House Tavistock Square London WC1H 9JP Tel: 020 7387 4499 www.bma.org.uk	National Institute for Clinical Excellence Mid City Place 71 High Holborn London WC1V 6NA Tel: 020 7067 5800 www.nice.org.uk
Fight for Sight Institute of Ophthalmology Bath Street London EC1V 9EL Tel: 020 7608 4000 www.fightforsight.org.uk	National Poison Information Service (London Centre) Guys and St. Thomas' Hospital NHS Trust Medical Toxicology Unit Avonley Road London SE14 5ER Tel: 0870 600 6266 www.spib.axl.co.uk
General Medical Council 178 Great Portland Street London W1W 5JE Tel: 020 7580 7642 www.gmc-uk.org	Royal College of Ophthalmologists 17 Cornwall Terrace London NW1 4QW Tel: 020 7935 0702 www.rcophth.ac.uk

Guidedogs for the Blind Association Burghfield Common Reading RG7 3YG Tel: 0870 600 2323 www.guidedogs.org.uk	Royal College of Surgeons (Edinburgh) Nicolson Street Edinburgh EH8 9DW Tel: 0131 527 1600 www.rcsed.ac.uk
Institute of Optometry 56–62 Newington Causeway London SE1 6DS Tel: 020 7407 4183 www.ioo.org.uk	RNIB (Royal National Institute for the Blind) 105 Judd Street London WC1H 9NE Tel: 0845 330 3723 www.rnib.org.uk
Macular Disease Society PO Box 247 Haywards Heath West Sussex RH17 5FF Tel: 0990 143 573 www.maculardisease.org	Vision 2020 London School of Hygiene and Tropical Medicine Keppel Street London WC1E 7HT Tel: 020 7927 2974/3 www.v2020.org

Index

A